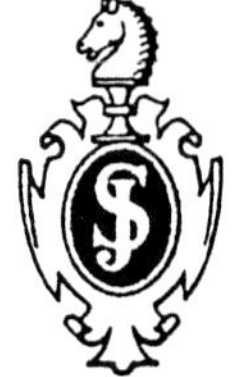

David E. Neal (Ed.)

Tumours in Urology

With 39 Figures

Springer-Verlag
London Berlin Heidelberg New York
Paris Tokyo Hong Kong
Barcelona Budapest

David E. Neal MS FRCS
Professor, Department of Surgery, The Medical School, University of
Newcastle upon Tyne, Newcastle upon Tyne NE2 4HH, UK

On the front cover is a colour illustration showing staging of bladder cancer and a
DNA Southern blot probed with c-*erb*B-2

ISBN 3–540–19867–9 Springer-Verlag Berlin Heidelberg New York
ISBN 0–387–19867–9 Springer-Verlag New York Berlin Heidelberg

British Library Cataloguing in Publication Data
Tumours in Urology: Biology and Clinical Management
I. Neal, David E.
616.9926
ISBN 3–540–19867–9

Library of Congress Cataloging-in-Publication Data
Tumours in urology : biology and clinical management / David E. Neal (ed.).
p. cm.
Includes bibliographical references and index.
ISBN 3–540–19867–9 (alk. paper). – ISBN 0–387–19867–9 (alk. paper)
1. Genitourinary organs–Tumors. I. Neal, David E., 1951–
[DNLM: 1. Bladder Neoplasms. 2. Prostatic Neoplasms. 3. Kidney
Neoplasms. WJ 504 T925 1994]
RC280.U74T85 1994
616.99'461–dc20
DNLM/DLC
for Library of Congress 94–14579

Typeset by The Electronic Book Factory Ltd, Fife, Scotland
Printed by The Alden Press Ltd, Osney Mead, Oxford
28/3830–543210 Printed on acid-free paper

Preface

The growth of uro-oncology has been one of the dramatic features of the past decade in urology. Basic science research into the immunology and molecular biology of cancer is beginning to impact on clinical urology and this poses a number of problems, both for practising urologists and basic scientists. If they are going to contribute to future research in this area they will have to communicate with each other: at present there is a gap which is widening at an increasingly rapid rate. One of the aims of this book is to bridge this gap by collating the views of a group of internationally distinguished scientists and clinicians in order to make this information more easily accessible. It is intended that the book will be useful to any urologist interested in recent developments in uro-oncology both at the clinical and basic science level. I believe the book has a useful function not otherwise fulfilled by present texts.

The first section of the book is directed towards bladder cancer. Progress is being made in understanding risk factors for progression; mucosal abnormalities are still a source of continuing controversy, but flow cytometry and the use of monoclonal antibodies to label specific subsets of tumour cells may improve our ability to assess these risks. The use of BCG may allow some patients to preserve bladder function who would otherwise require cystectomy. On the other hand, systemic chemotherapy has yet to find a role in standard management of locally advanced, non-metastatic disease. Whether it will be shown to augment survival in patients treated either by radiotherapy or cystectomy or whether it will permit bladder preservation in selected patients remains uncertain. However, recent progress in bladder reconstruction is allowing patients to be treated radically, but to retain voiding function. The role of molecular biology in assessing bladder cancer behaviour and improving our understanding of tumour formation is proceeding at a great pace and the time is not far off when the use of toxins directed at specific receptors will be tried.

Prostate cancer remains a difficult topic, for although techniques of radical prostatectomy have been refined its role has yet to be defined clearly. In addition, many patients present with advanced disease and the use of new medical methods of androgen deprivation is reviewed along with the role of "complete androgen blockade".

The final section reviews renal and testis cancer. The role of conservative surgery for specific patients with renal cancer is discussed together with immunotherapy for advanced renal cell cancer – both topics of immense interest to urologists. Early biochemical abnormalities in Wilms' tumour and hereditary forms of renal cancer are leading to a better understanding of sporadic forms of the disease. Finally, the role of radical retroperitoneal lymphadenectomy in the treatment of advanced testis tumours is reviewed.

The intended audience will include urologists in Europe and North America. Those basic scientists interested in clinical tumour work should find this book a useful reference.

Newcastle, March 1994   *D. E. Neal*

Contents

PART THREE: RENAL CANCER

PART FOUR: TESTIS CANCER

Contributors

P. M. Alken
Department of Urology, Klinikum Mannheim, Ruprecht-Karls-
Universität Heidelberg, 68135 Mannheim, Germany

G. L. Andriole
Division of Urologic Surgery, Washington University School of
Medicine, St Louis, Missouri 63110, USA

M. C. Benson
J Bentley Squier Urologic Clinic, Columbia Presbyterian Medical
Centre, Department of Urology, Columbia University College of
Physicians and Surgeons, New York, USA

J. Franklin
J Bentley Squier Urologic Clinic, Columbia Presbyterian Medical
Centre, Department of Urology, Columbia University College of
Physicians and Surgeons, New York, USA

N. J. R. George
Withington Hospital, West Didsbury, Manchester M20 8LR, UK

K. Griffiths
Tenovus Building, University of Wales College of Medicine,
Cardiff, South Glamorgan, UK

F. K. Habib
University Department of Surgery, Western General Hospital,
Edinburgh EH4 2XU, UK

R. R. Hall
Department of Urology, Freeman Hospital, Newcastle upon Tyne
NE7 7DN, UK

W. F. Hendry
149 Harley Street, London W1N 2DE, UK

J. Lunec
Cancer Research Unit, University of Newcastle upon Tyne,
Framlington Place, Newcastle upon Tyne NE2 4HH, UK

E. R. Maher
Department of Pathology, Cambridge University, Tennis Court
Road, Cambridge CB2 1QP, UK

J. K. Mellon
Department of Surgery, University of Newcastle upon Tyne, NE2 4HH
and Department of Urology, Freeman Group of Hospitals Trust,
Newcastle upon Tyne, UK

D. E. Neal
Department of Surgery, The Medical School, University of Newcastle
upon Tyne, Newcastle upon Tyne NE2 4HH, UK

A. C. Novick
Department of Urology, Cleveland Clinic Foundation, Cleveland,
Ohio, USA

W. B. Peeling
St Woolos Hospital, Newport, Gwent NP9 2UB, UK

K. B. Pittman
Institute of Cancer Studies, St James's University Hospital, Beckett
Street, Leeds LS9 7TF, UK

A. W. S. Ritchie
Urology Department, Gloucestershire Royal Hospital, Great
Western Road, Gloucester GL1 3NN, UK

J. T. Roberts
Northern Centre for Cancer Treatment, Newcastle General
Hospital, Westgate Road, Newcastle upon Tyne NE4 6BE, UK

O. Seeman
Department of Urology, Klinikum Mannheim, Ruprecht-Karls-
Universität Heidelberg, 68135 Mannheim, Germany

P. J. Selby
Institute for Cancer Studies, St James's University Hospital, Beckett
Street, Leeds LS9 7TF, UK

H. Wasan
Department of Clinical Oncology, Royal Postgraduate Medical
School, Hammersmith Hospital, Du Cane Road, London
W12 0NN, UK

J. Waxman
Department of Clinical Oncology, Royal Postgraduate Medical
School, Hammersmith Hospital, Du Cane Road, London
W12 0NN, UK

H. Wolf
Department of Urology, Skejby University Hospital,
Brendstrupgaardsvej, DK-8200 Aarhus N, Denmark

Chapter 1

Advances in Bladder Cancer

D. E. Neal

Introduction

The purpose of this chapter is to highlight areas of research into bladder cancer which have either developed significantly over recent years or remain areas of persistent controversy. Several key factors have been instrumental in making bladder cancer one of the most exciting growing points in urology. A better understanding of the genetic mechanisms which may predispose certain individuals to the development of cancer is being achieved by means of biochemical and pharmacogenetic studies; and molecular biological studies when applied to the tumours themselves are leading to increased knowledge about the mechanisms of tumour formation, progression and metastasis.

Detailed clinical follow-up studies of patients with non-muscle invasive bladder cancer have demonstrated the differences between tumours confined to lamina propria (Ta) and those invading the lamina propria (T1) in their ability to progress and metastasise (Anderström et al. 1980). This realisation has led to the clinical need to be able to identify T1 tumours which have an increased risk of progression. The combination of carcinoma in situ (Althausen et al. 1976) with a primary T1 tumour of high grade is particularly dangerous (Wolf et al. 1987), although it is difficult for pathologists to be consistent in their grading of tumours (Ooms et al. 1983) and in their diagnosis of in situ change. It is to be expected that future studies of the biology of those T1 tumours which subsequently become invasive will lead to a clearer understanding of the factors which are responsible and may permit earlier and more aggressive treatment of a subset of patients.

Trials of the use of intravesical chemotherapy have shown that small, but statistically significant, reductions in recurrence rate can be achieved in patients with Ta and T1 tumours (Herr et al. 1987); it is a major disappointment that they have not yet answered the clinically important question of whether intravesical treatment decreases the risk of progression, for the studies have neither been pursued for long enough nor have they yet been carried out in groups of patients at high enough risk of tumour progression. Systemic chemotherapy in the neo-adjuvant setting is now being formally evaluated in Phase III studies in patients undergoing conventional treatment either by means of cystectomy or radiotherapy (overseen by the Medical Research Council of Great Britain and the EORTC). Finally, the ability of surgeons to reconstruct the bladder after cystectomy is a major surgical advance in patients requiring cystectomy, but who are assessed as being at low risk of urethral recurrence.

Aetiology

The incidence and mortality of transitional cell cancer (TCC) of the urinary bladder are 15/100 000 and 4/100 000 respectively, but increase steeply between 50 and 55 years of age and are 4–5-fold higher in the male. It is the seventh most common cause of cancer death in men in England and Wales. The incidence of bladder cancer is increasing partly because of the ageing population.

Genetic Polymorphism in the Aetiology of Bladder Cancer

The factors which lead some patients to develop a tumour include influences derived from the environment such as diet, occupation, smoking and alcohol use and genetic differences between individuals. Recent studies have shown how the latter may interact with other factors to put an individual at greater or lesser degrees of risk of carcinogenesis. It is now clear that genetic polymorphism (somatic genetic differences found in individuals of a population; among the best known being the class I MHC antigens) for several enzymes which are responsible for detoxification can increase the risk of carcinogenesis. These enzymes include two of the 57 types of cytochrome *P*-450 enzymes: namely debrisoquine 4-hydroxylase (encoded by the CYP2D6 gene) and inducible aryl hydrocarbon hydroxylase (AHH) activity (encoded by the CYP1A1 gene). Other enzymes which are important are the glutathione *S*-transferase I and arylamine *N*-acetyltransferse (NAT). These enzymes are likely to be important in the metabolism of several known carcinogens. For example, CYP1A1 is involved in the metabolism of certain polycyclic hydrocarbons; individuals who are of the high inducibility type are at increased risk of lung cancer (for review see Idle 1991) with 30% of cases and 9% of controls being of this type compared with 4% of cases and 48% of controls found in the low inducible type. It is proposed that a similar excess of bladder cancer is found for both CYP1A1 and CYP2D6. About 10% of Caucasians inherit in a recessive fashion an inborn error of debrisoquine 4-hydroxylation. This poor metaboliser (PM) type is at increased risk of toxic reactions from certain drugs whereas the extensive metaboliser (EM) type is at increased risk of tumours because the enzyme converts a procarcinogen into a carcinogen. It has been proposed that the EM is at increased risk of lung and bladder cancer, although the number of PM in a given population will usually be small (Caporaso et al. 1991). Kaisery et al. (1987) reported that EM for debrisoquine were more likely to develop aggressive bladder tumours.

The best evidence of an association between such polymorphism and bladder cancer is for *N*-acetyltransferase. This enzyme is responsible for the metabolism of arylamines which include such carcinogens as benzidine and 2-aminofluorene; and arylamines are found in cigarette smoke. In 1982, Cartwright and colleagues described a case control study of 111 patients with bladder cancer and 207 controls. The *N*-acetylation phenotype was measured using dapsone; they found that 57% of the controls and 67% of the cases were slow acetylators. However, 22 of the 23 occupationally acquired (benzidine) bladder cancers were of the slow acetylator type. Most studies, including an earlier one from Denmark (Wolf et al. 1980), have found about a 30% excess risk for bladder cancer in those with a slow acetylator phenotype. This represents about a fifth of the excess risk associated with cigarette smoking (a 1.5–2-fold excess risk). However, few of the studies have been properly controlled for confounding variables such as smoking, alcohol use and occupation in addition to genetic factors. These studies have used standard pharmacological techniques for measurement of these phenotypes, although recent studies have used molecular biological techniques which will facilitate future studies as this technique requires only small amounts of somatic DNA derived from leucocytes. Such studies show that in addition to gross changes owing to major mutations in the gene encoding cytochrome *P*-450s leading to a deficient protein, more subtle alterations may result in failure of insertion of a relatively normal protein product in microsomal membranes (Tyndale et al. 1991).

Clonal Origin of Metachronous Bladder Cancer

A recent report on the clonal origin of metachronous (concomitant) tumours of the bladder (Sidransky et al. 1992) has significantly increased the understanding of the genetic changes occurring in the early phases of neoplasia in the human urinary bladder. As pointed out previously in this chapter, the aetiology is multifactorial, but exposure to chemical carcinogens – whether derived from cigarette smoke or encountered in the workplace – is thought to be of particular importance. Between 60% and 70% of all newly diagnosed bladder cancers are confined to the urothelium (Ta) or lamina propria (T1). It is well known that metachronous recurrence distant from the site of the primary tumour occurs in well over 60% of Ta and T1 tumours. The rate of tumour progression associated with invasion of the muscular wall of the bladder is discussed at length in a later section in the chapter, but develops in about 5% of Ta tumours and about 25% of T1 tumours. About 30% of newly diagnosed tumours are muscle invasive at the time of presentation.

Another feature of bladder cancer in man and animal models (Hicks 1980) is its multifocal nature. Furthermore, abnormalities of the urothelium lining the bladder are common in patients with bladder cancer and range from dysplasia to frank carcinoma in situ (Schade and Swinney 1968; see Chapter 3). The question of a "field change" of in situ tumour formation in the urothelium preceding primary and recurrent urothelial cancer has been widely supported; such changes being found near the base of 25% of primary superficial bladder cancers and being associated with subsequent tumour recurrence and invasion (Wolf and Højgaard 1983). These findings have led some authors to suggest that chemical carcinogens initiate many clones of cells and subsequent promotion may lead to the formation of multifocal tumours which may be synchronous or metachronous. In the language of the new biology, multiclonal oncogene activation or loss of tumour suppressor genes may be sustained from chemical insult and subsequent further allelic loss will result in the formation of separate tumours of more or less malignant behaviour depending on the type of genetic change.

However, a monoclonal origin has also been supported by many biologists studying chromosomal banding patterns in human bladder cancer (Sandberg, 1977). The multifocal nature of bladder cancer may be a reflection of intraluminal dispersion of single clones of viable tumour cells or lateral intraepithelial migration – perhaps facilitated by inflammatory changes within the bladder. One such possible cause is endoscopic resection. However, several factors suggest that multifocality commonly occurs prior to endoscopic resection. First, multiplicity is a presenting feature of 30% of newly diagnosed bladder cancers (Lutzeyer et al. 1982) and is a major risk factor for future multiple tumour recurrence and more importantly of progression. Second, distant in situ changes at first tumour presentation are associated with future multiple recurrence and progression of Ta and T1 bladder cancers and are found in over 50% of newly diagnosed patients with muscle invasive tumours (Olsen et al. 1988) undergoing cystectomy (Kazikoe et al. 1985). Third, in patients with pTa and T1 tumours, where in situ changes near to the primary lesion are common, recurrent tumours are found near the site of the primary lesion in between 50% and 70% of cases (Jakse et al. 1987). Also, in patients with T1 cancer, re-resection only 8–14 days after the first operation, detects persistent cancer in 44% which must have arisen well before any effects of implantation following resection could become apparent (Klän et al. 1991) and suggests that prior in situ change is the more important factor. These findings together with those of Lunec et al. (1992) and Sidransky et al. (1992) suggest that monoclonality is common in multiple bladder cancers and that multiplicity or multiple areas of intraepithelial neoplasia often occurs prior to endoscopic resection. Subsequent genetic change in cells in these areas of intraepithelial neoplasia will then be associated with frank neoplasia of a more or less malignant degree.

Several other pieces of evidence support this view. Tumours of the renal pelvis and ureter account for only 4%–5% of cases of transitional cell cancer. Such patients have a 40% risk of developing bladder cancer (Kazikoe et al. 1980), but only a 2%–3% risk of developing a contralateral upper tract TCC whereas only 2%–3% of patients with primary bladder cancer ever develop upper tract tumours. In addition, in patients with Ta tumours of the bladder, most recurrent tumours are found at sites distant from the primary. In combination, these findings support the suggestion of monoclonal tumour development with implantation or intraepithelial spread as a cause of multiplicity or widespread in situ change which may be monoclonal in origin.

The study reported by Sidransky et al. (1992) addressed the question of genetic changes in multifocal bladder tumours presenting concomitantly in four females undergoing cystectomy. Two had muscle invasive disease and two had tumours invading lamina propria; each had multifocal tumours. In the tissues of the female, one X chromosome (either the paternal or maternal copy) is inactivated during embryogenesis (genomic imprinting) and the inactive copy is differentially methylated compared with the active chromosome. On average, 50% of cells have the paternal copy activated and 50% have the maternal copy activated, although it is known that particular zones of cells within the tissue have the same chromosome activated – presumably owing to clonal expansion during embryogenesis and it is also known that for some particular genes in animals the maternal or paternal copy only is activated throughout the body. By studying polymorphic markers on the X chromosome in DNA before and after treatment with an endonuclease whose cleavage pattern is sensitive to methylation sites it can be determined whether both copies of the chromosome are activated in a tumour. If multifocal bladder cancer were derived from a single clone of cells one would expect the same X chromosome to be activated in all the tumours. In the human bladder it is not known how large the zones of urothelium are in which the same X chromosome is activated as a consequence of embryonal and neonatal clonal expansion during morphogenesis. Sidransky and his colleagues studied restriction fragment length polymorphism (RFLP) for the HPRT and PGP gene on the X chromosome before and after treatment with a methylation site sensitive endonuclease to determine the question of X chromosome inactivation and also looked at allelic deletion of 9q, 17p, 18q, 2q, 13q, 5q and 1q. Deletions of whole or part of a chromosome are common in many types of cancer, but the deletions are not random. Particular chromosomes are deleted in bladder cancer and their presence is related to stage (Tsai et al. 1990).

Urothelium which was apparently normal was isolated from two patients and a heterogenous pattern of X chromosome activation was observed (Sidransky et al. 1992), although we do not know how large the pieces of tissue were. In a total of ten tumours from three patients, it was found that the same X chromosome was activated, suggesting that each tumour arose from a single clone of cells. A similar clonal pattern was found for allelic loss of chromosome 9q reinforcing suggestions that this is a relatively early event in bladder tumorigenesis (Tsai et al. 1990). On the other hand, allelic losses of 17p containing the site of the p53 gene (see Chapter 2) are considered to be late events in tumour formation (Sidransky et al. 1991) often being associated in bladder cancer with the development of muscle invasion (Wright et al. 1991). Recent work (Lunec et al. 1992) also supports the suggestion of monoclonality. A patient with multifocal TCC of the kidney, ureter and bladder who underwent cystectomy was found to have in each of the tumours amplification for the c-*erb*B-2 gene and identical point mutations in codon 282 of the p53 gene with no such abnormalities in the normal kidney and bladder. This finding reinforces suggestions of a common clonal origin of these concomitant urothelial tumours.

Such genetic studies performed on multifocal TCC are shedding light on the early events which take place in tumour formation. It therefore seems likely that a single clone of cells is subject to tumour initiation with genetic changes such as loss of chromosome 9q. At an early stage, these cells may spread elsewhere in the bladder by lateral migration or intravesical implantation – perhaps lying dormant for many years and being morphologically normal. Subsequent genetic events may allow frank tumour formation and mechanisms such as allelic losses, mutations (Wright et al. 1991; Lunec et al. 1992) and overexpression of peptide growth factor receptors (Neal et al. 1990) may then permit the formation of carcinoma in situ or invasive cancer. It seems certain that in many patients with bladder cancer, cells from which new tumours can arise are already present at the time of clinical presentation within the urothelium distant from the primary tumour. The clinical role of mucosal abnormalities elsewhere in the bladder in predicting future behaviour has been uncertain because of variability between pathologists in interpreting these changes. The study reported by Sidransky points out the direction which clinical pathology will have to take in the future if it is to play its full part in clinical oncology.

Basic Diagnosis, Management and Staging

Over 90% of patients with bladder cancer present with haematuria and most patients present quickly to their doctor. Some authors have studied whether a screening service looking for dip-stick positive haematuria is worthwhile (Britton et al. 1989). This is time consuming and leads to large numbers of patients who have no abnormality undergoing upper urinary tract imaging and investigation of the lower tract with urine cytology and ultrasound scanning at least and possibly also by means of cystoscopy and biopsy. As with so many issues connected with cancer screening, the cost–benefit balance is uncertain – in part because the screening method is not specific. The question of whether a delay before the initiation of appropriate treatment can worsen the outcome has been addressed by several studies (Turner et al. 1977; Hendry 1988), although the results remain inconclusive (Gulliford et al. 1991). In one study which is often quoted to demonstrate the benefit of reducing delay in diagnosis, the introduction of a haematuria service increased the proportion of T2 tumours (from 9% to 15%) and decreased the proportion of T3 tumours (from 19% to 14%), but these changes were statistically insignificant. Probably the only patients who will really benefit from early treatment are those with primary carcinoma in situ, T1 tumours which are going to progress to muscle invasion and T2 tumours or T3 tumours which have not yet developed blood borne or lymphatic metastatic disease. It is likely that many of the facets of an individual tumour's behaviour are already present when the patient first develops haematuria partly because of the long natural history prior to this event and partly because the tumours are already genetically programmed with their pattern of future clinical behaviour. The commonest tumours are well differentiated or moderately well differentiated Ta tumours; it is not likely that a delay of a few weeks before treatment will impact on the eventual outcome for such patients. Likewise, most patients with T4 tumours who form about 5% of cases with primary bladder cancer and many of the patients with large T3 tumours are likely to have already metastasised before referral. Having said this, it is certain that there will a be a window of time in certain patients with bladder cancer when appropriate intervention will be curative, but procrastination will lead to a lost opportunity.

Flexible Cystoscopy

The use of flexible cystoscopy under local anaesthetic is very useful in the initial evaluation of patients with haematuria, for it allows better and more focused use of valuable general anaesthetic sessions. This procedure is well tolerated (Powell et al. 1984) as a diagnostic procedure, but not many patients will permit biopsy of an obvious tumour or treatment by cystodiathermy of even small recurrent Ta tumours. I restrict the use of flexible cystoscopy in the follow-up of patients with transitional cell bladder cancer to those with low or moderate grade Ta tumours with a low risk of progression because patients with T1 tumours are at greater risk of tumour progression and may develop associated in situ changes. Patients with T1 bladder cancer who are not to be treated radically for some reason and are being followed-up after intravesical treatment therefore require bladder washings, cytology and random urothelial biopsy and cystoscopy and examination under general anaesthetic.

Urine Cytology

The use of urinary cytology is very important in the assessment of patients with haematuria or with bladder cancer, for it may permit the detection of carcinoma in situ which cannot otherwise be diagnosed – even multiple biopsies may fail in this setting because the surface urothelial cells which are not adherent in carcinoma in situ are washed off. Bladder washing usually gives a higher yield of satisfactory cells for either diagnostic cytological examination or for flow cytometry (Mellon et al. 1991). It should be remembered, however, that the unwary urologist can be caught out by reports from the cytological examination of bladder washings because this technique can produce clumps of cells from normal urothelium which can be difficult to distinguish from the spontaneously shed cells from a well-differentiated Ta tumour. In addition, the cytological examination of several specimens of urine may be necessary to detect carcinoma in situ – a high index of suspicion is necessary in patients presenting with marked irritative lower urinary tract symptoms of dysuria, frequency and urgency accompanied by suprapubic pain.

The T1 Tumour

The prognostic impact of severe dysplasia or carcinoma in situ has been shown in many studies (Schade and Swinney 1968; Althausen et al. 1976; Wolf et al.

1987) in terms of both recurrence and progression to muscle invasion of Ta or T1 tumours. One area of great controversy at present is the T1 tumour. Clearly, on pathological grounds such tumours have the potential for invasion, for they have already begun to lyse the basement membrane and grow into the lamina propria. The relatively poor outcome of such tumours has been well shown (Table 1.1) since the initial studies by Anderström et al. (1980) who showed a death rate from bladder cancer of 4% in Ta tumours and 24% in T1 tumours. This was confirmed in a recent study from Newcastle (Abel et al. 1988) which showed a progression rate to muscle invasion of 0 in Ta tumours and 33% in T1 tumours with no fewer than 50% of grade

Table 1.1. Progression rates in pTa and pT1 tumours

Reference	Follow-up	pTa progression/death	pT1 progression/death
Anderström et al. 1980	5 years	Died: gI – 0/22 (0%) gII – 1/46 (2%) gIII – 0/9 (0%)	Died: gII – 6/41 (15%) gIII – 14/48 (29%) gIV – 4/10 (40%)
Lutzeyer et al. 1982	3 years	Died: gI – 7/225 (3%) gII – 4/36 (11%)	Died: gI – 8/99 (8%) gII – 38/135 (28%) gIII – 8/18 (44%)
Heney et al. 1983	3 years	Progression: gI – 2/85 (2%) gII – 3/50 (6%) gIII – 1/4 (25%)	Progression: gI – 0/7 (0%) gII – 6/29 (21%) gIII – 13/27 (48%)
Jakse et al. 1987	9 years	Death rates: gI – 5% gII – 11% gIII – 16% Progression to muscle invasion: pTa – 2/89 (2%)	Death rates: gI – gII – 22% gIII – 50% Progression to muscle invasion: pT1; gIII – 11/31 (35%)
Malmström et al. 1987	5 years	Progression to pT1 or muscle invasion: gI – 5/45 (11%) gII – 9/46 (20%) gIII – 0/2 (0%)	Progression to muscle invasion (22 other patients with T1 gIII disease treated by cystectomy or DXT): gI – 0/3 (0%) gII – 5/18 (28%) gIII – 3/9 (33%)
Abel et al. 1988	3 years	Progression to pT1: gI – 0/6 (0%) gII – 8/42 (19%) gIII – 1/3 (33%)	Progression to muscle invasion: gII – 7/20 (35%) gIII – 4/6 (67%)

III tumours in the T1 category progressing to muscle invasion at 2 years. Three years after initial diagnosis the progression rate to muscle invasion in all T1 tumours was 46%. At least in some cases, subsequent muscle invasion represents a failure of initial staging, for muscle may not be included in the initial biopsy, but this criticism cannot be levelled at the previous study. The rate of tumour progression of high grade Ta and T1 tumours averages 40% at 5 years (Birch and Harland, 1989). However, the policy of determining treatment of T1 bladder cancer on the basis of grade is open to question because pathologists are unreliable in this regard. For instance, in a series of 57 cases of bladder cancer reviewed by six pathologists, the proportion of high grade cases varied from 10% in the hands of one pathologist to over 25% in another. Moreover, on review of the same cases by the same pathologist, 50% of sections were re-graded and 15% of cases shifted by more than one grade (Ooms et al. 1983).

In patients with recurrent Ta and T1 tumours, the recurrent tumours are found at the site of the primary lesion in between 50% and 70% of cases (Table 1.2; Jakse et al. 1987; Klän et al. 1991). This is unlikely to represent tumour implantation following transurethral resection of bladder tumour (TURT) and probably is a reflection of *in situ* change near to the tumour (Althausen et al. 1976). Whereas most urologists would be unhappy with the suggestion that this is persistent gross disease, a recent study of patients with T1 cancer demonstrated that re-resection only 8–14 days after the first resection detected persistent cancer in 44% of patients (Klän et al. 1991).

One commonly quoted fallacy is that patients with Ta or T1 tumours who progress to muscle invasion can be salvaged by timely radical surgery: in the Newcastle series 10 of the 11 patients who progressed to muscle invasion died of bladder cancer. Most such patients who develop muscle invasive tumours die of bladder cancer and to improve survival, radical treatment at the time of initial presentation would be necessary if these patients could be identified. Muscle invasion is the first sign of recurrence in 43% of patients with T1 tumours who develop recurrence (Malmström et al. 1987). There is little comfort for the urologist or the patient in the results of treatment with intravesical chemotherapy in patients with G3 disease who have a progression rate of about 40% (Smith et al. 1986); a rate which does not differ greatly from untreated patients. Some authors have supported the use of initial intravesical treatment with chemotherapy or BCG (Soloway 1988) in patients with T1 disease before cystectomy. In this small series of 18 patients with T1 disease treated by mitomycin who were followed-up for three years, only four were alive and free of disease; two patients died of bladder cancer, two had positive cytology, two had superficial recurrences, three underwent cystectomy, three died of other causes and two were lost to follow-up. In my view these figures

Table 1.2. Site of superficial tumour (pTa, pT1) recurrence

Reference	Same site only	Distant site only	Same + distant site
Jakse et al. 1987 – pTa	39%	48%	13%
Jakse et al. 1987 – pT1	53%	28%	14%
Klän et al. 1991 – pT1 (at 10 days)	44%	not recorded	not recorded

are not encouraging. Similarly 15 of 29 patients (52%) with T1 disease before BCG treatment developed progression about 29 months after treatment; the risks were even greater in patients with persistent T1 disease 3 months after BCG (82%; Herr 1991).

The results of radiotherapy for this disease are poor with a progression rate of about 40% at about 3 to 4 years (Table 1.3; Sawczuk et al. 1988; Greven et al. 1990) – results not markedly different from patients treated by means of resection alone. Although some authors have supported the use of radiotherapy for the control of this disease, their results are not reassuring on critical review (Duncan and Quilty 1986; Jenkins et al. 1989). The results of these latter two studies showed 5-years survival rates of about 60%. Furthermore, it was observed that survival did not differ in patients with or without a complete local response to radiotherapy. These results are in marked contrast to those of cystectomy which is associated with a 5-year cure rate of 85%–90% (Bracken et al. 1981; Stöckle et al. 1987; Malkowicz et al. 1990). These data argue that in the fitter younger patient, early cystectomy should be considered; they also suggest that if BCG is tried, then cystectomy should be advised if tumour is still present after the first 6-week course.

The options for patients with T1 bladder cancer are variable. There is a case to be made for offering immediate cystectomy to those with G3 disease particularly if carcinoma in situ (cis) is present. Others would offer one or two six-week courses with BCG and carry out cystectomy in those who failed to achieve a complete response. In my view, endoscopic treatment alone for patients with T1 G3 disease could hardly ever be justified because of the high rate of later progression. Even in patients who achieve a complete response to intravesical treatment, later recurrence may occur; the problems of adequate

Table 1.3. Response to treatment of pTa and pT1 tumours

Reference and treatment	Follow-up	Response and survival
Duncan and Quilty 1986 Radiotherapy for pTa and pT1	5 years	Complete response (CR; 83/174; 48%) CR – 63% survival rate not CR – 66% survival rate
Sawczuk et al. 1988 Radiotherapy for pTa and pT1	not stated	Died of cancer – 14/37 (38%) Overall survival rate – 21/37 (67%)
Jenkins et al. 1989 Radiotherapy for G3 pT1	5 years	Survival rate – 64%
Greven et al. 1990 Radiotherapy for pTa/pT1	5 years	Permanent local control – 9/35 (26%) Overall survival rate – 14/35 (40%)
Bracken et al. 1981 Cystectomy for pT1 G3	5 years	Overall survival rate – 26/29 (89%)
Stöckle et al. 1987 Cystectomy for pT1 (mainly G3)	5 years	Overall survival rate – 49/55 (89%) for cystectomy on diagnosis Overall survival rate – 11/18 (61%) if surgery delayed until muscle invasive recurrences present
Malkowicz et al. 1990 Radical cystectomy	5 years	Survival for pT1 – 80%

surveillance in patients with T1 disease should not be underestimated. Frequent follow-up cystoscopies in patients with T1 disease should be carefully performed with regular mucosal biopsies and cytological examination of bladder washings – flexible cystoscopyy under local anaesthesia may not be the ideal method in these high risk patients. My own practice is to offer immediate cystectomy to fit young patients with multiple G3 T1 tumours and cis and to patients with solitary G3 T1 tumours plus cis. In other patients with T1 disease, I carry out a repeat cystoscopy at 6 weeks and re-resect the area of the primary tumour and carry out random biopsies and bladder washings. In fitter younger patients with persistent disease at this 6-week cystoscopy, I again offer cystectomy. Other patients with T1 tumours, are treated with Bacillus Calmette–Guérin (BCG) given for one or two six-week cycles. In patients with a complete response, careful follow-up is carried out as outlined above. Patients with recurrent disease after two complete cycles are again offered cystectomy.

Reconstruction after Cystectomy

Several key factors have been instrumental in improving the outcome of urinary tract reconstruction for the urologist. These include a better understanding of urodynamics, the advent of artificial urinary sphincters (AUS), the use of clean intermittent self-catheterisation (CISC; Lapides et al. 1972; Webb et al. 1990), the construction of compliant, large capacity urinary reservoirs from bowel segments (Goodwin et al. 1959) and improvements in the design of continent urinary diversion (Thüroff et al. 1986; Skinner et al. 1987). It is now possible in most motivated patients to produce a continent bladder of satisfactory capacity which can be emptied by means of CISC, provided the urethra is present: these principles are now being applied to patients undergoing cystectomy. In patients in whom the urologist feels it to be important to remove the urethra, advances in techniques now make it possible to construct a continent diversion. The Mitrofanoff principle (Mitrofanoff 1980; Woodhouse et al. 1989) consists of providing from the urinary reservoir a narrow conduit which is tunnelled submucosally to provide continence; emptying being achieved by means of CISC. One example of this is the use of the appendix tunnelled into a de-tubularised ileocaecal segment to provide a method of continent external urinary diversion. If the stoma is brought out through the umbilicus it is almost invisible. One problem in the long term is skin level stenosis which can be minimised by reversing the appendix so that its base with a segment of caecum is brought onto the skin; the apex being tunnelled into the caecum (Barker 1991). The main difficulty is if the appendix is missing: in such cases, the ureter or fallopian tube can be used and there have been reports of the use of narrowed segments of intestine, including the greater curvature of the stomach (Bihrle et al. 1991).

However, the standard technique of continent diversion – if there is such a thing – is probably the Kock pouch developed and refined by Skinner and associates, but it remains with a high rate of re-operation rate mainly owing to problems with the continence mechanism (Skinner et al. 1987). Other techniques which have been used if the appendix is absent are the construction of a continence mechanism using the plicated terminal ileum (Rowland et al. 1987) or the use of the terminal ileum invaginated in an aboral direction through the ileocaecal valve with the spout covered by peritoneum on its outer surface being brought to the abdominal wall (Benchekroun et al. 1989).

The option of orthotopic reconstruction of the urinary bladder after cystectomy remains controversial mainly because of the risk of urethral recurrences in such patients, although only those urologists who routinely carry out urethrectomy in conjunction with cystectomy should perhaps argue this point with any conviction. Many series of cystectomies have shown that the risk of urethral recurrence increases with length of follow-up, but is about 5%–10% at 5 years (Stöckle et al. 1990). Various factors are associated with an increased risk of urethral recurrence. In situ change in the urethra was found in 19% of men with multifocal papillary disease who died of bladder cancer (Hendry et al. 1974), being found only rarely in patients with solid solitary tumours. It might seem that multifocal tumours and cis of the bladder would represent a significant risk, but Levinson et al. (1990) showed that prostatic involvement poses the major risk of subsequent urethral recurrence. However, in this study, most men with a previous history of cis or multifocal disease underwent a prophylactic urethrectomy. In another study of a series of men who had been pretreated rather heavily with intravesical chemotherapy (Hardeman and Soloway, 1990), urethral recurrence was also associated with prostatic tumour; 11 of 30 men (37%) developed a urethral recurrence and 20 of these 30 men also had multifocal disease or cis. Only one of 29 patients (3%) with a tumour at the bladder neck or with multifocal tumour or cis, but without prostatic involvement developed a urethral recurrence and only one of 27 patients with a solitary tumour away from the bladder neck developed a urethral tumour. This is helpful information in deciding whether to preserve the urethra or to carry out a urethrectomy. It is of note that Skinner et al. (1991) consider that the only contraindication to bladder reconstruction after cystectomy is the presence of urethral tumour, or tumour or carcinoma in situ involving the prostate; carcinoma *in situ* of the bladder is apparently not regarded as a contraindication.

The technique of total bladder reconstruction has varied from the use of a hemi-Kock ileal reservoir (Skinner et al. 1991), a "W" ileal reservoir (Hautmann et al. 1988), the intact ileum (Lilien and Camey 1984), the detubularised ileocaecal segment (Marshall et al. 1991), the use of the detubularised sigmoid colon (Reddy et al. 1991) to the intact right colon (Mundy et al. 1986). We do not yet know which of these procedures is best, although detubularised ileum provides a reservoir with the least amount of pressure activity during filling. In theory, this should result in a diminished rate of nocturnal incontinence. In my opinion, the use of intact colon or ileum is not the best option because of the high pressures which can develop, which put the upper tracts at risk of damage and possibly result in an increased rate of urinary leakage. It is best if the surgeon is familiar with several techniques because not all patients are suitable for one type of operation – the ileal mesentery may be too short, the caecum may not reach the urethra or the sigmoid colon may be affected with diverticular disease. The method of implanting the ureters has also varied, but most authors agree than an antireflux procedure is sensible; the Leadbetter/Cordonnier procedure and the Camey/le Duc technique are the simplest to use in the colon or ileum respectively (Le Duc et al. 1987).

The recent report by Skinner et al. (1991) has emphasised the advantages of this approach. The in-patient death rate was 1.6% (2 of 126). The age range of patients undergoing this technique was not clear, although the implication was that it was offered to all suitable patients. Some studies have suggested that elderly patients may not achieve as satisfactory urinary control as younger patients. The average length of the operation was 4.5 h. Early complications were similar to those seen after comparable major surgery; thromboembolic disease was surprisingly infrequent. I have seen several patients with this complication despite the use of perioperative heparin and early mobilisation and one of my patients had biopsy proven osteitis pubis (Robertson et al. 1991). The other satisfactory aspect of this series was the low incidence of incontinence: 95% being dry during the day and about 85% dry at night if they woke to void. Voiding was accomplished by straining in about 90%; with the remainder practising CISC. This has not been my experience – either in these patients or in those undergoing enterocystoplasty for idiopathic instability (Sethia et al. 1991) in whom, in the long term, residual urine volumes tend to increase with a resultant predisposition to urinary infection and incontinence. Many of these patients need to practice CISC.

In conclusion, these changes in management of patients who in the past would have undergone ileal conduit urinary diversion, are likely to offer major improvements in quality of life. In particular, these changes are likely to alter the way that patients with bladder cancer and urologists view cystectomy and may result in more patients with early stage disease being offered this treatment.

References

Abel PD, Hall RR, Williams G (1988) Should pT1 transitional cell cancers of the bladder still be classified as superficial? Br J Urol 62:235–239

Anderström C, Johansson S, Nilsson S (1980) The significance of lamina propria invasion on the prognosis of patients with bladder cancer. J Urol 124:23–26

Althausen AF, Prout GR, Daly JJ (1976) Non invasive papillary carcinoma associated with carcinoma *in situ*. J Urol 116:575–580

Barker SB (1991) Continent diversion with an appendix conduit and an ileocecal bladder. J Urol 146:754–755

Benchekroun A, Essakalli N, Marzouk M, Hachimi M, Abakka T (1989) Continent urostomy with hydraulic ileal valve in 136 patients: 13 years of experience. J Urol 142:46–51

Bihrle R, Klee LW, Adams MC, Foster RS (1991) Early clinical experience with the transverse colon-gastric tube continent urinary reservoir. J Urol 146:751–753

Birch BRP, Harland SJ (1989) The pT1 G3 bladder tumour. Br J Urol 64:109–116

Bracken RB, McDonald MW, Johnston DE (1981) Cystectomy for superficial bladder cancer. Urology 18:459–463

Britton JP, Dowell AC, Whelan P (1989) Dipstick haematuria and bladder cancer in men over 60: results of a community study. Br Med J 299:1010–1012

Caporaso N, Landi MT, Vineis P (1991) Relevance of metabolic polymorphisms to human carcinogenesis: evaluation of epidemiologic evidence. Pharmacogenetics 1:4–19

Cartwright R, Ahmed RA, Barham-Hall D et al. (1982) Role of *N*-acetyltransferases in bladder carcinogenesis: a pharmacogenetic epidemiological approach to bladder cancer. Lancet ii:842–845

Duncan W, Quilty PM (1986) The results of a series of 963 patients with transitional cell carcinoma of the urinary bladder primarily treated by radical megavoltage X-ray therapy. Radiother Oncol 7:299–310

Goodwin WE, Winter CC, Barker WF (1959) "Cup-patch" technique of ileocystoplasty for bladder enlargement or partial substitution. Surg Gynecol Obstet 108:240–245

Greven KM, Solin LJ, Hanks GE (1990) Prognostic factors in patients with bladder carcinoma treated with definitive irradiation. Cancer 65:908–912

Gulliford MC, Petruckevitch A, Burney PGJ (1991) Survival with bladder cancer, evaluation of delay in treatment, type of surgeon and modality of treatment. Br Med J 303:437–440

Hardeman SW, Soloway MS (1990) Urethral recurrence following radical cystectomy. J Urol 144:666–669

Hautmann H, Egghart G, Frohneberg D, Miller K (1988) The ileal neobladder. J Urol 139:39–42

Heney NM, Ahmed S, Flanagan MJ et al. (1983) Superficial bladder cancer: progression and recurrence. J Urol 130:1083–1086

Hendry WF (1988) Diagnosis and management of primary bladder cancer: a British perspective. In: Raghavan D (ed) The management of bladder cancer. E. Arnold, London, pp 69–93

Hendry WF, Gowing NFC, Wallace DM (1974) Surgical treatment of urethral tumours associated with advanced bladder cancer. Proc R Soc Med 67:304–307

Herr HW (1991) Progression of stage T1 bladder tumors after intravesical bacillus Calmette–Guérin. J Urol 145:40–44

Herr HW, Laudone VP, Whitmore WF (1987) An overview of intravesical therapy for superficial bladder tumors. J Urol 138:1363–1368

Hicks RM (1980) Multistage carcinogenesis in the urinary bladder. Br Med Bull 36:39–46

Idle JR (1991) Is environmental carcinogenesis modulated by host polymorphism? Mutat Res 247:259–266

Jakse G, Loidl W, Seeber G, Hofstädter F (1987) Stage T1, grade 3 transitional cell carcinoma of the bladder: an unfavourable tumour. J Urol 137:39–42

Jenkins BJ, Nauth-Misr RR, Martin JE, Fowler CG, Hope Stone HF, Blandy JP (1989) The fate of G3pT1 bladder cancer. Br J Urol 64:608–610

Kaisery A, Smith P, Jaczq E et al. (1987) Genetic predisposition to bladder cancer: ability to hydroxylate debrisoquine and mephentoin as risk factors. Cancer Res 47:5448–5493

Kazikoe T, Fujita J, Murase T, Matrumoto K, Kishi K (1980) Transitional cell carcinoma of the bladder in patients with renal pelvic and ureteral cancer. J Urol 124:17–19

Kazikoe T, Matumoto K, Nishio Y, Ohtani M, Kishi K (1985) Significance of carcinoma in situ in association with bladder cancer. J Urol 133:395–398

Klän R, Loy V, Huland H (1991) Residual tumor discovered in routine second transurethral resection in patients with stage pT1 transitional cell carcinoma of the bladder. J Urol 146:316–318

Lapides J, Diokno AC Silber SJ, Lowe BS (1972) Clean intermittent self catheterization in the treatment of urinary tract disease. J Urol 107:458–461

Le Duc A, Camey M, Teillac P (1987) An original anti-reflux uretero-ileal implantation technique: long term follow up. J Urol 137:1156–1158

Levinson AK, Johnson DE, Wishnow KI (1990) Indications for urethrectomy in an era of continent urinary diversion. J Urol 144:73–75

Lilien OM, Camey M (1984) 25 year experience with replacement of the human bladder (Camey procedure). J Urol 132:886–891

Lunec J, Challen C, Wright C, Mellon K, Neal DE (1992) Amplification of c-erbB-2 gene and mutation of p53 in concomitant transitional carcinomas of renal pelvis and urinary bladder. Lancet 339:439–440

Lutzeyer W, Rüben H, Dahm H (1982) Prognostic parameters in superficial bladder cancer: an analysis of 315 patients. J Urol 127:250–252

Malkowicz SB, Nichols P, Lieskovsky G, Boyd SD, Huffman J, Skinner DG (1990). The role of radical cystectomy in the management of high grade superficial bladder cancer. J Urol 144:641–645

Malmström P, Busch C, Norlen BJ (1987) Recurrence, progression and survival in bladder cancer. Scand J Urol Nephrol 21:185–195

Marshall FF, Mostwin JL, Radebaugh LC, Walsh PC, Brendler CB (1991) Ileocolic neobladder post-cystectomy: continence and potency. J Urol 145:502–504

Mellon K, Shenton BK, Neal DE (1991) Is voided urine suitable for flow cytometric DNA analysis? Br J Urol 67:48–53

Mitrofanoff P (1980) Cystostomie continente trans-apendiculaire dans le traitment des vessies neurologiques. Chir Ped 21:297

Mundy AR, Nurse DE, Dick JA, Murray KHA (1986) Continence and potency preserving cystoprostatectomy and substitution cystoplasty for patients with bladder cancer. Br J Urol 58:664–668

Neal DE, Sharples L, Smith K, Fennelly JA, Hall RR, Harris AL (1990) The epidermal growth factor receptor and the prognosis of bladder cancer. Cancer 65:1619–1625

Olsen PR, Wolf H, Schroeder T, Fischer A, Højgaard K (1988) Urothelial atypia and survival rate of 500 unselected patients with primary transitional cell tumour of the urinary bladder. Scand J Urol Nephrol 22:257–263

Ooms ECM, Anderson WAD, Alons CL, Boon ME, Veldhuizen RW (1983) Analysis of the performance of pathologists in the grading of bladder tumors. Hum Pathol 14:140–143

Powell PH, Manohar V, Ramsden PD, Hall RR (1984) A flexible cystoscope. Br J Urol 56:622–644

Reddy PK, Lange PH, Fraley EE (1991) Total bladder replacement using de-tubularized sigmoid colon: technique and results. J Urol 145:51–55

Robertson AS, Davies JB, Webb RJ, Neal DE (1991) Bladder augmentation, substitution and replacement using bowel segments: a clinical and urodynamic review of 25 patients. Br J Urol 68:590–597

Rowland RG, Mitchell ME, Bihrle R, Kahong RJ, Piser JE (1987) Indiana continent reservoir. J Urol 137:1136–1139

Sandberg AA (1977) Chromosome markers and progression in bladder cancer. Cancer Res 37:2950–2956

Sawczuk IS, Olsson CA, de Vere White R (1988) The limited usefulness of external beam radiotherapy in the control of superficial bladder cancer. Br J Urol 61:330–332

Schade ROK, Swinney J (1968) Pre-cancerous changes in bladder epithelium. Lancet ii:943–945

Sethia KK, Webb RJ, Neal DE (1991) A urodynamic study of ileocystoplasty in the treatment of idiopathic detrusor instability. Br J Urol 67:286–290

Sidransky D, von Eschenbach A, Tsai YC et al. (1991) Identification of p53 gene mutations in bladder cancer and urine samples. Science 252:706–708

Sidransky D, Frost P, von Eschenbach A, Oyasu R, Preisinger AC, Vogelstein B (1992) Clonal origins of metachronous tumors of the bladder. N Engl J Med 326:737–740

Skinner DG, Leiskovsky G, Boyd SD (1987) Continuing experience with the continent ileal reservoir (Kock pouch) as an alternative to cutaneous urinary diversion: an update after 250 cases. J Urol 137:1140–1144.

Skinner DG, Boyd SD, Lieskovsky G, Bennett C, Hopwood B (1991) Lower urinary tract reconstruction following cystectomy: experience and results in 126 patients using the Kock ileal reservoir with bilateral ureteroileal urethrostomy. J Urol 146:756–760

Smith G, Elton RA, Chisholm GD et al. (1986) Superficial bladder cancer: intravesical chemotherapy and tumour progression to muscle invasion or metastasis. Br J Urol 58:659–663

Soloway MS (1988) The management of superficial bladder cancer, with emphasis on intravesical chemotherapy. In: Raghavan D (ed) The management of bladder cancer. E. Arnold, London, pp 118–139

Stöckle M, Alken P, Englemann U, Jacobi GH, Riedmiller H, Hohenfellner R (1987) Radical cystectomy – often too late. Eur Urol 13:361–367

Stöckle M, Gökcebay E, Riedmiller H, Hohenfellner R (1990) Urethral tumor recurrences after radical cystoprostatectomy: the case for primary cystoprostatourethrectomy. J Urol 143:41–43

Thüroff JW, Alken P, Riedmiller H, Engelmann U, Jacobi CH, Hohenfellner R (1986) The Mainz pouch (mixed augmentation with ileum and cecum) for bladder augmentation and continent diversion. J Urol 136:17–21.

Tsai YC, Nichols PW, Hiti AL, Williams Z, Skinner DG, Jones PA (1990) Allelic loss of chromosomes 9, 11, and 17 in human bladder cancer. Cancer Res 50:44–47

Turner GA, Hendry WF, Williams GB, Wallace DM (1977) A haematuria diagnostic service. Br Med J ii:29–31

Tyndale R, Aoyama T, Broly F et al. (1991) Identification of a new variant CYP2D6 allele lacking the codon Lys-281: possible association with the poor metabolizer phenotype. Pharmacogenetics 1:26–32

Webb RJ, Lawson AL, Neal DE (1990) Clean intermittent catheterisation in 172 adults. Br J Urol 65:20–23

Wolf H, Højgaard K (1983) Urothelial dysplasia concomitant with bladder tumours as a determinant factor for future new occurrences. Lancet ii:134–138

Wolf H, Lower GM Jr, Bryan GT (1980) Role of N-acetyltransferase phenotype in human susceptibility to bladder carcinogenic arylamines. Scand J Urol Nephrol 14:161–165

Wolf H, Olsen PR, Fischer A, Højgaard K (1987) Urothelial atypia concomitant with primary bladder tumour. Scand J Urol Nephrol 21:33–38

Woodhouse CR, Malone PR, Cumming J, Reilly TM (1989) The Mitrofanoff principle for continent diversion. Br J Urol 63:53–57

Wright C, Mellon K, Johnston P et al. (1991) Expression of mutant p53, c-erbB-2 and the epidermal growth factor in transitional cell carcinoma of the human urinary bladder. Br J Cancer 63:967–970

Chapter 2

Molecular Biology and Bladder Cancer

J. Lunec and J. K. Mellon

Introduction

Recent advances in molecular biology have deepened our understanding of the mechanisms governing tumour initiation and subsequent progression. These advances hold out the promise of improving clinical management in two main ways; first by establishing molecular assays to predict the biological behaviour and therapeutic response of the tumour and second by identifying novel targets and approaches for improved therapies. Here we review the current state of knowledge on the molecular biology of cancer relevant to the genesis and progression of bladder neoplasms.

The development of antibody and recombinant DNA techniques has provided the foundation for advances in our knowledge of the molecular basis of cancer and has revolutionised the pathology of cancer. In particular the specificity and sensitivity of polymerase chain reaction (PCR) techniques for amplifying small amounts of a specific DNA sequence has allowed us to extend considerably the degree of information on altered gene structure and expression that can be extracted from limited clinical tumour samples.

The molecular biology of cancer has become a vast and complex area of research and no attempt is made to cover all aspects here. The emphasis is on the molecular pathology of bladder cancer, concentrating on the genetic alterations which are the primary events that are believed to be responsible for the loss of normal growth control and malignant progression that defines cancer; namely alterations associated with oncogenes and tumour suppressor genes, and peptide growth factors and their receptors.

Oncogenes

The term oncogene literally means a gene causing cancer and was originally used to describe genes carried by retroviruses found to be the agents of

certain transmissable forms of cancer in animals. It became apparent that
these retroviral oncogenes (v-*oncs*) were closely related to normal cellular
genes of the infected hosts. These normal cellular counterparts were termed
proto-oncogenes and were thought to become altered to an activated form
on incorporation into the viral genomes. With the development of DNA
transfection techniques it was demonstrated that human tumours contained
transforming genes, which on introduction into preneoplastic indicator cells
(such as NIH3T3 fibroblasts) could abrogate their normal patterns of growth
control and in some cases render them tumorigenic. Families of such cellular
oncogenes (c-*oncs*) were found by this and other means and shown to be
normal genes that had become "activated" by a variety of mechanisms.
These include point mutation, insertional mutagenesis, translocation and
overexpression, sometimes associated with gene amplification. Because the
techniques and systems involved, particularly the NIH3T3 transfection system and oncogenic retroviruses, tended to select for dominantly acting
transforming genes the term oncogene has come to be associated with
this class of transforming gene. What have sometimes been referred to as
"recessive oncogenes" are now more generally called tumour suppressor
genes.

As the list of known oncogenes has accumulated and the cellular location
and function of the gene products established they have been found to fall into
families which are defined by the role of their normal cellular counterparts in
the growth signal control pathways. These include growth factors and their
cell surface receptors, nuclear regulators of gene transcription and DNA
replication, and the growth signal transduction proteins which couple between
cell surface receptors and the nucleus. Although more than 60 oncogenes have
now been identified only a small number of these have been examined for their
role in bladder cancer.

Ras G-protein Family

The human *ras* gene family consists of three closely related genes: H-*ras*,
K-*ras* and N-*ras*. These encode related 21 kDa proteins which are members
of the G-protein class of signal transduction proteins that are involved in
the transmission of chemical signals from cell surface receptors to their
intracellular targets. Activation of the *ras* proteins to oncogene form occurs
as a result of a single amino acid change which is the consequence of single
nucleotide mutations at one of a small number of specific sites along the
gene. There is evidence of specificity of activation of the *ras* oncogenes in
particular tumour types; for example, activated H-*ras* has been predominantly
found in bladder carcinomas, K-*ras* in lung and colon carcinomas and N-*ras*
in haemopoietic malignancies (Bos 1989).

Earlier studies of *ras* oncogenes in bladder cancer used the NIH3T3
transfection assay. Indeed the discovery of the activation of *ras* proteins
to oncogene form by single specific point mutations was made as a result
of the isolation of the c-H-*ras* oncogene from the T24 bladder carcinoma
cell line using this technique (Reddy et al. 1982; Tabin et al. 1982; Capon
et al. 1983). This involves co-precipitating DNA from the tumour with
calcium phosphate and introducing this suspension into monolayer cultures

of NIH3T3 fibroblasts, followed by a transient membrane permeabilisation step to facilitate the uptake of DNA precipitate. Selection of clones which have taken up and express oncogenes is achieved by inspection of cultures for areas in which cells have lost normal contact inhibition of monolayer growth and are piled up to form readily visible foci. Although this has been a powerful technique for the discovery of oncogenes its use as a systematic screening method is limited. The overall incidence of mutated *ras* in human bladder tumours, determined by the NIH3T3 transfection assay, is approximately 5%–10% (Fujita et al. 1985; Malone et al. 1985). A subsequent variation of this assay has been to inject the transfected cells into nude mice in order to select directly for tumorigenicity. Using this method, Visvanathan et al. (1988) detected an activated c-H-*ras* gene in 4/24 (16.6%) human primary bladder carcinomas. Two of these were from superficial (Ta) and two from early stage invasive tumours (T1, T2). Only two of these cases showed up with the *in vitro* assay alone. These studies indicate that there is preferential activation of the c-H-*ras* gene and most of the reported mutations are at codon 12, although one codon 13 (Visvanathan et al. 1988) and two codon 61 mutations (Fujita et al. 1985) have also been found.

Some molecular characterisations using direct methods of identification have led to suggestions that the NIH3T3 DNA transfection assay may considerably underestimate the frequency of *ras* mutations (Bos 1989). The advent of the polymerase chain reaction (PCR) technique allows amplification of specific genes and has offered detection of an increasing number of specific DNA abnormalities associated with the development and progression of cancers. Recently a mutation frequency of 50% has been reported for human bladder tumour DNA samples using direct screening of PCR-amplified tumour DNA with sequence-specific oligonucleotide probes (Czerniak et al. 1990). However, these data were not validated by DNA sequencing and the results were markedly higher than the 7%–20% found in the earlier NIH3T3 transfection studies.

In a recent study of 152 human bladder tumours, single strand conformation polymorphism (SSCP) and restriction fragment polymorphism analysis were used to screen for mutations in the first two exons of the c-H-*ras* gene (Knowles and Williamson 1993). Only nine tumours (6%) were found to contain mutations; four in codon 12, two in codon 13 and four in codon 61. Eight of these mutations were confirmed by subsequent direct sequencing. No correlation was found with tumour stage or grade.

We have recently examined this further by analysing bladder tumour DNA samples for mutations at codons 12 and 13 of the H-*ras* gene using PCR-based direct sequencing methods without prior screening by SSCP analysis (Burchill et al. 1994). Point mutations were found in nine of 50 tumours (18%). As previously reported for bladder cancer, the most frequent mutation (8/9) was a G to T transversion within codon 12 converting GGC to GTC, which would result in a glycine to valine substitution in the protein. The remaining mutation was a G to A transition altering GGC to GAC, producing a glycine to aspartic acid substitution, not previously reported in bladder cancer. The frequency of mutations (18%) is comparable to that reported using the tumorigenesis modification of the NIH3T3 transfection assays, but lower than some recent reports using sequence-specific oligonucleotide hybridisation methods. No relationship between mutations and tumour grade and stage was apparent, indicating that *ras* mutations may be early events in the development of human bladder cancer.

In addition to activation by point mutations, over expression of the normal form of *ras* genes has been shown to be transforming. Viola et al. (1985) reported increased levels of p21^{ras} protein detected by immunohistochemistry in high grade bladder carcinomas and premalignant (dysplastic) urothelium. However, the specificity of the antibody used has been questioned and the results are not supported by other studies (Malone et al. 1985). An isolated case (1/21) of overexpression due to a 50-fold amplification of the normal c-Ki-*ras* gene was reported by Fujita et al. (1985).

Other Oncogenes

Apart from *ras* and those oncogenes related to growth factor receptors dealt with in the next section there has not been an extensive investigation of other known dominant oncogenes. Although there have been attempts to study expression of the nuclear oncoproteins *myc* and *fos* in bladder tumours by immunohistochemisty, doubt has been expressed about the interpretation of these observations made on archival paraffin-embedded material because of the short half-life of these proteins and the fact that they may merely be general indicators of cell proliferation (Neal and Mellon, 1992a,b).

An alternative approach to screening tumours for alterations to the structure or expression of known oncogenes is to use general methods to screen for gain or loss, or rearrangement of normal sequences. Kallioniemi et al. (1993) have developed a comparative genomic hybridisation method to produce a map of DNA sequence copy number as a function of chromosomal location. Test DNA and normal reference DNA are differentially labelled with distinguishable fluorophores and hybridised simultaneously to normal chromosome spreads. Deletions, duplications or amplifications are visualised as differences in the intensity ratio of the two labels. By applying this to tumour cell lines and primary bladder carcinomas they identified 16 different regions of gene amplification, many in loci not previously known to be amplified.

One area which is frequently found to be amplified in a range of tumours including bladder cancer is chromosome 11q13. The specific gene that is being selected for overexpression within this region is not known, although *bcl*1, *int*2 and *hst* map to this region and were found to be co-amplified in 20/97 (20.6%) of bladder tumours (Procter et al. 1991). Amplification at 11q13 showed no correlation with tumour grade or with *erb*B-2 amplification.

Growth Factors and Growth Factor Receptors

The establishment and propagation of mammalian cells in culture generally requires the supplementation of nutrient media with growth factors present in serum or tissue extracts. Searches for the active components have led to the discovery that these are generally small peptides which stimulate growth by binding to specific cell surface receptor proteins and in so doing activate a cascade of sequential intracellular biochemical events which constitute a growth signal transduction pathway that can couple the surface receptor activation to nuclear transcription and DNA replication systems. Not surprisingly, in view of their key role in cellular growth control, a subset of oncogenes has been found to be closely related to particular growth factors and growth factor receptors. A key observation has been that tumour cells often have a reduced demand for exogenously supplied growth factors because of the ability to produce peptide growth factors to promote their own growth in what is known as the autocrine mechanism of growth stimulation. In addition the growth of tumour cells can be stimulated by circulating growth factors secreted by distant tissues or by growth factors from nearby stromal tissues; the latter method is referred to as the paracrine mechanism of stimulation.

Epidermal Growth Factor (EGF) and the EGF Receptor

EGF is a 53 amino acid peptide with mitogenic activity whose action is mediated by binding to a membrane-bound receptor. It was originally isolated from murine submaxillary gland extracts and its presence is widespread in human tissues, with high levels in milk, prostatic fluid and urine. The detection of high levels of EGF in urine has prompted surveys of EGF receptor levels in bladder cancers to establish whether EGF has a significant role in supporting the growth of these tumours.

The EGF receptor is a 175 kDa transmembrane protein with an extracellular EGF binding domain, a small hydrophobic region which spans the plasma membrane and an intracellular domain which has tyrosine kinase activity as well as target tyrosine residues for autophosphorylation. These overall features are shared by a family of related proto-oncogenes. Because of considerable sequence homology to the gp65^{erbB} transforming protein product of the avian erythroblastosis virus, the EGF receptor gene is also referred to as the c-*erb*B-1 proto-oncogene. The EGF receptor has also been found to be the target for the peptide growth factor TGF-α, which is structurally related to EGF and appears to be synthesised by a wide range of common epithelial tumours including transitional cell carcinomas of the urinary bladder. Activation of the receptor by the binding of EGF or the alternative ligand TGF-α can produce both autophosphorylation of tyrosine residues and phosphorylation of target proteins.

EGF receptors are distributed in many sites throughout the body and are present in normal tissues including fibroblasts, corneal cells, kidney cells as well as basal cell layers of normal urothelium. The significance of EGF receptors in neoplasia stems from the fact that overexpression of the EGF receptor has been demonstrated to be transforming and that a proportion of human solid tumours as well as some transitional cell cancers (TCCs) have been found to possess extremely high levels of EGF receptor as a result of elevated expression of the gene by a variety of mechanisms, including gene amplification and upregulation of expression at both the transcriptional, translational or post-translational levels.

Studies of EGF/TGF-α in Bladder Cancer

Several studies have looked at EGF levels in the urine of patients with bladder cancer (Kristensen et al. 1988; Ishikura et al. 1991; Fuse et al. 1992). There appears to be a consensus that the level of EGF in the urine is reduced in patients with bladder tumours of increasing stage with levels rising again following tumour ablation (Kristensen et al. 1988; Fuse et al. 1992).

In addition, EGF has been examined in tumour tissue of renal and urothelial origin as well as normal tissue using immunocytochemistry (Lau et al. 1988). Typical granular staining was noted in the cytoplasm of all transitional cell and squamous carcinomas of the bladder. Staining of normal urothelium was limited to superficial cells only. Subjectively, the staining intensity of transitional cell carcinomas correlated inversely with tumour differentiation. In view of the fact that internalised, receptor-bound EGF is known to be rapidly degraded, the results from this immunohistochemical study suggest that there is active synthesis of EGF within the cytoplasm, perhaps being involved in autocrine mechanisms of malignant proliferation.

We have looked at the levels of EGF and TGF-α in non-neoplastic and neoplastic bladder tissue using a standard radioimmunoassay technique (Mellon 1993). There were two significant findings. First, tumour samples had much higher TGF-α levels compared to EGF. The mean TGF-α of malignant tissue was 9.5 ng/g (range of 0.34–46.4 ng/g) compared to mean EGF of 0.8 ng/g (range of 0–5.4 ng/g, $P < 0.0001$). Second, the mean TGF-α level of malignant tissue was significantly greater than that of benign bladder tissue which had a mean TGF-α of 2.6 ng/g ($P = 0.016$). There was, in addition, a difference in mean EGF levels of four normal bladder samples from non-tumour bearing areas of bladder in patients with bladder cancer (1.6 ± 0.5 ng/g) compared with three samples of bladder tissue obtained from normal bladders at the time of organ retrieval surgery (0.40 ± 0.3 ng/g, $P = 0.05$). There was no statistical difference in mean TGF-α content of normal bladder tissue from bladder cancer patients (3.2 ± 3 ng/g) compared with samples obtained at organ retrieval (1.9 ± 1.8 ng/g, $P = 0.86$).

In a study by Messing et al. (1987) it was demonstrated that intravesical EGF induced *in vivo* activity of ornithine decarboxylase and DNA synthesis in rat bladder, with nuclear thymidine incorporation which was limited to the basal epithelial cell layer. These studies indicated that urothelium could potentially respond to intravesical urinary EGF and that this response parallels the distribution of EGF receptors on normal urothelial cells and neoplastic cells.

The effect of TGF-α on bladder tumour cells has been studied by Gavrilovic et al. (1990). NBT-II rat carcinoma cells were transfected with a gene encoding human TGF-α. Subsequently, it was noted that the cells became motile and vimentin positive and secreted significant levels of a 95 kDa gelatinolytic metalloproteinase. These results suggest that expression of TGF-α in an epithelial tumour cell results in the development of a motile, fibroblast-like phenotype with matrix-degrading potential, which could result in a more aggressive tumour in vivo.

EGF Receptor Expression in Bladder Cancer

EGF receptor expression has now been extensively studied in transitional cell carcinoma of the bladder. In 1984 Messing reported that the growth and division of certain malignant transitional cell lines was stimulated by EGF (Messing, 1984). In the same year the first reports appeared of EGF receptor detection in bladder cancer by immunohistochemistry (Gusterson et al. 1984). In the first clinical study of EGF receptors in TCC (Neal et al. 1985), a significantly higher expression of EGF receptors detected by immunohistochemistry was found in tumours of high grade and advanced stage. These initial observations suggested that EGF receptor status reflected elements of the clinical behaviour of the tumour and the overall prognosis of the patient.

Subsequent DNA studies revealed that, unlike sarcomas, c-*erb*B-1 gene amplification is not the mechanism responsible for EGF receptor over-expression in the majority of bladder cancers (Berger et al. 1987; Wood et al. 1992). In the latter study of a small number of bladder tumours no evidence of altered gene copy number or rearrangements of the c-*erb*B-1 gene were found. However, elevated levels (4–15-fold) of EGF receptor messenger RNA were detected in 5/14 (36%) compared to normal urothelium from the same bladder (Wood et al. 1992). Further studies have reported on quantitative assessment of EGF receptor in bladder tumours (Smith et al. 1989) and on the correlation between different methods of assessment (Neal et al. 1989).

EGF Receptor Expression and Other Genes Involved in Tumorigenesis

EGF receptor expression has been studied in relation to other genes involved in tumour initiation and progression. It has been shown that transfection and overexpression of normal or mutated c-Ha-*ras* gene into a non-invasive transitional cell carcinoma cell line results in acquisition of an invasive phenotype and up-regulation of EGF receptor expression (Theodorescu et al. 1991). Evidence has recently emerged of a positive association between EGF receptor and c-*jun* oncogene expression in bladder cancer (Tiniakos et al. 1994). Other studies have failed to demonstrate any relationship between EGF receptor expression and either that of c-*erb*B-2 (discussed below) or the p53 tumour suppressor gene (Wright et al. 1991).

In an immunohistochemical study of nine bladder cancers the expression of p-glycoprotein, the protein product of the multidrug resistance (MDR1) gene and that of the EGF receptor was examined. No association was found in this limited sample (Kageyama et al. 1991). Further studies of this nature are required to establish whether there is a link between oncogenes and growth factors and the expression of genes associated with drug-resistance mechanisms.

In collaboration with the Oncology Group at the ICRF, we have carried out an immunohistochemical study of EGF receptor, c-*erb*B-2 and TGF-α expression in a series of paraffin-embedded human tissues (Gullick et al. 1991). Two antibodies raised to short synthetic peptides from the cytoplasmic domain of the EGF receptor molecule gave concordant staining in a series of bladder cancers known to express or lack EGF receptors. Approximately 30%

of the tumours were also found to overexpress the c-*erb*B-2 protein with no evidence of coexpression. Cancers with EGF receptor expression were also noted to have high levels of TGF-α, consistent with an autocrine regulation of growth.

The Regulation of Proteinase Expression by EGF

The expression of the closely related serine proteinases, urokinase (u-PA) and tissue plasminogen activator (t-PA) have been investigated in both cultured normal and neoplastic urothelial cells (Dubeau et al. 1988). These enzymes have been implicated in tumour invasion and malignancy. Both were found to be synthesised by normal urothelial cells grown in vitro under chemically defined conditions. The level of t-PA activity was found to decrease when normal urothelial cells reached saturation density but was stimulated more than tenfold by the addition of EGF to the culture medium. On the other hand u-PA activity was regulated to a lower degree by EGF and was not affected by cell density. In comparison the tumour cells made only u-PA under all conditions tested and the levels of this expression were either unaffected or slightly decreased by EGF. These differences were reflected by the ability of cells to degrade subendothelial and smooth muscle matrices, particularly in the presence of plasminogen (Allen et al. 1990). A subsequent study showed that TGF-β reduced total secreted PA activity by log phase normal urothelium, but not transformed cells (Hiti et al. 1990). Further analysis showed this effect to be due to the stimulated expression of plasminogen activator inhibitor (PAI-1).

EGF and Stromal–Epithelial Interactions

Much discussion at present centres on the stromal–epithelial interaction in both benign and malignant disease. A report has suggested that in a rodent tissue culture model EGF or an EGF-like substance produced by rat urothelial cells is released into the tissue medium and stimulates growth in the rat stromal cells (Noguchi et al. 1990). This interaction is possibly mediated by EGF receptors.

Prognostic Significance of EGF Receptor Expression in Bladder Cancer

We have now studied the prognostic significance of EGFr status, as determined by immunohistochemistry, in a group of 212 patients with primary bladder cancer with a mean follow-up of 26.5 months (SD: 23.6 months, range 1 to 96 months). This study has confirmed the strong association between EGFr positivity and high tumour stage $\chi^2 = 50.6$, $P < 0.0001$) and high tumour grade ($\chi^2 = 23.5$, $P < 0.0001$) (unpublished data).

Sixty-two patients died during the study due to bladder cancer and of these 47 (76%) were EGFr positive. A multivariate analysis showed that the factors which were significant predictors of death were stage ($P = 0.004$), grade ($P = 0.005$) and EGF receptor status ($P = 0.004$). The difference in survival for EGF receptor-positive and EGF receptor-negative tumours just failed to

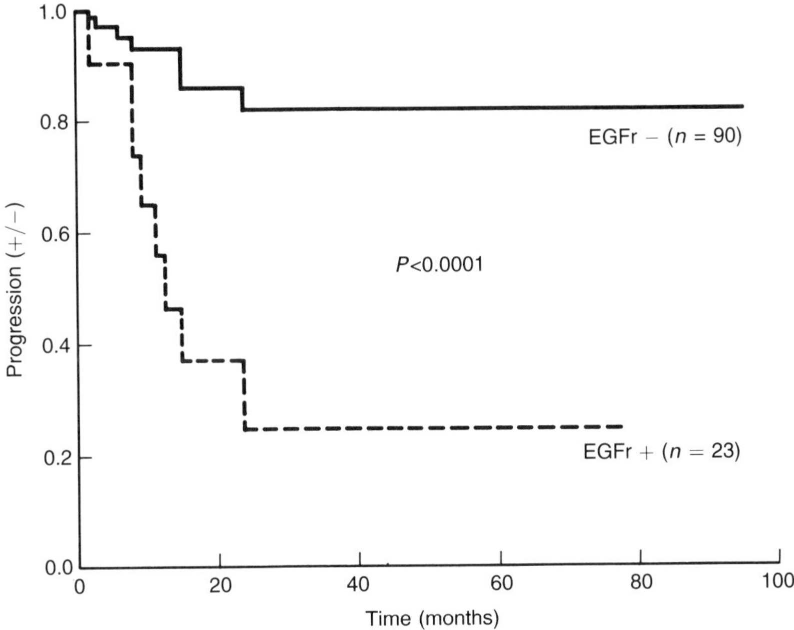

Fig. 2.1. Progression and EGFr status (pTa and pT1 tumours).

reach statistical significance when the data from patients with muscle-invasive tumours were analysed separately ($P = 0.06$).

For Ta tumours, the mean recurrence rate was significantly higher for EGF receptor-positive tumours, 18.1/100 patient months (CI = 8.4–27.8/100 patient months, $n = 9$) compared with those which were EGF receptor negative, 7.6/100 patient months (CI = 5.4–9.8/100 patient months, $n = 61$, $P = 0.012$). The recurrence rate of pT1 tumours was similar regardless of EGF receptor status. On multivariate analysis EGF receptor status was not found to be a significant predictor of tumour recurrence. Of the parameters assessed (sex, stage, grade, size, multiplicity, EGF receptor status and age) only size of tumour was found to be a significant independent predictor of recurrence.

Stage progression occurred in 19 of 113 pTa/pT1 tumours and was more likely in EGF receptor-positive tumours (10/23) compared with EGF receptor-negative tumours (9/90) $\chi^2 = 14.7$, $P < 0.001$) (Fig. 2.1). Of twenty T1G3 tumours five progressed, four of which were EGF receptor positive. Of fifteen T1G3 tumours which did not progress, only one was EGF receptor positive. Multivariate analysis showed EGF receptor status to be an independent predictor of stage progression.

Therapeutic Approaches Based on EGF Receptor Status

The question then arises as to how EGF receptor overexpression might be exploited in the clinical setting. Therapeutic strategies which have been suggested include the use of peptide antagonists which might block EGF stimulation of growth or high concentrations of EGF which have been shown to be growth inhibitory. Dioxin has been found to bind to EGF receptors, suggesting this may be a lead compound for designing non-peptide antagonists.

The targeting of radioisotopes or toxins to EGF receptor-positive tumours has also been explored. The EGF receptor has been used to target bladder tumour cells for radioimmunoscintigraphy (Harney et al. 1991). Recently a hybrid protein (TP-40) consisting of TGF-α fused to a segment of Pseudomonas exotoxin-A protein has been shown to bind selectively to tissues rich in EGFr. In studies using the bladder carcinoma cell lines, 5637, J82, RT4, Scaber, T-24, MBT-2 and TCC-SUP, TP-40 has been shown to have a significant growth inhibitory effect. A phase I clinical trial to assess the use of intravesical TP-40 is currently under way in the USA.

Other EGF receptor-based approaches include the use of retinoic acid to delay bladder tumour recurrence (Nutting and Chowaniec 1992), based on the observation that retinoic acid reduces the EGF-induced increase in anchorage-independent growth in bladder tumour cell lines. An alternative suggestion to exploit EGF receptors on tumour cells has been to use EGF or TGF-α to stimulate cell proliferation prior to treatment with radiotherapy or chemotherapy.

c-*erb*B-2

The proto-oncogene c-*erb*B-2 (also known as *neu* or HER2) encodes a transmembrane glycoprotein which is similar to the EGF receptor. Structural homology with the EGF receptor (Bargmann et al. 1986; Yamamoto et al. 1986), possession of tyrosine kinase activity (Akiyama et al. 1986; Stern et al. 1986) and its ability to generate mitogenic responses (Lee et al. 1989) all point to the function of the c-*erb*B-2 protein being akin to that of the EGF receptor. Several groups have recently reported candidate ligands for the c-*erb*B-2 receptor and elucidation of the primary structure of one of these molecules (*neu* differentiation factor, NDF or Heregulin-α, HRG-α) reveals it to be an additional member of the EGF family (Lee et al. 1992; Wen et al. 1992). Two further members of the *erb*B receptor family have also recently been discovered, HER3/p160*erb*B-3 and HER4/p180*erb*B-4 (Plowman et al. 1990, 1993).

The largest and most comprehensive studies of the c-*erb*B-2 gene have been conducted in breast carcinomas in which gene amplification was found to be a significant predictor of both disease-free survival and overall survival in node-positive patients in a univariate analysis (Slamon et al. 1989). Amplification of the c-*erb*B-2 gene in patients with ovarian cancer has also been reported to have a direct relationship with survival (Slamon et al. 1989).

There are now several studies concerning the incidence of c-*erb*B-2 overexpression in bladder cancer although the results of these have been conflicting (Wright et al. 1990; McCann et al. 1990; Asamoto et al. 1990; Wright et al. 1991; Moriyama et al. 1991). In an immunohistochemical study of c-*erb*B-2 oncoprotein expression in 82 primary bladder tumours, we have found evidence of strong positive staining in 12/81 (15%) primary bladder tumours and weak positive staining in a further 19 (23%) (Wright et al. 1991).

We noted a weak association between staining for c-*erb*B-2 and tumour stage but none with histological grade, unlike the study by Moriyama et al. (1991). Our finding that c-*erb*B-2 protein is expressed by 15% of transitional cell tumours of the bladder differs from the results of McCann et al. (1990), in which the reported incidence of strong staining was only 2% (1/48 tumours). It must be pointed out that in the latter study paraffin-embedded tumours were assessed for c-*erb*B-2 protein using the 21N antibody (Gullick et al. 1987). These conflicting results underline the importance of methodological factors in immunohistochemical analyses.

Although DNA amplification of c-*erb*B-2 has been reported as a frequent mechanism of overexpression for this gene in breast cancer, this does not seem to be the case in bladder cancer. Coombs et al. (1991) reported Southern blotting studies in which amplification of the c-*erb*B-2 gene was found in 1/37 grade 1, 5/32 grade 2 and 6/13 grade 3 tumours. Zhau et al. (1990) reported 2/24 cases of c-*erb*B-2 gene amplification, which only accounted for a small proportion of the increased p185^{erbB-2} protein expression detected by Western blotting. From 24 tumour DNA samples analysed for c-*erb*B-2 gene copy number only one case of gene amplification was found (Mellon et al. 1991). Recently, Sauter et al. (1993) examined 141 bladder tumour specimens for c-*erb*B-2 gene amplification using fluorescence *in situ* hybridisation (FISH) on frozen and formalin fixed tissues. Amplification of c-*erb*B-2 was detected in only 10/141 cases and overexpression without amplification was present in 51 tumours. The amplification was more frequent in invasive tumours and considerable heterogeneity of amplification was observed within a given sample.

Bladder Cancer Prognosis Related to c-erbB-2 Status

We have assessed the prognostic value of determining c-*erb*B-2 status by immunohistochemistry in 95 primary bladder tumours of which 20 (21%) were positive for c-*erb*B-2, i.e. eight superficial and 12 muscle-invasive tumours. From the 95 patients in this study group, there were 16 bladder cancer-related deaths (four patients with c-*erb*B-2 positive tumours and 12 with c-*erb*B-2 negative tumours). c-*erb*B-2 status was not a significant factor in predicting death.

Of 33 pTa and 20 pT1 tumours assessed for c-*erb*B-2, three pTa and five pT1 tumours were c-*erb*B-2 positive. There was no significant difference between the mean recurrence rate of c-*erb*B-2 positive Ta tumours, 9/100 patient months (CI = 0–36/100 patient months, *n* = 3) and c-*erb*B-2 negative Ta tumours, 11/100 patient months (CI = 7–15/100 patient months, *n* = 30, *P* = 0.85). However a significant difference was detected between the mean recurrence rate of T1 tumours which were positive for c-*erb*B-2, 25/100 patient months (CI = 18–32/100 patient months, *n* = 5) and those which were negative, 13/100 patient months (CI = 8–19/100 patient months, *n* = 15, *P* = 0.04). c-*erb*-2 was not a significant factor in predicting time to recurrence.

Seven tumours developed stage progression (Ta = 3 and T1 = 4): two were c-*erb*B-2 positive and five were c-*erb*B-2 negative. Three Ta tumours progressed to T1 (one c-*erb*B-2 positive), two T1 tumours progressed to T3 (one c-*erb*B-2 positive), one T1 tumour progressed to T4b G3 disease at 15 months and developed a rib metastasis at 21 months (c-*erb*B-2 negative) and one T1 tumour developed hepatic metastases at 20 months (c-*erb*B-2 negative).

Fibroblast Growth Factor

In essence the only other group of growth factors to be examined in bladder cancer to any significant degree is the fibroblast growth factor (FGF) family. The FGFs are a family of peptides related by sequence similarity which have been implicated in the regulation of cell proliferation, embryonal development, differentiation and motility. The family includes acidic fibroblast growth factor (aFGF), basic fibroblast growth factor (bFGF), *int* 2 (FGF3), *hst* (FGF4), FGF5 and *hst* 2 (FGF6). They bind with varying degrees of specificity to a family of tyrosine kinase receptors (FGFRs). bFGF has been shown to transform mouse fibroblasts in vitro and the family includes *int* 2 and *hst* oncogenes. *int* 2 (FGF3) is the human homologue to one of the common integration sites of mouse mammary tumour virus (MMTV). *hst* (FGF4) is the most frequently detected human transforming gene, after *ras* genes, in the NIH3T3 focus assay. Both *int* 2 and *hst* are located on chromosome band 11q13 which is found amplified in a wide range of common tumours. Theillet et al. (1989) reported these two genes to be amplified in 3/43 (7%) of bladder tumours and 41/238 (17%) of breast carcinomas. Gene amplification at the 11q13 locus involving *int* 2 and *hst* co-amplification has also been reported by Procter et al. (1991) in 20/97 (20.6%) bladder tumours.

An FGF-like factor has previously been reported in raised amounts in the urine of patients with bladder cancer (Chodak et al. 1988). In a small-scale immunohistochemical study of aFGF (12 TCCs), strong immunostaining was found in high-grade urothelial tumours with little staining of normal tissues (Ravery et al. 1992). In the same study, basic FGF was found in basement membranes and blood vessels but not in urothelium.

It has been observed that treatment of rat NBT-II bladder carcinoma cells in culture with aFGF induced morphological changes from epithelial to a more fibroblastic appearance and promoted cell dissociation and dispersion (Valles et al. 1990). In a further study, aFGF or *hst* (FGF4)-producing NBT-II cells were produced by transfection resulting in increased cell dispersal, gelatinase activity and tissue invasion in organ co-culture (Jouanneau et al. 1991). These observations suggest that FGFs can act in an autocrine manner to amplify the invasive and metastatic potential of bladder tumour cells and merit further investigation in the human clinical context.

Transforming Growth Factor Beta

The TGFβ peptides are of interest because they appear to have opposite effects to TGF-α and aFGF, in that they inhibit the growth of normal epithelial cells and many transformed cells, as well as promoting differentiation and extracellular matrix formation. Coombs et al. (1993) have analysed 40 transitional cell carcinomas for the structure and expression of the TGFβ1 and TGFβ2 genes. No altered copy number or rearrangement of either gene was found. However, there was some association between reduced TGFβ1 expression and advanced disease.

Tumour Suppressor Genes

Early studies based on the analysis of acutely transforming retroviruses and the NIH3T3 transfection system had led to an emphasis on the role of dominant acting oncogenes in models of the molecular basis of cancer. However, more recently it has become apparent that there is an equally important group of recessive oncogenes or tumour suppressor genes which are transforming as a consequence of loss of function. This is perhaps not surprising given that biochemical pathways, including those that govern cellular growth, are controlled by both positive and negative regulators. Evidence for the existence of tumour suppresssor genes has come from several sources, although in some cases the significance of the observations was not widely appreciated at the time. Experiments dating back to the 1960s involving the fusion of normal and transformed cells had clearly shown that factors in normal cells could suppress transformation and malignancy, suggesting these can be recessive characteristics in some circumstances.

The second major line of evidence came from an analysis of the patterns of inheritance for rare hereditary childhood cancers. Based on an analysis of familial and sporadic retinoblastoma, Knudson (1971) proposed a two-hit inactivation process in which both copies of a critical gene had to be inactivated for the disease to be manifested. On this model individuals with the familial form of retinoblastoma had inherited one inactivated and one normal gene from their parents, with a second mutation inactivating the remaining normal allele having a high probability of occurring in one of the "at risk" retinoblasts at some point during the development of the eye. In the case of the sporadic form, individuals inherit two normal alleles and inactivating mutations have to knock out both copies of the critical gene in the same retinoblast to produce the tumour. This requirement for two somatic mutations in the same gene in the same cell explains the much lower incidence of the sporadic tumours compared with the familial case, where inheritance of a germ-line mutation only requires a single somatic mutation in any one of the developing retinoblasts, all of which carry the germ-line mutation. This seminal analysis has become a paradigm by which a wide spectrum of hereditary predispositions to cancer have been interpreted on the basis of inherited germ-line mutations of tumour suppressor genes.

The additional fact that these hereditary cancers are often associated with predisposition to a wide range of sporadic tumours of other tissues led to the further suggestion that somatic mutation or loss of these same genes were probably involved in the genesis of a wider range of common cancers including bladder cancer. This provided a possible explanation for the observation of non-random chromosome deletions often seen in sporadic tumours, and established the third major line of evidence for the existence of tumour suppressor genes. This in turn ultimately led to the identification of the p53 gene as a tumour suppressor gene as a result of detailed mapping of frequent chromosome 17p losses in colorectal cancer.

Non-random Chromosome Losses in Bladder Cancer: Novel Tumour Suppressor Genes to be Discovered?

Reports of non-random chromosome losses in tumour cells have gained added significance as it has become apparent that these may be part of the two-hit mechanism required to inactivate both copies of a tumour suppressor gene. Mutations of the p53 tumour suppressor gene in bladder cancer, as well as other tumours, are often associated with the loss or deletion of chromosome 17p. The combination of a subtle point mutation combined with removal of the remaining gene copy by a gross deletion of all or part of chromosome 17 seems to be more common than the alternative of both copies of the gene being inactivated by point mutations. This is likely to be a mechanism extending to other tumour suppressor genes and therefore the mapping of non-random chromosome deletions offers the promise of discovering the location of novel tumour suppressor genes. This is a particularly pertinent strategy in bladder cancer since the absence of cases of strong familial predisposition to this tumour type precludes the use of linkage analysis to locate putative bladder-specific tumour suppressor genes.

Early studies of chromosome losses and deletions by classical cytogenetic methods have more recently given way to analysis by recombinant DNA techniques for visualising mapped polymorphic regions of DNA, which allow the two copies of a chromosome in normal tissue, and the possible loss of one of them in a tumour, to be distinguished by either Southern blotting or PCR methods. One spin-off from the Human Genome Mapping Project is that a rapidly increasing number of such markers is becoming available, allowing deletion mapping to be pursued to higher resolutions than hitherto possible.

Cytogenetic studies have shown that frequent non-random chromosome alterations occur in bladder cancer, particularly involving chromosomes 1p, 3p, 9q, 10q, 11, 13q, 17p and 18q (Smeets et al. 1987; Hopman et al. 1991; Presti et al. 1991). Notably, loss of one copy of chromosome 9 was found as an early event in low-stage low-grade tumours, unlike other chromosome losses which appeared more prevalent in advanced tumours. Tsai et al. (1990) examined a panel of 25 bladder tumours for loss of heterozygosity for nine polymorphic markers located on five chromosome arms (11p, 9q, 14q, 17p and 6p) and found a high rate of chromosome deletions for markers on chromosomes 9q (67%), 11p (40%) and 17p (63%). The high frequency of chromosome 9q losses in bladder cancer is of particular interest as it is not seen in other tumour types and suggests possible location of a tumour suppressor gene which is specific to bladder cancer. Subsequent studies have also shown that loss of chromosome 9 markers is the only frequent genetic alteration seen in low-grade superficial (Ta) bladder tumours, suggesting that loss of a tumour suppressor gene on this chromosome is a candidate initiating event in bladder carcinogenesis (Cairns et al. 1993; Habuchi et al. 1993). More detailed mapping of chromosome 9q deletions by Cairns et al. (1993) has defined a minimum area of deletion between the chromosome markers *D9S22* at 9q22 to *D9S18* at 9p12–13, suggesting the target tumour suppressor gene resides within this region. This conclusion is supported in a preliminary report by Lin et al. (1993) who found the most common subchromosomal deletion in bladder tumours to be for marker *D9S15* which is located within the region 9q22.1–9q22.3.

The absence of a familial form of bladder cancer suggests that inactivated forms of the putative bladder-specific tumour suppressor gene on chromosome 9q are rarely or never carried in the germ-line. This may be because two viable copies of the gene are required for normal development and that the level of expression is critical.

The p53 Tumour Suppressor Gene

The human p53 gene, located on the short arm of chromosome 17 (Miller et al. 1986), encodes a nuclear phosphoprotein which binds specific DNA sequences in the human genome (Kern et al. 1991) and appears to play a key role in the control of DNA replication and hence cellular proliferation. Non-random chromosome 17 losses involving the p53 locus are commonly found in human tumours, including bladder cancer, and loss of one copy of the p53 gene has been found to be frequently accompanied by mutation of the remaining allele (Nigro et al. 1989). Transfection studies have shown that the wild type protein is able to suppress cell proliferation and transformation (Finlay et al. 1989). It thus acts in such circumstances as a tumour suppressor gene which can contribute to tumour formation by deletions or loss of function mutations. However, in other situations a subset of p53 mutations can result in dominant transforming properties. Germ-line mutations of the p53 gene have been found in certain inherited predispositions to cancer (Li-Fraumeni syndrome) and somatic cell mutations have frequently been detected in a wide range of common sporadic tumours, including breast, colon, brain and lung tumours as well as bladder cancer (Nigro et al. 1989; Iggo et al. 1990). These mutations are predominantly of the point missense type and occur at many different locations within four highly conserved regions of the gene (codons 117–142, 171–181, 234–258 and 270–286) located in exons 4 to 9 of the p53 gene (Hollstein et al. 1991).

The p53 protein has a short half-life, measured in the order of minutes, and is normally present at low levels that are not detectable by immunohisto-chemistry. One of the remarkable features of the p53 gene is that a broad spectrum of mutations can lead to an altered conformation of the protein product with an increased cellular half-life, resulting in accumulation in the cell to levels that are readily detectable by immunohistochemical staining. Although this initially led to suggestions that positive detection of p53 by immunohistochemistry was synonymous with the detection of mutations, a concept eagerly grasped at by histopathologists, this has to be qualified by more recent observations that other mechanisms for increasing p53 expression exist, such as the effect of DNA damage and the action of other oncogenes. Furthermore, it has become evident that some mutations do not result in accumulation of the altered protein product and these have to be screened for by alternative complementary methods such as single-strand conformation poymorphism (SSCP) to obtain a more complete picture. However, even combined, these techniques are at best a way of trawling for mutations rather than a way of systematically screening for all possible mutations. The definitive method of establishing the presence of a mutation in a sample is by DNA sequencing procedures. If a mutation is present in greater than 25% of the cells in the sample then PCR-based direct sequencing methods will pick these up with a high probability; for lower proportions subcloning the PCR products and sequencing a representative sample of the individual subclones are required.

Immunohistochemical p53 Studies

The first reported study of p53 expression in bladder cancer was by Wright et al. (1991), who examined frozen sections of 82 primary transitional cell carcinomas of the bladder using the PAb240 monoclonal antibody, believed to be specific for mutant forms of the protein. Strong or moderate staining was found in 18% of tumours with weak staining evident in an additional 36%. Tumours invading the bladder muscle were found to show a higher frequency of staining compared with superficial tumours, suggesting that tumours with a high risk of progression may contain elevated levels of mutant p53 protein and that high intensities of staining may provide useful prognostic information. This study also examined the relationship between p53 expression and that of c-*erb*B-2 and epidermal growth factor receptor (EGFr) proteins. No association between p53 and EGFr expression was evident, but a weak positive correlation was found between c-*erb*B-2 and p53 staining.

More recently an extensive study on 212 archival paraffin-embedded samples using the CMI polyclonal antibody has confirmed and extended these observations (Lipponen 1993). In this study 29% of tumours stained positively for p53 protein and over-expression was reported to be associated with stage of tumour progression, histological grade, non-papillary growth architecture, dense inflammatory reaction, DNA aneuploidy, high S-phase fraction and mitotic frequency. Over-expression of p53 was found to predict poor outcome in muscle-invasive but not superficial tumours. However, in a multivariate survival analysis over-expression of p53 was found to have no independent prognostic value over clinical stage and mitotic index.

Analysis of p53 Mutations by DNA Sequencing

Following the discovery of mutations of the p53 gene in a diverse range of common tumour types, data have been accumulating from several laboratories on the specific pattern of p53 mutations in bladder cancer. Sidransky et al. (1991) reported alterations of the p53 gene in 11 out of 18 invasive bladder carcinomas examined by direct PCR-based DNA sequencing for exons 5 to 9. Ten cases involved point mutations resulting in a single amino acid substitution and one 24 bp deletion. In all but one case these mutations were accompanied by loss of the wild-type sequence as a result of chromosome 17p allelic deletions, consistent with p53 behaving as a tumour suppressor in bladder cancer. In addition these authors were able to demonstrate the presence of cells carrying these same mutations in a small proportion of the cells (1%–7%) of the urine sediment from each of three patients tested.

A subsequent study (Fujimoto et al. 1992) examined 25 bladder carcinomas from 23 patients and included 13 superficial tumours. In this study, unlike that of Sidransky et al. (1991), the samples were initially screened for the presence of mutations in exons 4 to 11 of the gene by SSCP analysis and then those showing evidence of conformational shifts, indicating the presence of mutations, were subjected to PCR-based direct sequencing to confirm and identify the mutation. The results indicated that the incidence of p53 mutations was much higher in invasive compared with superficial tumours. Only one of 13 superficial tumours (Tis, Ta and T1) was found to have a p53 mutation, whereas six of 12 invasive bladder cancers (T2, T3 and T4) were found with mutations. Notably, two of the mutations were found in exon 4, a region not generally covered by other studies. The mutations found did not show any specific pattern of distribution along the gene.

The largest and most recent study reported to date is that of Spruck et al. (1993), who screened 80 tumours and examined the relationship of the p53 mutations found to tobacco usage by the patients. This study was restricted to exons 5 to 8 of the p53 gene and SSCP screening was used to identify sets of samples for sequencing. Mutations were found in 16/40 (40%) of bladder tumours from smokers and 13/40 (33%) of those from non-smokers. In six tumours identical point mutations at codon 280 were observed, suggesting a mutational hot-spot for bladder cancers at this position. There was no obvious difference in the type or position of mutations found in smoking and non-smoking groups. Although there was no significant difference in the overall frequency of cases with mutations between the smoking and non-smoking groups, interestingly all five cases in which multiple mutations were found in the same sample came from the group of patients who smoked. This suggests a subset of smokers may have a particularly high predisposition to the carcinogenic effects of tobacco smoking. This could be due to differences in the metabolic activation of procarcinogens or defects in the repair of the DNA adducts and base changes produced by exposure to circulatory carcinogens resulting from cigarette smoking. The authors proposed that the unusually high rate of G:C to C:G transversions found could be generated by oxygen free radicals and suggested these reactive species may have an important role in the aetiology of bladder cancer.

A DNA sequencing study has been carried out by our Newcastle group to follow on from the initial immunohistochemical analysis (Challen et al. 1993). This is the only bladder cancer study which was based on prior screening of samples by immunohistochemistry. PCR-based direct sequencing was used to analyse the p53 tumour suppressor gene in DNA extracts from 35 bladder tumours, 24 of which were selected for positive immunohistochemical staining for p53 and 11 were negative. Full sequence analysis was carried out for exons 4–9 of the p53 gene, covering the major highly conserved domains. Point mutations were detected in 10 of the 35 samples analysed. In one of the samples three mutations were found, making a total of 12 muta-tions: 8/12 (66%) mutations were transitions and 4/12 (33%) transversions.

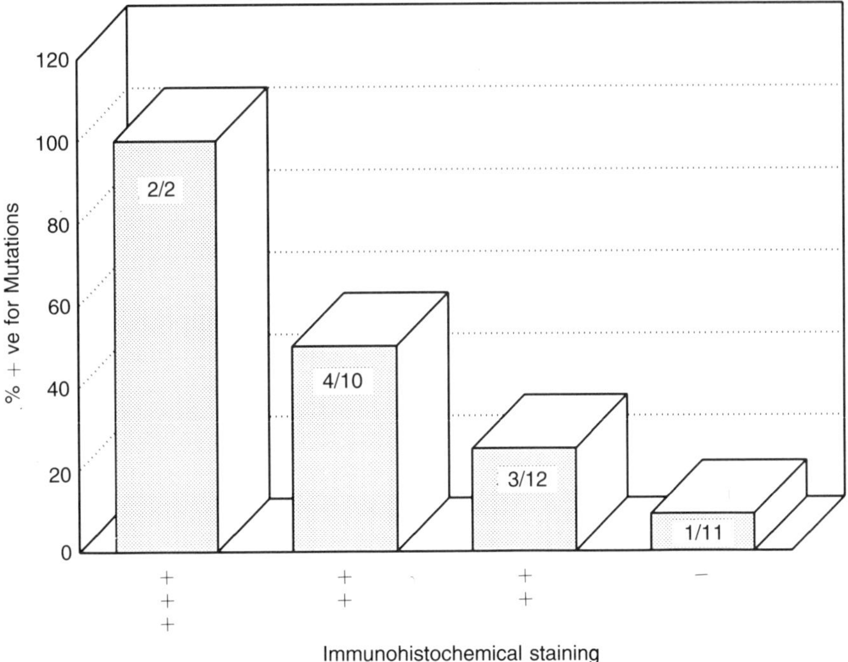

Fig. 2.2. p53 mutations and immunohistochemistry.

The proportion of transitions was not significantly different from that for spontaneous mutations.

A marked clustering in exons 7 and 8 was evident, corresponding to conserved domains IV and V. This probably reflects the binding site for a host factor which has a key role in cellular growth control. Mutations in this region may prevent binding of this host factor, mimicking the effect of certain tumour viruses such as SV40, which encode transforming proteins that are known to interact with this region of p53. There was a significant association between the detection of mutations and positive staining for p53 protein by immunohistochemistry (Fig. 2.2). This was consistent with studies which have shown that a broad spectrum of p53 mutations lead to an increase in the half-life of the protein and a consequent accumulation in the cell to readily detectable levels. The relationship between p53 mutations and smoking habits in bladder cancer patients was examined. For the group of 35 samples sequenced, information on smoking habits was available for 19 male patients; of these the five for which mutations were detected were all smokers rather than non- or ex-smokers. Although the numbers were small there was a significant positive association between the detection of mutations and smoking which merits further investigation. The detection of p53 mutations in tumour samples was associated with poor patient survival. Only 50% of patients whose tumours showed evidence of p53 mutations survived beyond 18 months compared with 89% survival beyond this time in the group without mutations. However, the mutations were found more frequently in high stage invasive tumours and it remains to be established whether the detection of p53 mutations by direct sequencing has any independent prognostic significance in the early stages of tumour invasion. This study included both superficial and invasive tumours and reinforces the observation that p53 mutations are a late event in the progression of bladder cancer, being rare in superficial tumours and common in high grade invasive tumours.

More recently the Newcastle study has been extended by SSCP screening of those tumours which were negatively staining for p53 on immunohistochemical screening. A further five cases of p53 mutation were detected from 35 tumours screened in this way, with multiple mutations found in the same tumour in two cases, involving a further total of eight mutations. In contrast to the mutations found in samples which had stained positive for p53 overexpression, which were predominantly found in exons 7 and 8 of the p53 gene, those discovered by following-up SSCP screening were found to be more evenly distributed along the p53 gene, with three located in exon 4, a region not generally covered in other studies. The mutations revealed by SSCP shifts revealed a higher proportion of transversions and insertional mutations. This suggests that the initial method of screening for mutations can bias the spectrum and position of mutations detected.

A compilation plot of the position of mutations along the p53 gene which is based on all the published mutations and those recorded in the Newcastle study is shown in Fig. 2.3. The striking feature of this is that the strongest clustering of mutations is seen in exon 8 of the p53 gene between codons 280 and 287. This appears to be a particular feature of bladder cancer and is distinct from the overall pattern of mutations found for a range of different tumour types. This suggests that in bladder urothelium there is a

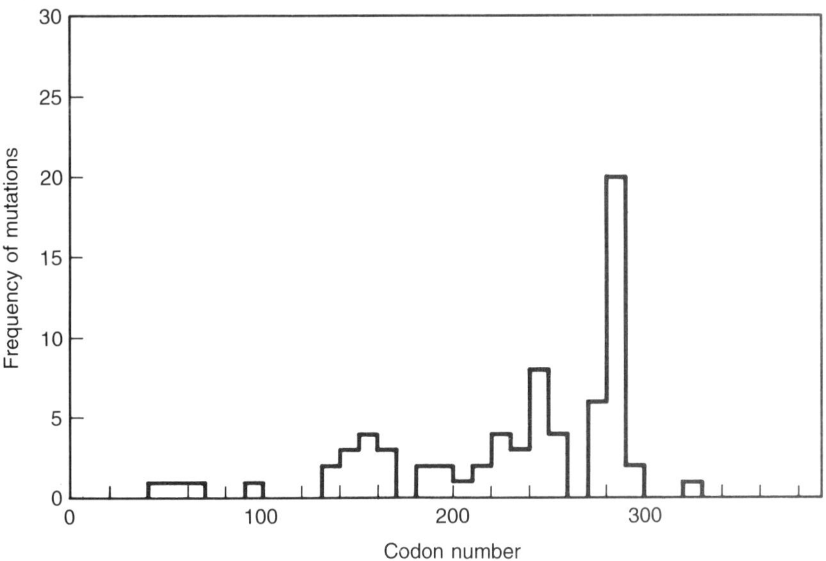

Fig. 2.3. p53 mutations in bladder cancer.

Table 2.1. Proportion of p53 mutations found in bladder tumours of different stage complied from three separate studies. A highly significant association with stage is seen for the combined data (P=0.00114; χ^2 test)

	Ta	T1	T2	T3	T4
Sidransky et al. (1991)	–	1/3	0/2	10/12	0/1
Fujimoto et al. (1992)	0/7	0/5	1/1	5/10	1/1
Newcastle	1/8	2/7	2/8	6/17	4/4
Total	1/15	3/15	3/11	21/39	5/6
Proportion	6.7%	20%	27.3%	53.8%	83.3%

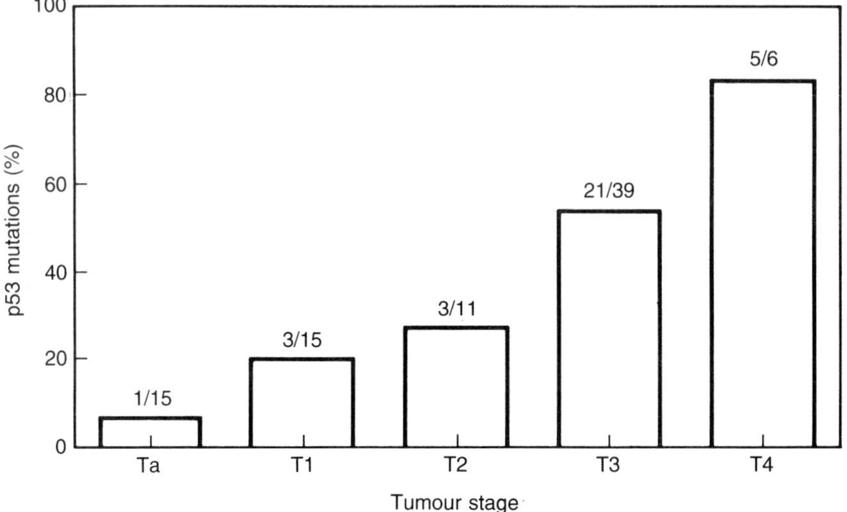

Fig. 2.4. p53 mutations in bladder cancer: association with tumour stage.

tissue-specific factor involved in normal growth control which interacts with p53 by a specific binding which is disrupted by mutations in the 280–287 region.

An overall comparison of the reported incidence of mutations with respect to tumour stage is summarised in Table 2.1 and Fig. 2.4. This clearly shows that p53 mutations are late events in bladder tumour progression being associated predominantly with invasive tumours. The largest proportional increase in the incidence of mutations is seen between the superficial Ta and the early invasive T1 groups, with successive increases rising to an incidence of over 83% in the late stage metastatic T4 group. This clearly shows that the incidence of p53 mutations is strongly associated with invasive progression in this tumour system and that p53 mutations are not involved in the loss of normal growth control that defines the initial formation of superficial bladder tumours. It remains to be established whether p53 mutations are causally involved in the process of tumour invasion or merely markers of progression without direct involvement, although clearly they must be associated with some selective clonal growth advantage to become present in the majority of cells in late stage tumours.

Retinoblastoma Gene

Retinoblastoma is a malignant embryonal eye tumour diagnosed at a median age of two years. In 30%–40% of cases the predisposition to retinoblastoma is inherited as an autosomal dominant trait, being associated with the inheritance of a defective allele (Rb1) which has been mapped to the q14 band of chromosome 13. A wider role for the Rb1 gene was suggested by the observation that those who inherit the mutant allele have a higher incidence of a wide range of non-ocular second tumours, particularly osteosarcomas but also lung, melanoma and bladder cancer (Sanders et al. 1989). Since the cloning of the gene the extent of its possible involvement as a tumour suppressor in the development and progression of a subset of common sporadic adult human tumours has become directly apparent.

The Rb1 gene encodes a 105–115 kDa nuclear phosphoprotein which binds to DNA and appears to be involved in growth regulation in a wide variety of cell types. The Rb1 gene product binds to transforming proteins of several DNA tumour viruses, including adenovirus E1A, SV40 large T antigen and human papilloma virus E7 proteins. Initial studies with the Rb1 cDNA probe, based mainly on tumour cell lines, reported frequent structural abnormalities of the gene and absence of Rb1 mRNA. Subsequent extensions of these studies with polyclonal antisera indicated that absence or abnormal forms of the Rb protein are almost universal in SCLC cell lines and in one-third of bladder carcinoma cell lines surveyed, but infrequent in colonic, breast and melanoma cell lines (Horowitz et al. 1990).

Studies on primary bladder tumours have shown that loss of heterozygosity for Rb1-linked markers is associated with the development of invasive lesions (Cairns et al. 1991; Ishikawa et al. 1991). Combining the data from these studies shows overall frequencies of Rb1 allele loss for the retinoblastoma gene of 3/63 (4.8%) for superficial (Ta/T1) and 30/58 (51.7%) for invasive (T2–T4) tumours. Major rearrangements of the remaining Rb1 gene were detected in only a small proportion of these cases, suggesting that generally more subtle small deletions or point mutations are involved, which have yet to be characterised.

The prognostic significance of altered retinoblastoma protein expression has been investigated. Logothetis et al. (1992) in a study of 43 patients with locally advanced bladder carcinoma reported altered Rb protein expression detected by immunohistochemistry in 37% of the tumour specimens and a significantly poorer tumour-free survival rate was noted for patients with tumours showing altered Rb protein expression. Rb protein alterations did not correlate with other known prognostic factors examined, suggesting that it is an independent indicator of tumour progression. Cordon-Cardo et al. (1992) examined Rb protein levels by immunohistochemistry in 48 primary bladder tumours and reported undetectable or heterogeneous expression in 14/38 muscle-invasive tumours, but only 1/10 superficial tumours. The five-year survival frequency was significantly reduced in the group of patients whose tumours showed altered patterns of Rb protein expression. Both these studies indicate that reduced Rb protein expression is associated with more aggressive tumours. The causal role of Rb protein expression in bladder carcinoma cell malignancy has been tested by transfection studies in which it has been shown that the introduction of an expressed normal Rb gene into bladder carcinoma cells suppresses their tumorigenicity without reducing growth rate (Goodrich et al. 1992).

The Multistep Multistage Model

Genetic Alterations and the Clonal Origin of Multiple Tumours of the Urinary Tract Epithelium

It has become a central tenet of cancer molecular biology that tumours are monoclonal in origin. However it has not been clear how this concept of clonal origin from a single transformed cell applies to neoplasia in organs such as bladder where multiple tumours of the urothelium are common, often accompanied by diffuse areas of dysplasia. In some cases this can involve concomitant transitional cell carcinomas of the renal pelvis, ureter and urinary bladder. These clinical observations have led to the notion of "field defects" where exposure to a carcinogen results in the independent transformation of many epithelial cells. The alternative hypothesis is that only a single cell is initially transformed which by clonal expansion, cell detachment and dispersion then gives rise to spatially separate, but genetically related, multiple tumours.

Techniques which allow the detection of genetic alterations at the molecular level have recently been used to test these alternative hypotheses. Lunec et al. (1992) reported identical p53 mutations and c-*erb*B-2 gene amplification in a case of concomitant transitional carcinomas of the renal pelvis and urinary bladder. The high level of c-*erb*B-2 amplification found is rare in bladder cancer and it is most unlikely that the identical point mutation found at the same codon of the p53 gene could have arisen by chance from separate independent mutation events. These observations showed that the renal pelvis and bladder TCCs had the same clonal origin. The most likely interpretation was that the bladder cancer had arisen as a result of distal tumour cell spread from the primary renal pelvis tumour.

The use of molecular genetic markers to investigate the clonal origin of multiple tumours of the bladder has also recently been reported by Sidransky et al. (1992). In this case the authors employed polymorphic markers on the X-chromosome and the fact that the cells of adult tissues in females have either one of the two X-chromosomes randomly inactivated by methylation. Thus if multiple tumours arose from different single cells they would be heterogeneous with respect to which X-chromosome remained active. For each of four female patients with multiple tumours it was found that all the tumours from an individual had inactivation of the same X-chromosome, whereas the normal bladder urothelium showed the expected random pattern of inactivation. In addition the authors examined patterns of allele loss in these tumours using markers for chromosomes 9q, 17p and 18q. Each tumour for a given patient showed loss of the same chromosome 9q allele, consistent with chromosome 9q losses being early events in bladder cancer initiation and preceding the spread of neoplastic cells to form multiple tumours. Losses of chromosome 17p and 18q alleles, which are known to be late events in bladder tumour progression, were not common to different tumours from the same individual, showing that these events occurred subsequent to the seeding of secondary tumours from the primary. These observations indicate that multiple bladder tumours can arise from a single transformed cell by clonal expansion and early spread and that subsequently the individual tumours can follow different paths of progression by independent additional genetic alterations. Studies are in progress in several centres to extend this type of analysis to address the question of the clonal origin of recurrent tumours.

Multiple Alterations Involving Dominant Oncogenes and Tumour Suppressor Genes

Although for the purposes of presentation we have traced development of knowledge in these areas separately, it is clear that a comprehensive molecular model for the initiation and progression of bladder cancer, as with other cancers, must involve a multistep process which is a multifactorial synthesis of all these elements. For instance it has been found that mutated *ras* and p53 genes together can transform primary cells in culture, whereas either alone fails. Reznikoff et al. (1989) have shown that immortalised normal urothelial cells transfected with an activated *ras* oncogene only become tumorigenic when the p21^{ras} product is overexpressed and other genetic alterations, such as chromosomal loss, have taken place. The late onset and age-related incidence of bladder cancer is consistent with the requirement for an accumulation of multiple events over an extended period of time. By analogy with analyses of such data for colorectal cancer one can conclude that as many as four or five genetic alterations may be required. Of course the rate at which such events accumulate can vary considerably for individuals depending on the exposure to carcinogens and variations in individual abilities to metabolise carcinogens or repair the DNA damage they produce. Direct evidence for the presence of multiple genetic events in human bladder tumour samples can be found in detailed molecular pathology studies, such as the case study discussed above in which both c-*erb*B-2 gene amplification and p53 mutations were found in the same tumour sample.

As more detailed analyses of alterations in a range of oncogenes, growth factors and tumour suppressor genes in the same tumour samples are built up, the presence of multiple changes is being substantiated. Further studies of this nature will define which of these genetic alterations appear to cooperate, whether any particular combinations are associated with a worse prognosis and whether a particular order of events is important. The loss of a tumour suppressor gene on chromosome 9 is probably a particularly critical event in the initiation of bladder cancer and the identification of the specific gene involved is a major goal at present.

Finally it must be said that, in spite of the considerable advances in our knowledge which have firmly established genetic alterations at the somatic cell level as central to the general mechanisms of tumour initiation and progression, the detailed picture for bladder cancer is far from clear. Some of the pieces of the puzzle and their connections have been established – the task of completing the picture remains and may yet yield further surprises that challenge our current view.

References

Akiyama T, Sudo C, Ogawara H, Toyoshima K, Yamamoto T (1986) The product of the human c-*erb*B-2 gene: a 185-kilodalton glycoprotein with tyrosine kinase activity. Science 232:1644–1646

Allen LE, Dubeau L, Alvarez O, Jones PA (1990) Rapid degradation of extracellular matrix proteins by normal human uroepithelial cells. Cancer Res 50:1897–1904

Asamoto M, Hasegawa R, Masuko T et al. (1990) Immunohistochemical analysis of c-*erb*B-2 oncogene product and epidermal growth factor receptor expression in human urinary bladder carcinomas. Acta Pathol Jpn 40:322–326

Bargmann CI, Hung M-C, Weinberg RA (1986) The *neu* oncogene encodes an epidermal growth factor receptor-related protein. Nature 319:226–230

Berger MS, Greenfield C, Gullick WJ et al. (1987) Evaluation of epidermal growth factor receptors in bladder tumours. Br J Cancer 56:533–537

Bos JL (1989) *ras* oncogenes in human cancer: a review. Cancer Res 49:4682–4689

Burchill SA, Neal DE, Lunec J (1994) Frequency of H-*ras* mutations in human bladder cancer detected by direct sequencing. Br J Urol (in press)

Cairns P, Proctor AJ, Knowles MA (1991) Loss of heterozygosity at the RB locus is frequent and correlates with muscle invasion in bladder carcinoma. Oncogene 6:2305–2309

Cairns P, Shaw ME, Knowles MA (1993) Preliminary mapping of the deleted region of chromosome 9 in bladder cancer. Cancer Res 53:1230–1232

Capon DJ, Chen EY, Levinson AD, Seeburg PH, Goeddel DV (1983) Complete nucleotide sequences of the T24 human bladder carcinoma oncogene and its normal homologue. Nature 309:33–37

Challen C, Mellon K, Neal DE, Lunec J (1993) p53 mutations in human bladder cancer: association with smoking and poor prognosis. Br J Cancer 67(Suppl XX):58 (Abs)

Chodak GW, Hospelhorn V, Judge SM, Mayforth R, Koeppen H, Sasse J (1988) Increased levels of fibroblast growth factor-like activity in urine from patients with bladder or kidney cancer. Cancer Res 48:2083–2088

Coombs LM, Pigott DA, Eydmann ME, Proctor AJ, Knowles MA (1993) Reduced expression of TGFβ is associated with advanced disease in transitional cell carcinoma. Br J Cancer 67:578–584

Coombs LM, Pigott DA, Sweeney E et al. (1991) Amplification and overexpression of c-*erb*B-2 in transitional cell carcinoma of the urinary bladder. Br J Cancer 63:601–608

Cordon-Cardo C, Wartinger D, Petrylak D et al. (1992) Altered expression of the retinoblastoma gene product: prognostic indicator in bladder cancer. J Natl Cancer Inst 84:1251–1256

Czerniak B, Deitch D, Simmons H, Etkind P, Herz F, Koss LG (1990) Ha-*ras* gene codon 12 mutation and DNA ploidy in urinary bladder carcinoma. Br J Cancer 62:762–763

Dubeau L, Jones PA, Rideout WM 3rd, Laug WE (1988) Differential regulation of plasminogen activators by epidermal growth factor in normal and neoplastic human urothelium. Cancer Res 48:5552–5556

Finlay CA, Hinds PW, Levine AJ (1989) The p53 proto-oncogene can act as a suppressor of transformation. Cell 57:1083–1093

Fujimoto K, Yamada Y, Okajima E et al. (1992) Frequent association of p53 gene mutation in invasive bladder cancer. Cancer Res 52:1393–1398

Fujita J, Srivastava SK, Kraus MH, Rhim JS, Tronick SR, Aaronson SA (1985) Frequency of molecular alterations affecting *ras* protooncogenes in human urinary tract tumours. Proc Natl Acad Sci USA 82:3849–3853

Fuse H, Mizuno I, Sakamoto M, Katayama T (1992) Epidermal growth factor in urine from the patients with urothelial tumour. Urol Int 48:261–264

Gavrilovic J, Moens G, Thiery JP, Jouanneau J (1990) Expression of transfected transforming growth factor alpha induces a motile fibroblast-like phenotype with extracellular matrix-degrading potential in a rat bladder carcinoma cell line. Cell Regul 1:1003–1014

Goodrich DW, Chen Y, Scully P, Lee WH (1992) Expression of the retinoblastoma gene product in bladder carcinoma cells associates with a low frequency of tumor formation. Cancer Res 52:1968–1973

Gullick WJ, Berger MS, Bennett PLP, Rothbard JB, Waterfield MD (1987) Expression of the c-*erb*B-2 protein in normal and transformed cells. Int J Cancer 40:246–254

Gullick WJ, Hughes CM, Mellon K, Neal DE, Lemoine NR (1991) Immunohistochemical detection of the epidermal growth factor receptor in paraffin-embedded human tissues. J Pathol 164:285–289

Gusterson B, Cowley G, Smith JA, Ozanne B (1984) Cellular localisation of human epidermal growth factor receptor. Cell Biol Int Rep 8:649–658.

Habuchi T, Ogawa O, Kakehi Y et al. (1993) Accumulated allelic losses in the development of invasive urothelial cancer. Int J Cancer 53:579–584

Harney JV, Liebert M, Wedemeyer G et al. (1991) The expression of epidermal growth factor receptor on human bladder cancer: potential use in radioimmunoscintigraphy. J Urol 146:227–231

Harris AL (1991) Cancer genes: telling changes of base. Nature 350:377–378

Hiti AL, Rideout WM 3rd, Laug WE, Jones PA (1990) Plasminogen activator regulation by transforming growth factor-beta in normal and neoplastic human urothelium. Cancer Commun 2:123–128

Hollstein M, Sidransky D, Vogelstein B, Harris CC (1991) p53 mutations in human cancers. Science 253:49–53

Hopman AHN, Moesker O, Smeets AWGB, Pauwels RPE, Vooujs GP, Ramaekers FCS (1991) Numerical chromosome 1, 7, 9 and 11 aberrations in bladder cancer detected by *in situ* hybridisation. Cancer Res 51:644–651

Horowitz JM, Park S-H, Bogenmann E et al. (1990) Frequent inactivation of the retinoblastoma anti-oncogene is restricted to a subset of human tumour cells. Proc Natl Acad Sci USA 87:2775–2779

Iggo R, Gatter K, Bartek J, Lane D, Harris AL (1990) Increased expression of mutant forms of p53 oncogene in primary lung cancer. Lancet 335:675–679

Ishikawa J, Xu HJ, Hu SX et al. (1991) Inactivation of the retinoblastoma gene in human bladder and renal cell carcinomas. Cancer Res 51:5736–5743

Ishikura K, Hasegawa M, Nomura K et al. (1991) Epidermal growth factor in the urine of patients with renal cell carcinoma and bladder tumor. Hinyokika Kiyo 37:1229–1234

Jouanneau J, Gavrilovic J, Caruelle D et al. (1991) Secreted or non-secreted forms of acidic fibroblast growth factor produced by transfected epithelial cells influence cell morphology, motility and invasive potential. Proc Natl Acad Sci USA 88:2893–2897

Kageyama Y, Katoh M, Okada K, Yoshida K, Tsuruo T (1991) Detection of P-glycoprotein in human urogenital carcinomas and its relationship to epidermal growth factor receptor expression. Eur Urol 20:58–61

Kallioniemi A, Kallioniemi OP, Sudar D et al. (1993) Comparative genomic hybridisation for molecular cytogenetic analysis of solid tumours. Science 258:818–821

Kern SE, Kinzler KW, Bruskin A et al (1991) Identification of p53 as a sequence-specific DNA binding protein. Science 252:1708–1711

Knowles MA, Williamson M (1993) Mutation of H-*ras* is infrequent in bladder cancer: confirmation by single-strand conformation polymorphism analysis, designed restriction fragment length polymorphisms, and direct sequencing. Cancer Res 53:133–139

Knudson AG (1971) Mutation and cancer: statistical studies of retinoblastoma. Proc Natl Acad Sci USA 68:820

Kristensen JK, Lose G, Lund F, Nexo E (1988) Epidermal growth factor in urine from patients with urinary bladder tumors. Eur Urol 14:313–314

Lau JL, Fowler JE Jr, Ghosh L (1988) Epidermal growth factor in the normal and neoplastic kidney and bladder. J Urol 139:170–175

Lee J, Dull TJ, Lax I, Schlessinger J, Ullrich A (1989) HER2 cytoplasmic domain generates normal mitogenic and transforming signals in a chimeric receptor. EMBO J 8:167–173

Lin C-W, Zhang D-S, Kwiatkowski DJ, Yandell DW (1993) Allelic deletions on chromosome 9q in bladder tumours detected by VNTR polymorphism. Proc Am Assoc Cancer Res 34:514 Abstract 3065

Lipponen PK (1993) Over-expression of p53 nuclear oncoprotein in transitional-cell bladder cancer and its prognostic value. Int J Cancer 53:365–370

Logothetis CJ, Xu HJ, Ro JY et al. (1992) Altered expression of retinoblastoma protein and known prognostic variables in locally advanced bladder cancer. J Natl Cancer Inst 84:1256–1261

Lunec J, Challen C, Wright C, Mellon K, Neal DE (1992) c-erbB-2 amplification and identical p53 mutations in concomitant transitional carcinomas of renal pelvis and urinary bladder. Lancet 339:439–440

Malone PR, Visvanathan KV, Ponder BA, Shearer RJ, Summerhayes IC (1985) Oncogenes and bladder cancer. Br J Urol 57:664–667

McCann A, Dervan PA, Johnston PA, Gullick WJ, Carney DN (1990) c-erbB-2 oncoprotein expression in primary human tumours. Cancer 65:88–92

Mellon K (1993) c-erbB oncogenes and cell cycling in human bladder cancer. MD Thesis, University of Newcastle upon Tyne

Mellon K, Wright C, Lunec J et al. (1991) p53, c-erbB-2 and EGFr in bladder cancer. Br J Cancer 63:834 (Abs)

Messing E (1984) Growth factors and human bladder tumors. J Urol 131:111A

Messing EM, Hanson P, Ulrich P, Erturk E (1987) Epidermal growth factor – interactions with normal and malignant urothelium in vivo and in situ studies. J Urol 138:1329–1335

Miller C, Mohandas T, Wolf D, Prokocimer M, Rotter V, Koeffler HP (1986) Human p53 gene is localised to short arm of chromosome 17. Nature 319:783–784

Moriyama M, Akiyama T, Yamamoto T et al. (1991) Expression of c-erbB-2 gene product in urinary bladder cancer. J Urol 145:423–427

Neal DE, Mellon K (1992a) Oncogenes and growth factors in genitourinary tract tumours. In: Waxman J, Williams G (eds) Urological oncology. Edward Arnold, London. pp 137–153

Neal DE, Mellon K (1992b) Epidermal growth factor receptor and bladder cancer: a review. Urol Int 48:365–371

Neal DE, Marsh C, Bennett MK et al. (1985) Epidermal-growth-factor receptors in human bladder cancer: comparison of invasive and superficial tumours. Lancet i:366–368

Neal DE, Smith K, Fennelly JA, Bennett MK, Hall RR, Harris AL (1989) Epidermal growth factor receptor in human bladder cancer: a comparison of immunohistochemistry and ligand binding. J Urol 141:517–521

Neal DE, Sharples L, Smith K, Fennelly J, Hall RR, Harris AL (1990) The epidermal growth factor receptor and the prognosis of bladder cancer. Cancer 65:1619–1625

Nigro JM, Baker SJ, Preisinger AC et al. (1989) Mutations in the p53 gene occur in diverse tumour types. Nature 342:705–708

Noguchi S, Yura Y, Sherwood ER, Kakinuma H, Kashihara N, Oyasu R (1990) Stimulation of stromal cell growth by normal rat urothelial cell-derived epidermal growth factor. Lab Invest 62:538–544

Nutting C, Chowaniec J (1992) Evaluation of the actions and interactions of retinoic acid and epidermal growth factor on transformed urothelial cells in culture: implications for the use of retinoid therapy in the treatment of bladder cancer patients. Clin Oncol 4:51–55

Plowman GD, Whitney GS, Neubauer MG et al. (1990) Molecular cloning and expression of an additional epidermal growth factor receptor-related gene. Proc Natl Acad Sci USA 87:4905–4909

Plowman GD, Culouscou J-M, Whitney GS et al. (1993) Ligand-specific activation of HER4/p180erbB4, a fourth member of the epidermal growth factor receptor family. Proc Natl Acad Scl USA 90:1746–1750

Presti JC, Reuter VE, Galan T, Fair WR, Cordon-Cardo C (1991) Molecular genetic alterations in superficial and locally advanced human bladder cancer. Cancer Res 51:5405–5409

Procter AJ, Coombs LM, Cairns JP, Knowles MA (1991) Amplification at chromosome 11q13 in transitional cell carcinomas of the bladder. Oncogene 6:789–795

Ravery V, Jouanneau J, Gil Diez S, Abbou CC, Caruelle JP, Barritault D (1992) Immunohistochemical detection of acidic fibroblast growth factor in bladder transitional cell carcinoma. Urol Res 20:211–214

Reddy EP, Reynolds RK, Santos E, Barbacid M (1982) A point mutation is responsible for the acquisition of transforming properties by the T24 human bladder carcinoma oncogene. Nature 300:149–152

Reznikoff CA, Kingelhutz AJ, Kao C et al. (1989) A new *in vitro* model system to examine genetic events in multistep uroepithelial carcinogenesis. Proc Am Assoc Cancer Res 30:662 Abstract

Sanders BM, Jay M, Draper GJ, Roberts EM (1989) Non-ocular cancer in relatives of retinoblastoma patients. Br J Cancer 60:358–365

Sauter G, Moch H, Moore D et al. (1993) Heterogeneity of *erb*B-2 amplification in bladder cancer. Cancer Res 53:2199–2203

Sidransky D, von Eschenbach A, Tsai YC et al. (1991) Identification of p53 gene mutations in bladder cancers and urine samples. Science 252:706–709

Sidransky D, Frost P, Von Eschenbach A, Oyasu R, Preisinger AC, Vogelstein B (1992) Clonal origin of metachronous tumors of the bladder. N Engl J Med 326:737–740

Slamon DJ, Godolphin W, Jones LA et al. (1989) Studies of the HER-2/*neu* proto-oncogene in human breast and ovarian cancer. Science 244:707–712

Smeets W, Pauwels R, Laarakkers L, Debruyne F, Geraedts J (1987) Chromosomal analysis of bladder cancer. III. Cancer Genet Cytogenet 29:29 41

Smith K, Fennelly JA, Neal DE, Hall RR, Harris AL (1989) Characterization and quantitation of the epidermal growth factor receptor in invasive and superficial bladder tumors. Cancer Res 49:5810–5815

Spruck CH, Rideout WM, Olumi AF et al. (1993) Distinct pattern of p53 mutations in bladder cancer: relationship to tobacco usage. Cancer Res 53:1162–1166

Stern DF, Heffernan PA, Weinberg RA (1986) p185, a product of the *neu* proto-oncogene, is a receptor-like protein associated with tyrosine kinase activity. Mol Cell Biol 6:1729–1740

Tabin CJ, Bradley SM, Bargmann CI et al. (1982) Mechanism of activation of a human oncogene. Nature 300:143–149

Theillet C, Le-Roy X, De Lapeyriere et al. (1989) Amplification of FGF-related genes in human tumours: possible involvement of HST in breast carcinomas. Oncogene 4:915–922

Theodorescu D, Cornil I, Sheehan C, Man MS, Kerbel RS (1991) Ha-ras induction of the invasive phenotype results in up-regulation of epidermal growth factor receptors and altered responsiveness to epidermal growth factor in human papillary transitional cell carcinoma cells. Cancer Res 451:4486–4491

Tiniakos DG, Mellon JK, Anderson JJ, Robinson MC, Neal DE, Horne CHW (1994) c-*jun* oncogene expression in transitional cell carcinoma of the urinary bladder. Br J Urol (in press)

Tsai YC, Nichols PW, Hiti AL, Williams Z, Skinner DG, Jones PA (1990) Allelic losses of chromosomes 9, 11 and 17 in human bladder cancer. Cancer Res 50:44–47

Valles AM, Boyer B, Badet J, Tucker GC, Barritault D, Thiery JP (1990) Acidic fibroblast growth factor is a modulator of epithelial plasticity in a rat bladder carcinoma cell line. Proc Natl Acad Sci USA 87:1124–1128

Viola MV, Fromowitz F, Oravez S, Deb S, Schlom J (1985) *ras* oncogene p21 expression is increased in premalignant lesions and high grade bladder carcinoma. J Exp Med 161:1213–1218

Visvanathan KV, Pocock RD, Summerhays IC (1988) Preferential and novel activation of H-*ras* in human bladder carcinomas. Oncogene Res 3:77–86

Wen D, Peles E, Cupples R et al. (1992) Neu differentiation factor: a transmembrane glycoprotein containing an EGF domain and an immunoglobulin homology unit. Cell 69:559–572

Wood DP Jr, Fair WR, Chaganti RS (1992) Evaluation of epidermal growth factor receptor DNA amplification and mRNA expression in bladder cancer. J Urol 147:274–277

Wright C, Mellon K, Neal DE, Johnston P, Corbett IP, Horne CH (1990) Expression of c-erbB-2 protein product in bladder cancer. Br J Cancer 62:764–765

Wright C, Mellon K, Johnston P et al. (1991) Expression of mutant p53, c-*erb*B-2 and the epidermal growth factor receptor in transitional cell carcinoma of the human urinary bladder. Br J Cancer 63:967–970

Yamamoto T, Ikawa S, Akiyama T et al. (1986) Similarity of protein encoded by the human c-*erb*B-2 gene to epidermal growth factor receptor. Nature 319:230–234

Zhau HE, Zhang X, von-Eschenbach AC et al. (1990) Amplification and expression of the c-*erb*B-2/neu proto-oncogene in human bladder cancer. Mol Carcinog 3:254–257

Chapter 3

Tumour Progression in Superficial Bladder Cancer

H. Wolf

Introduction

Superficial bladder cancer can be considered as two separate clinical entities, one with a biological potential for invasion and progression, the other without this potential (Wolf et al. 1986). At presentation, superficial bladder cancer is either non-invasive (Ta) or invasive (T1). In addition to tumour category (T stage), there are other features which may predict the future course of the disease. The other type of superficial bladder cancer is intraepithelial neoplasia (carcinoma in situ, cis) which often develops into muscle invasive disease. An understanding of the behaviour of cis, Ta and T1 bladder cancer and the factors which may modify tumour progression is important for the proper care of patients. The most important question is to try to determine the risk of future tumour progression to muscle invasion or metastatic disease.

Definition of Superficial Bladder Cancer

In this chapter, superficial bladder cancer is defined as primary carcinoma in situ (cis), non-invasive bladder tumour (Ta) and tumours with lamina propria invasion (T1). Ta and T1 tumours may be accompanied by concomitant cis (secondary cis) or other less dedifferentiated types of intraepithelial neoplasia or atypia. Ta and T1 tumours cannot be separated on clinical grounds, but can only be distinguished by means of histological examination (Hermanek and Sobin 1987). Unfortunately, when different pathologists are faced with the same tumour, they may disagree about the diagnosis of superficial invasion of the papillary core or lamina propria (Robertson et al. 1990) – even histological examination has a subjective component.

Proportion of New Patients with Superficial/Advanced Cancer

In a series of 500 consecutive patients with bladder tumour from Copenhagen presenting over a period of seven years, 62% presented with superficial bladder cancer (Table 3.1: cis, Ta and T1 disease) (Wolf et al. 1987a). Thus, most primary bladder tumours are superficial. This figure is similar to other studies from the Western Hemisphere (Abel et al. 1988; Norming et al. 1989). Despite the potential histological difficulties of distinguishing Ta and T1 disease mentioned above (Robertson et al. 1990), T category remains the most important independent prognostic factor (Hendry et al. 1990). Therefore, it is essential for the pathologist to attempt to make a distinction between Ta and T1 disease. Most patients with superficial bladder cancer present with Ta disease (69%) as opposed to T1 disease (Abel et al. 1988: 71% versus 29%; Norming et al. 1989: 76% versus 24%).

Table 3.1. Distribution of T categories in 500 consecutive cases of primary bladder tumour (475 transitional cell tumours; 22 squamous cell carcinomas; 3 adenocarcinomas)

Category	No. of cases	%
Tis	6	1
Ta	210	42
T1	93	19
T2	55	11
T3	72	14
T4	62	12
Unknown	2	1
Total	500	100

Wolf et al. (1987a).

Impact of T Category on Recurrence, Progression and Survival

After transurethral resection of primary Ta and T1 tumours, the recurrence rate is between 40% and 75%.

Ta Disease

In a thorough review of 425 patients with Ta disease, Fitzpatrick et al. (1986) found that after 5–10 years of follow-up, 53% of patients had no recurrence, 20% had only one recurrence and 30% had more than one recurrence. In patients with solitary and small primary Ta tumours, recurrence is most likely to represent a new tumour (new occurrence) since most of these tumours should be removed completely by transurethral resection. Recurrence at three months follow-up is highly predictive of further recurrence (90% continue to recur), whereas no recurrence at three months is predictive of a permanently clear bladder (only 21% recur later). In addition, the longer the bladder is free from recurrent tumour, the smaller is the probability of future recurrence.

Among patients with Ta tumours who develop recurrence, about 15% progress; these comprise only 7% of the total group with Ta disease. Similar figures have been reported previously (Prior, 1973; Anderström et al. 1980; Lutzeyer et al. 1982; Heney et al. 1983; Hendry et al. 1990). In most instances Ta disease is a benign disease with little threat to the patient.

The benign behaviour of Ta disease is also apparent when looking at survival. We have found that the survival of patients with Ta disease was similar to that of an age and sex-matched control population (Fig. 3.1) (Olsen et al. 1988) despite these patients receiving no intravesical chemotherapy.

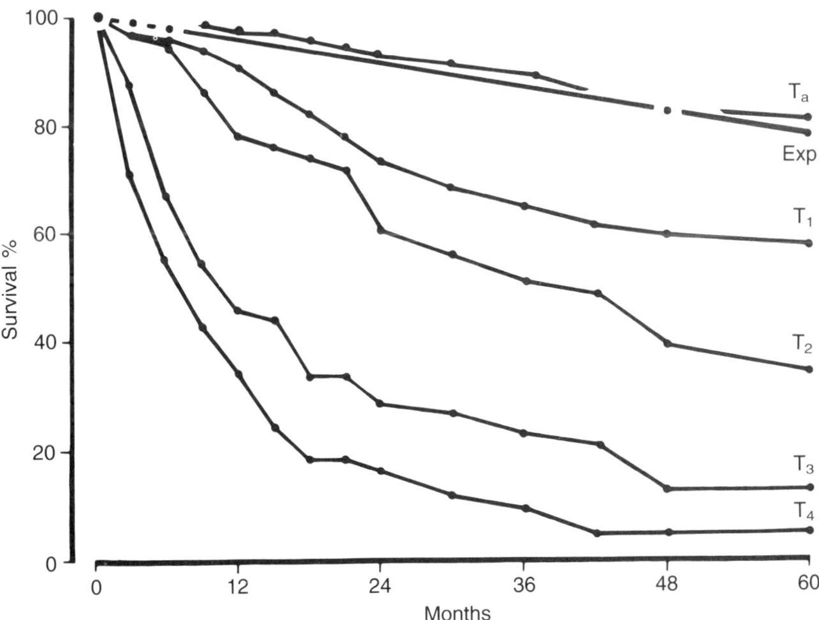

Fig. 3.1. Cumulative 5-year survival of 500 consecutive cases of newly detected primary bladder tumours according to T category of the primary tumour. (For the distribution of T categories see Table 3.1.) The survival of a sex- and age-matched control population is shown for comparison (Exp) (from Olsen et al. 1988).

T1 Disease

In contrast to patients with Ta disease, about 20% of patients with T1 disease will die from bladder cancer within five years (Fig. 3.1; Prior, 1973; Anderström et al. 1980; Lutzeyer et al. 1982; Heney et al. 1983). In patients with T1 disease (Wolf et al. 1987b), 74% develop recurrent tumours (Table 3.2). Thus in our studies, T category has been found to be predictive of recurrence, although others have shown similar recurrence rates in patients with or without lamina propria invasion (T1 and Ta disease). There are two types of recurrence, true recurrence, i.e. recurrence at the site of the original tumour and new occurrence, i.e. recurrence at sites distant from the original tumour. True recurrence may be due to tumour tissue not having been removed at the initial operation (Klan et al. 1991), unresected lymphatic vessel invasion (Anderström et al. 1980) or cis adjacent to the tumour. Cis near the site of the initial tumour is associated with decreased survival (Flamm and Havelec 1990). The survival of patients with early recurrence at the site of the initial T1 tumour is poor, being similar to patients with advanced bladder cancer, which may indicate that some of these tumours are understaged (Fig. 3.2).

From Table 3.2, it can be seen that during 5 years of follow-up, one third of patients presenting with a T1 tumour developed recurrent tumours of only

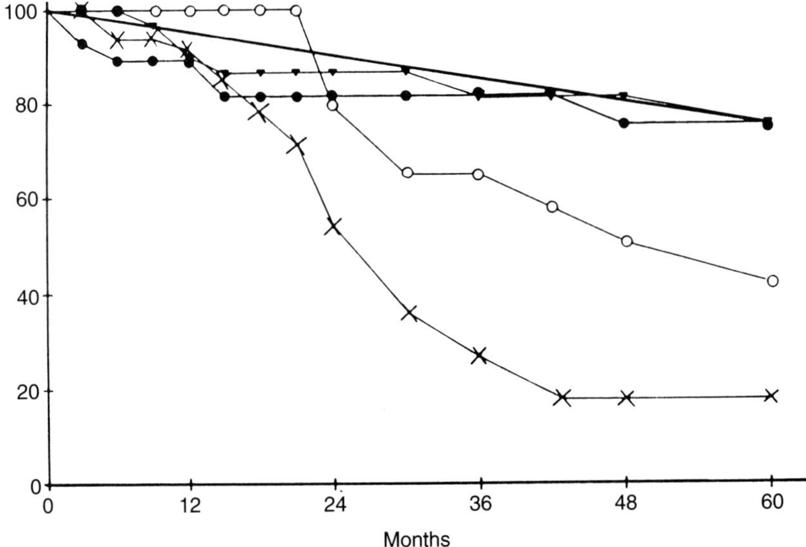

Fig. 3.2. Survival of patients with transitional cell bladder cancer of category T1 treated by transurethral resection. Bold line indicates the expected survival of an age- and sex-matched control population. ●-------●, patients with non-invasive new occurrence (see Table 3.2); ▼-------▼, patients without recurrence (see Table 3.2); o-------o, patients with a new invasive tumour growth (see Table 3.2); x-------x, patients with true recurrence (see Table 3.2) (from Wolf et al. 1987b).

Table 3.2. 5-year follow-up of patients with transitional cell tumour of category T1 treated by transurethral resection

No. of patients	No recurrence	True recurrence	New occurrence	
			Invasive	Non-invasive
77	20 (26%)	17 (22%)	15 (19%)	25 (33%)

Wolf et al. (1987b).

Ta stage. The survival of these patients was similar to those who had no recurrence and was similar to an age matched control population (Fig. 3.2) and was similar to that seen in patients with Ta tumours (Fig. 3.1). Non-invasive, Ta recurrences after primary T1 tumours have been found by others to occur in the same proportion (26%) and to behave similarly (Abel et al. 1988). It seems that either these tumours when they recurred had lost their ability to invade the lamina propria or that the original tumour was overstaged. One may also speculate whether Ta tumours that progress soon after diagnosis were understaged at presentation.

Impact of Differentiation (Grade) on Recurrence, Progression and Survival

There are a number of different grading systems. The most commonly used system is the WHO system (Mostofi et al. 1973). Another is that of Bergkvist et al. (1965) which utilises five grades (0–IV), where grade 0 is a true papilloma (papillary tumour with normal urothelium) and grade IV is the anaplastic type of urothelial carcinoma that has no resemblance to

Table 3.3. Histologic grading in relation to T category of 475 consecutive cases of primary transitional cell bladder tumour

Histologic grade	No. of cases	T category	No. of cases
0	1	Ta	1
I	34 (7%)	Ta	34 (100%)
II	223 (47%)	Tis	2 (1%)
		Ta	168 (75%)
		T1–4	53 (24%)
III	202 (43%)	Tis	4 (2%)
		Ta	6 (3%)
		T1–4	192 (95%)
IV	15 (3%)	T1–4	15 (100%)
Total	475		475

Wolf et al. (1987a).

urothelium. This system has the advantage that grade I tumours are never invasive (Bergkvist et al. 1965; Anderström et al. 1980; Table 3.3). About 24% of grade II tumours are invasive whereas 95% of grade III tumours are invasive and all grade IV tumours are invasive. In many reports the grading system is not clearly defined, although in such reports three grades are usually used. In addition, the interpretation of grades among different pathologists and also by the same pathologist varies considerably (Ooms et al. 1983; Robertson et al. 1990), so that it is difficult to make a direct comparison of the impact of grade on recurrence, progression and survival. Also tumour heterogeneity is a factor contributing to variation in tumour grading.

Despite these difficulties, most authors report that tumour grade has a pronounced influence on progression (Heney et al. 1983; Table 3.4). Similarly, a number of authors (Jakse et al. 1987; Abel et al. 1988; Jenkins et al. 1989; Kaubisch et al. 1991) have stressed the very poor prognosis of T1 grade III tumours. These reports are consistent with that of Fitzpatrick et al. (1986) who found that 70% of patients presenting with a Ta tumour of grade III progressed. Several authors have found that tumour grade is the second most important independent variable predicting outcome (Malmström et al. 1989; Hendry et al. 1990).

Since grading is subjective, a number of investigators have searched for more objective methods. Grade II tumours, in particular, are a heterogeneous group, including both non-invasive (Ta) and invasive (T1–T4) disease (Table 3.3), which progress in an appreciable number of cases (Table 3.4). On standard histopathological evaluation it is not possible to identify grade II tumours that are likely to progress and those that are not. A modified combination of the WHO and the Bergkvist grading systems has recently been used to classify grade II tumours into grade IIa and grade IIb tumours (Carbin et al. 1991a). By doing so, the authors were able to separate grade II tumours into a group (grade IIa) with a prognosis similar to grade I tumours and a group (grade IIb) with a prognosis similar to grade III tumours (Fig. 3.3) (Carbin et al. 1991b).

Others have proposed systems based on morphometry (Ooms et al. 1981; DeSanctis et al. 1987; Lipponen et al. 1991) which have been shown to have prognostic significance. These morphometric measurements correlate well with tumour grade (Nielsen et al. 1986) and were associated with risks of progression and recurrence (Table 3.5) (Nielsen et al. 1989).

Flow-cytometric DNA analysis correlates in general with grade, recurrence rate, risk of progression and survival (Gustafson et al. 1982; Hofstadter et al. 1984; Tribukait 1987). It represents an objective method which may be used to improve the reproducibility of tumour characterisation in the future. The question is whether flow-cytometric DNA analysis adds further information

Table 3.4. Progression by grade within each stage of superficial bladder cancer

Stage	Grade no. (%)		
	I	II	III
Ta	2/85 (2)	3/50 (6)	1/4 (25)
T1	0/7	6/29 (21)	13/27 (48)

Heney et al. (1983).

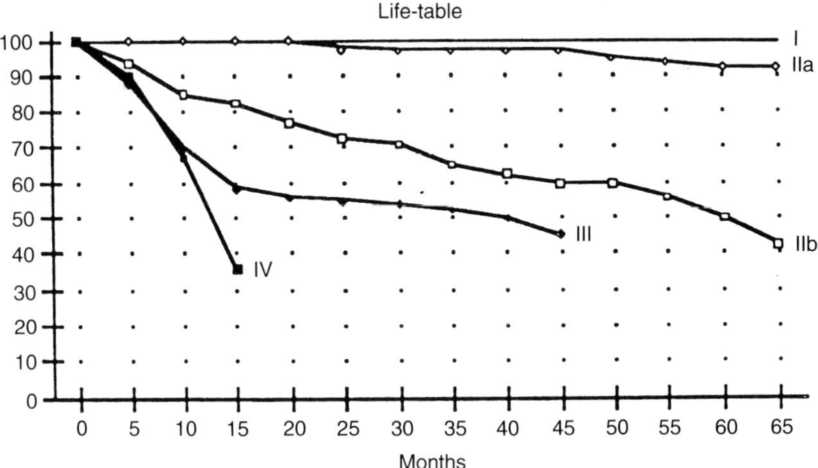

Fig. 3.3. Corrected survival rates according to tumour grade in modified Bergkvist system: – grade I; ◇ grade IIa; ☐ grade IIb; ▼ grade III; ■ grade IV. (From Carbin et al. (1991b), with permission of The Journal of Urology.)

to grading. In one study, the recurrence rate in Ta and T1 tumours of grade I and II was higher in non-tetraploid aneuploid tumours than in diploid tumours (Gustafson et al. 1982). Similarly, tumour progression in grade II tumours was linked to aneuploidy (Blomjous et al. 1988). However, in other studies DNA ploidy did not prove to be an independent prognostic variable (Malmström et al. 1989).

Table 3.5. Mean nuclear volume in presenting Ta grade II tumours in relation to recurrence and progression

	No. of patients		
	Below 165 μm^3	Above 165 μm^3	Total
No recurrence	9	1	10
Recurrence without progression	7	4	11
Recurrence with progression	2	12	14
Total	18	17	35

Nielsen et al. (1989).

Carcinoma in situ (cis)

Carcinoma in situ (intraepithelial carcinoma of the bladder) is usually classified into primary and secondary cis. In primary cis, there is no history of previous

a

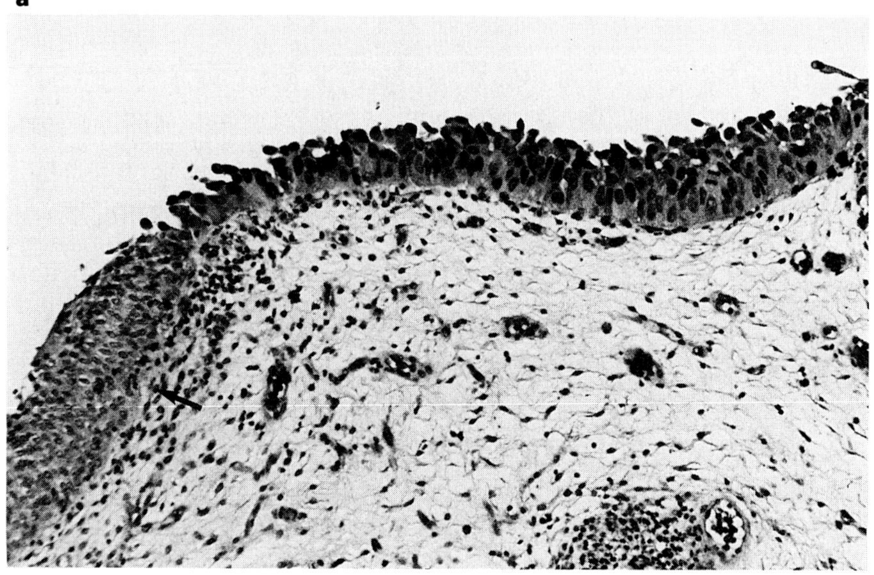

b

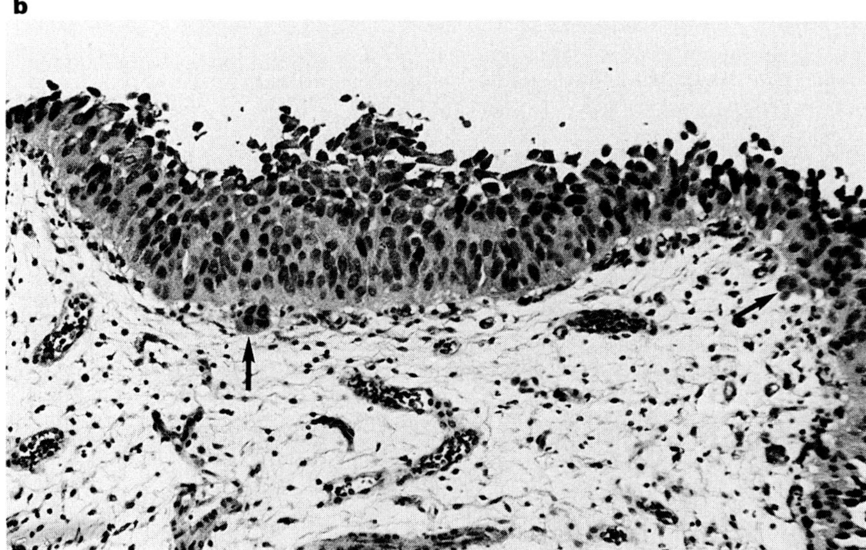

Fig. 3.4. Grade III neoplasia. The celluar deviation is considerable, individual cells and epithelial cords are in disarray. The transitional character of the epithelium is preserved. The cells and the nuclei vary greatly in size and shape, with occasional multinucleated giant cells being encountered (Bergkvist et al. (1965). **a** Flat intraepithelial neoplasia grade III (cis ×125). *Arrow* indicates normal transitional cell epithelium. **b** Flat (cis ×125). *Arrow* indicates minimal stromal invasion. **c** Papillary T1 grade III tumour. *Arrow* indicates subepithelial stromal invasion. (Slides were kindly provided by Henrik Barlebo MD, Department of Pathology, Aalborg Sygehus, 8000 Aalborg, Denmark.) (*continued opposite*)

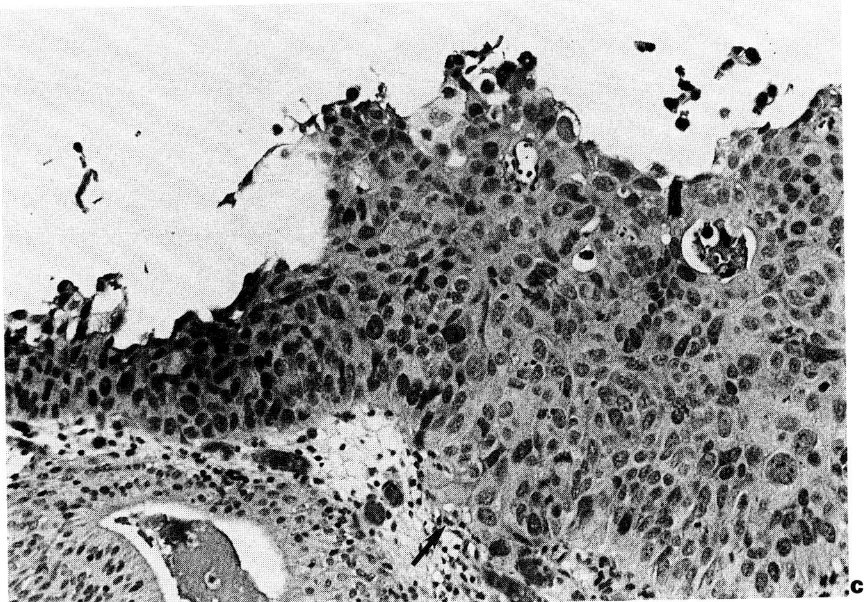

Fig. 3.4. (*continued*)

or concurrent tumour, whereas secondary cis is in patients with previous or concurrent tumour. The term concomitant cis is used when a tumour is present at the same time.

Cis is high grade (grade III) intraepithelial neoplasia. Intraepithelial neoplasia which is not poorly differentiated should be distinguished from cis and be referred to as intraepithelial dysplasia, atypia or neoplasia grade II (Figs. 3.4 and 3.5) (Bergkvist et al. 1965). Urologists need to be aware of the difficulty that pathologists have in diagnosing cis and distinguishing it from dysplasia and more minor degrees of atypia. The urothelial abnormalities referred to in this chapter are limited to cis and dysplasia grade II. Given this difficulty, it is not surprising that its clinical significance may be debated (Nagy et al. 1982; Richards et al. 1991). It is to be hoped that the use of more objective methods such as flow cytometry may help here (Norming et al. 1989).

Secondary cis

Primary cis is an infrequent finding (Table 3.1), but secondary cis is common. Its presence may be demonstrated by carrying out random or preselected site biopsies in patients with bladder cancer. The number of biopsies has varied; in our studies, we have taken seven or eight biopsies from preselected sites. In 1987 we reported on the incidence of concomitant cis or intraepithelial dysplasia in 397 patients (Table 3.6; Wolf et al. 1987a). No patients with grade I tumours had concomitant intraepithelial neoplasia, in agreement

a

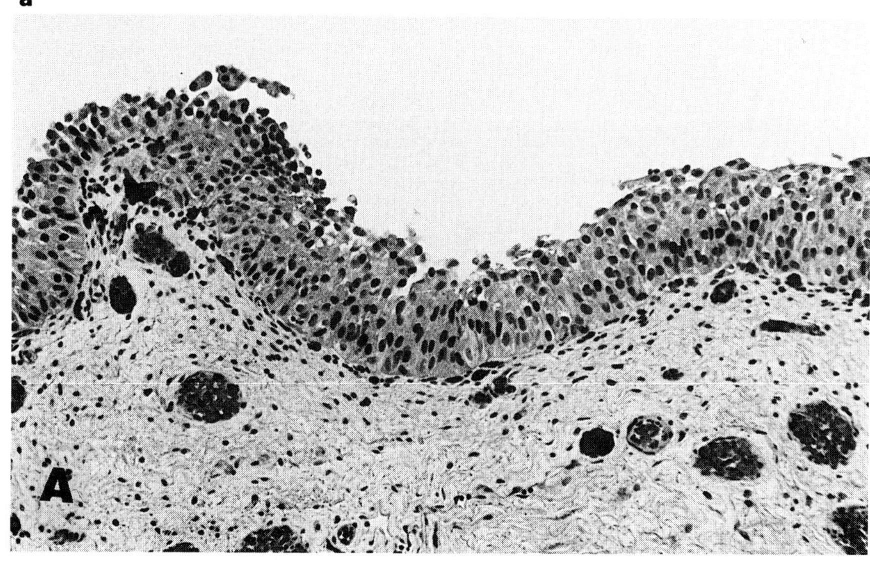

b

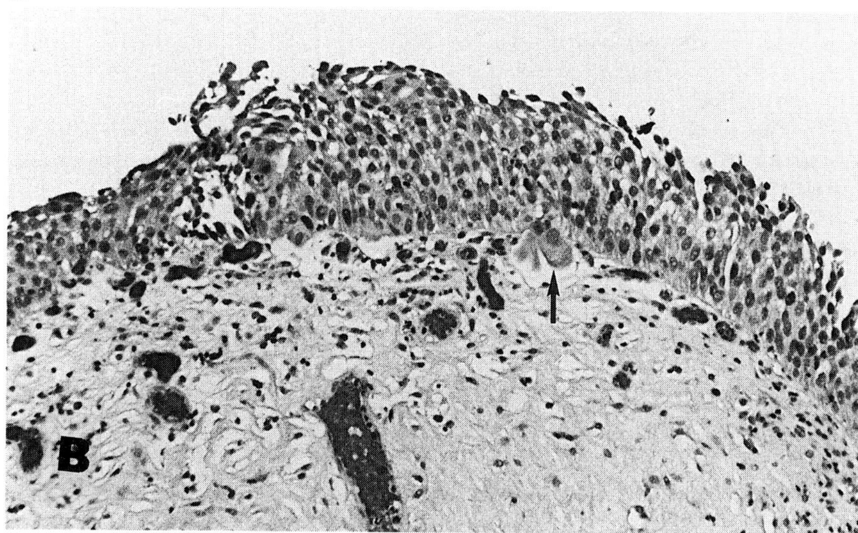

Fig. 3.5. Grade II neoplasia. The epithelium is thickened and displays moderate cellular **deviation with some variation in the size of the cells and nuclei and tendency to lose the normal polarity of individual cells (Bergkvist et al. 1965). a** Flat intraepithelial neoplasia grade II (dysplasia) (×125). **b** Flat intraepithelial dysplasia (×125). *Arrow* indicates subepithelial stromal invasion. **c** Papillary transitional cell tumour grade II (×125). (Slides were kindly provided by Henrik Barlebo MD, Department of Pathology, Aalborg Sygehus, 8000 Aalborg, Denmark.) (*continued opposite*)

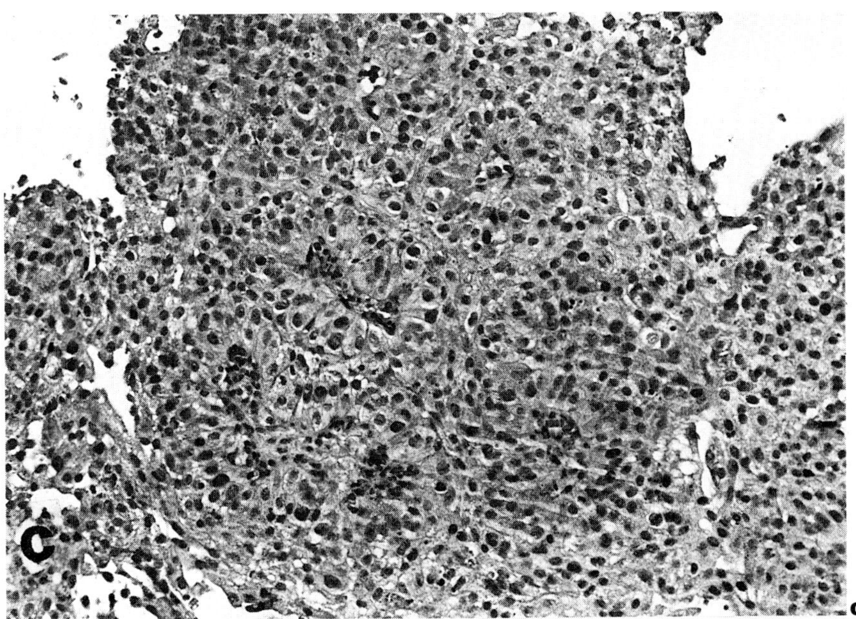

Fig. 3.5. (*continued*)

with subsequent studies (Norming et al. 1989). In patients with grade II tumours, we found a few patients with frank cis and 20% had concomitant intraepithelial dysplasia. The percentage of patients with cis differed in those with grade II Ta tumours (14%) compared with grade II T1 to T4 tumours (30%). In patients with grade III tumours, concomitant cis was found in 30% and a further 24% had intraepithelial dysplasia. Thus, urothelial abnormalities were found in more than 50% of patients with high grade disease. Patients with squamous cell carcinoma or adenocarcinoma generally had no concomitant intraepithelial neoplasia.

Table 3.6. Incidence of intraepithelial neoplasia in preselected site mucosal biopsies in relation to histologic type, grade and T category of primary bladder tumour

Histologic type	Grade, T-category	Biopsy findings			Total cases
		Carcinoma in situ	Grade II intra-epithelial neoplasia	Normal	
TCC	0, Ta	0	0	1	1
TCC	I, Ta	0	0	24	24
TCC	II, Ta	2 (2%)	17 (12%)	120 (86%)	139
TCC	II, T1–4	0	13 (30%)	31 (70%)	44
TCC	III	51 (30%)	40 (24%)	78 (46%)	169
Squamous cell carcinoma	0	1	11		12
Adenocarcinoma	0	0	2		2
Total		53	73	270	396

Wolf et al. (1987a).

Generalised Urothelial Disease in Superficial Bladder Cancer

One question is whether preselected site biopsies identify all patients with concomitant urothelial cis or dysplasia for in many patients only one biopsy showed abnormalities. Because primary cis results in the shedding of exfoliated cancer cells in the urine (Zincke et al. 1985), we theorised that patients with secondary or concomitant carcinoma would also have positive urinary cytology even if mucosal biopsies were negative. Among 60 patients with superficial bladder cancer studied, all patients with secondary cis had positive cytology as had 86% of those with intraepithelial dysplasia (Harving et al. 1988). Nineteen patients with a history of superficial bladder cancer and without any apparent bladder or upper tract tumour had positive cytology despite the fact that mucosal biopsies were negative. When followed up two years later, cis was identified in 16 of the 19 patients. We concluded that a combination of preselected site mucosal biopsies and cytology after tumour resection is the most accurate method of detecting secondary cis or dysplasia – provided the cytologist is expert (Table 3.6) (Gil-Salom et al. 1990).

Impact of Concomitant cis on Tumour Recurrence and Progression

The significance of concomitant cis or intraepithelial dysplasia has been investigated in T1 disease where it was found in 46% of patients (Wolf et al. 1987a).

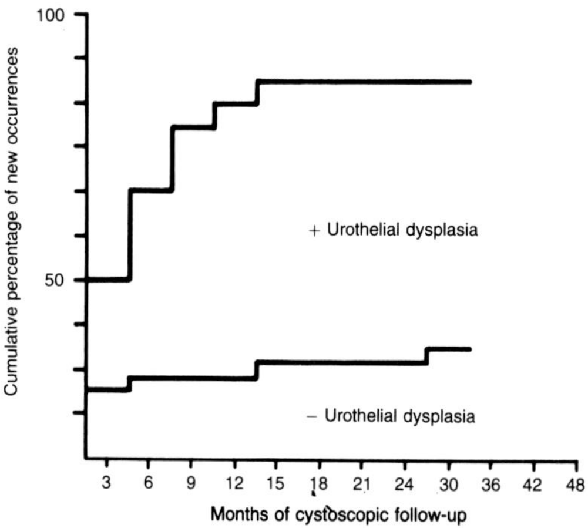

Fig. 3.6. Cumulative percentage at cystoscopic follow-up, of new occurrences in patients with T1 bladder cancer with or without cis or dysplasia (from Wolf and Höjgaard 1983).

In a group of 209 patients, 87% of those with cis or dysplasia developed a new tumour growth whereas only 26% of those without intraepithelial neoplasia developed recurrent disease (Fig. 3.6) (Wolf and Höjgaard 1983). Considering that some of the patients may have had undiagnosed cis, because at that time we were not using urine cytology routinely, it seems clear that the presence of cis is highly predictive of recurrent disease (Heney et al. 1983; Smith et al. 1983)

Concomitant cis also predicts progression of superficial bladder cancer (Smith et al. 1986; Flamm and Havelec 1990). A total of 209 patients with or without concomitant cis or dysplasia were studied. Of those with cis 50% progressed to muscle invasion whereas only 2%–3% of those without progressed (Fig. 3.7) (Smith et al. 1986). Many patients with cis eventually die of their tumour (Fig. 3.8) (Olsen et al. 1988).

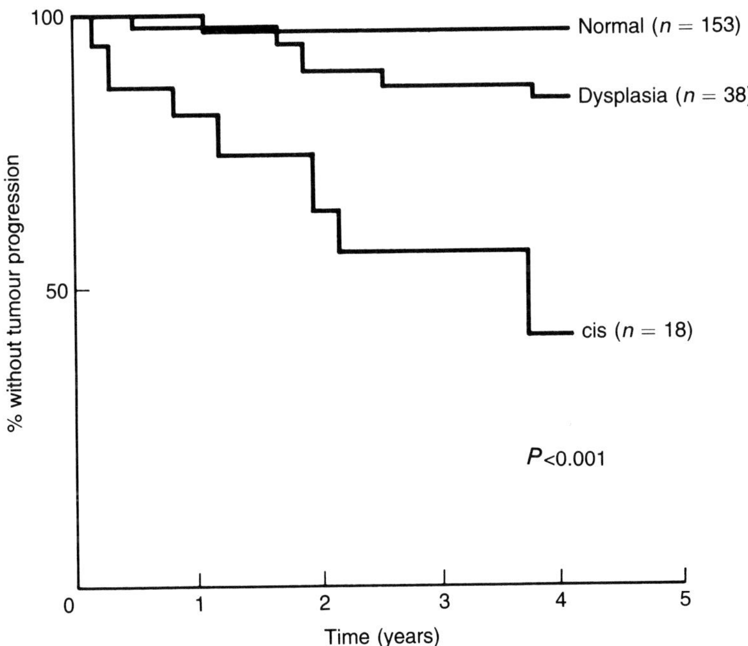

Fig. 3.7. Tumour progression (muscle invasion or metastases) in non-tumour-bearing urothelium. (From Smith et al. (1986), by permission of British Journal of Urology.)

Primary or Secondary Carcinoma in situ: the same disease?

The relationship between these two diseases is difficult to resolve. Weinstein et al. (1980) have proposed a scheme (Fig. 3.9) along which the development

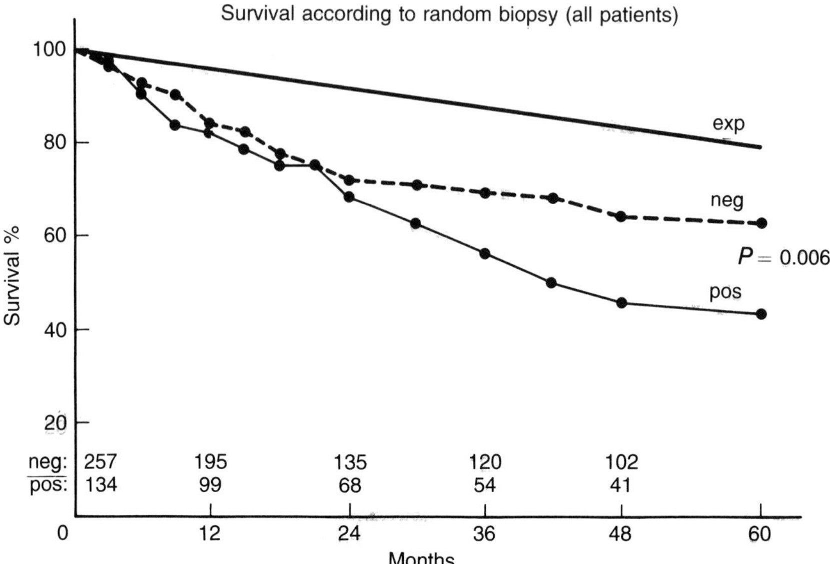

Fig. 3.8. Cumulative survival of patients with (pos) or without (neg) secondary cis at tumour presentation. exp: survival of an age- and sex-matched control population. (Patients at risk at indicated month of follow-up.) (From Olsen et al. 1988.)

of bladder cancer may proceed. Focal, grade II intraepithelial neoplasia may be the precursor of non-invasive grade I or II tumours as the grade of the recurrent tumour is most often similar to that of the primary. Only rarely does a recurrent tumour increase by grade (Fitzpatrick et al. 1986) and only rarely does a non-invasive grade II tumour change into a muscle-invasive grade II tumour. We do not know that invasive tumours are always preceded by cis, although we do know that primary or secondary cis often develops into

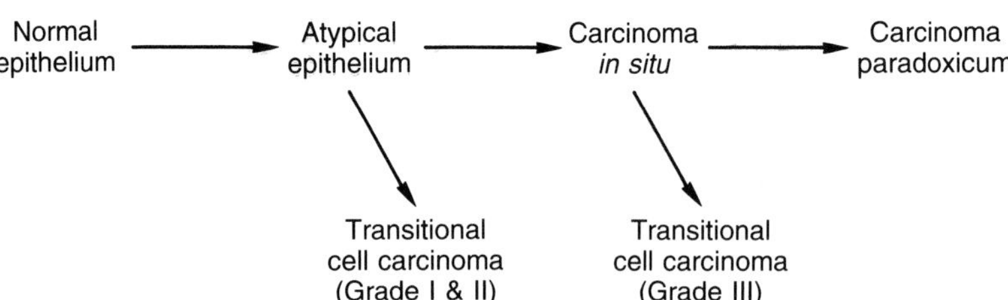

Fig. 3.9. A possible scheme for the origin of low and high grade transitional cell carcinomas. Cis may evolve into either a carcinoma of relatively high grade or a biologically innocuous lesion for which the term "carcinoma paradoxicum" has been coined (Weinstein et al. 1980). (Reproduced by permission of W.B Saunders Company, Philadelphia, PA, USA.)

invasive cancer. Paradoxically, one sees occasional patients who have cis for many years without developing invasive disease.

Our knowledge of the natural history of primary cis has been based on the follow-up of a few patients who for one reason or another have not received treatment. The Mayo Clinic (Zincke et al. 1985) summarised their experience as follows:

> The natural history of carcinoma in situ of the bladder is extremely variable. Carcinoma in situ probably develops from an area of atypical hyperplasia into an intra-epithelial malignant disease – carcinoma in situ. Carcinoma in situ is composed of cells with anaplastic features that grow in a disorderly pattern with loss of intracellular cohesiveness into flat areas of carcinoma. When not modified by treatment, carcinoma in situ is the precursor of most invasive cancers in an unknown percentage of patients. A small group of patients may have carcinoma in situ with malignant appearing, but biologically innocuous, intra-epithelial neoplasm ("carcinoma paradoxicum" a lesion with definite features of malignancy that may prove, however, to be biologically innocuous). Carcinoma in situ can coexist with papillary lesions, and it is a field disease with a potential to involve the entire urothelium, e.g. bladder, upper urinary tract, and urethra. At an early stage, cystoscopic localisation of carcinoma in situ might be difficult. Urinary cytology is the most reliable means for early detection. Microinvasion may be present at the time of cystectomy for clinical carcinoma in situ in a significant number of patients. Irritative bladder symptoms without evidence for infection may be one of the clinical clues of the disease.

Recently we were able to document the untreated natural history of primary (four patients) or secondary (27 patients) carcinoma in situ (excluding patients with intraepithelial neoplasia grade II or dysplasia). Thirty-one patients were followed-up from 15 to 109 months, either until death from other causes, until progression or until the end of the study. Sixteen patients progressed (T2 disease: five patients; T3, T4 disease: six patients; upper tract cancer: four patients; distant metastases: one patient). Of the patients who progressed, only six survived despite appropriate treatment; 15 patients did not progress. The conclusion is that the course of primary or secondary cis is highly unpredictable, with one half of patients experiencing progression.

Primary or secondary cis predicts tumour progression to muscle invasive or metastatic disease in about 50% of patients. Some authors in multivariate analysis have found that secondary cis is an independent prognostic variable (Smith et al. 1986). It is not yet possible to predict which patient will progress and which will not. Most urologists recommend that preselected site biopsies should be taken at tumour presentation and possibly at follow-up to identify patients who need intensive surveillance or more radical treatment.

Management of Patients with Superficial Bladder Cancer

Among patients with superficial bladder cancer, carcinoma in situ, Ta or T1 disease, there is a spectrum of tumour behaviour (Fig. 3.10). At one end, are

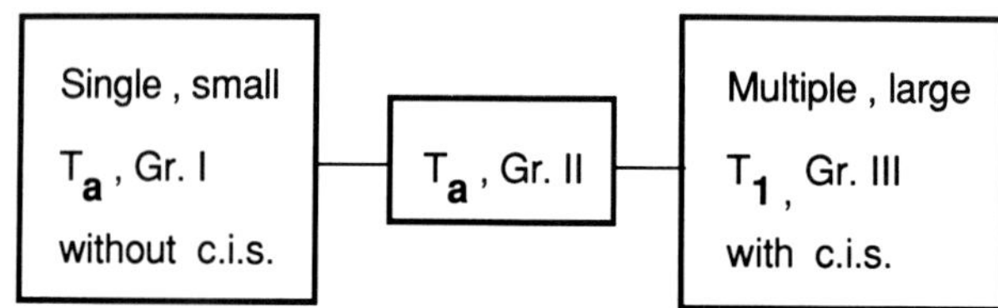

Fig. 3.10. Spectrum of types of superficial bladder tumours usually treated initially by transurethral resection.

single, papillary grade I Ta tumours with no intraepithelial neoplasia. At the other end, are multiple, solid, grade III/IV T1 tumours with cis or perhaps patients with primary cis. In the middle, are papillary grade II Ta tumours some of which have intraepithelial dysplasia. The potential of these tumours is difficult to predict. A number of other tumour characteristics including tumour size, appearance (papillary or solid), multiplicity, blood group antigen status, or the presence of other markers have been shown to have prognostic significance. It is debatable whether we should continue to group together tumours with such diverse biological potential (Wolf et al. 1986; Abel et al. 1988).

Solitary Ta tumours, particularly those without recurrence at their first follow-up, should be managed by means of transurethral resection alone; their follow-up can be performed by ultrasonography or flexible cystoscopy and urine cytology. Patients with multiple or recurrent Ta tumours should have a more careful follow-up. Histological examination should detect lamina propria invasion and cytology performed after resection may detect cis. Such patients may be candidates for intravesical chemotherapy or immunotherapy.

Patients with T1 grade III tumours with cis or patients with primary cis have a high rate of progression within 3 to 5 years. These patients should be offered one or two courses of BCG instillations. However, if the tumour recurs or the cis does not clear, early cystectomy should be undertaken. These patients should also be monitored by upper tract imaging and biopsies from the prostate to detect intraductal urothelial neoplasia. Full course radiotherapy does not clear primary cis (Zincke et al. 1985).

In patients with T3 and T4 tumours plus cis, we found that recurrent tumours developed in 70% after radiotherapy whereas patients without cis had a better outcome (Wolf et al. 1985). Although the significance of our study has been questioned (Quilty et al. 1987), others have also shown that cis is a significant determinant after radiotherapy of local tumour control (Gospodarowicz et al. 1989) and survival (Wijkström et al. 1992). These findings suggest that radiotherapy for most patients with T1 tumours and cis is inadequate treatment.

References

Abel PD, Hall RR, Williams G (1988) Should pT1 transitional cell cancers of the bladder still be classified as superficial? Br J Urol 62:235–239

Anderström C, Johansson S, Nilsson S (1980) The significance of lamina propria invasion on the prognosis of patients with bladder tumors. J Urol 124:23–26

Bergkvist A, Ljungquist A, Moberger G (1965) Classification of bladder tumours based on the cellular pattern. Preliminary report of a clinical–pathological study of 300 cases with a minimum follow-up of eight years. Acta Chir Scand 130:371–378

Blomjous CEM, Schipper NW, Baak JPA et al. (1988) Retrospective study of prognostic importance of DNA flow-cytometry of urinary bladder carcinoma. J Clin Pathol 41:21–25

Carbin C-E, Ekman P, Gustafson H et al. (1991a) Grading of human urothelial carcinoma based on nuclear atypia and mitotic frequency. Histological description. J Urol 145:968–971

Carbin C-E, Ekman P, Gustafson H et al. (1991b) Grading of human urothelial carcinoma based on nuclear atypia and mitotic frequency. Prognostic importance. J Urol 145:972–976

DeSanctis PN, Concepcion NB, Tannenbaum M et al. (1987) Quantitative morphometry measurement of transitional cell bladder cancer nuclei as indicator of tumour aggression. Urology 24:322–324

Fitzpatrick JM, West AB, Butler MR et al. (1986) Superficial bladder tumors (stage pTa, grades 1 and 2): the importance of recurrence pattern following initial resection. J Urol 135:920–922

Flamm J, Havelec L (1990) Factors affecting survival in primary superficial bladder cancer. Eur Urol 17:113–115

Gil-Salom M, Sanchez MC, Chuan P et al. (1990) Multiple mucosal biopsies and postoperative urinary cytology in patients with bladder cancer. Eur Urol 17:281–285

Gospodarowicz MK, Hawkins NV, Rawlings GA et al. (1989) Radical radiotherapy for muscle invasive transitional cell carcinoma of the bladder: failure analysis. J Urol 142:1448–1453

Gustafson H, Tribukait B, Eposti PL (1982) DNA pattern, histological grade and multiplicity related to recurrence rate in superficial bladder tumours. Scand J Urol Nephrol 16:135–139

Harving N, Wolf H, Melsen F (1988) Positive urinary cytology after tumour resection: an indicator for concomitant carcinoma in situ. J Urol 140:495–497

Hendry WF, Rawson NBS, Turney L et al. (1990) Computerisation of urothelial carcinoma records: 16 years experience with the TNM system. Br J Urol 65:583–588

Heney NM, Ahmed S, Flanagan MJ et al. (1983) Superficial bladder cancer: progression and recurrence. J Urol 130:1083–1086

Hermanek P, Sobin LH (1987) TNM classification of malignant tumours, 4th edn. Springer Verlag, New York

Hofstadter F, Jakse G, Lederer B et al. (1984) Biological behaviour and DNA cytophotometry of urothelial bladder carcinomas. Br J Urol 56:289–295

Jakse G, Loidl W, Sieber G et al. (1987) Stage T1 grade G3 transitional cell carcinoma of the bladder: an unfavourable tumour? J Urol 137:39–43

Jenkins BJ, Nauth-Misir RR, Martin JE et al. (1989) The fate of G3 pT1 bladder cancer. Br J Urol 64:608–610

Kaubisch S, Lum BL, Riese J et al. (1991) Stage T1 bladder cancer: grade is the primary determinant for risk of muscle invasion. J Urol 146:28–31

Klan R, Loy V, Huland H (1991) Residual tumour discovered in routine second transurethral resection in patients with T1 transitional cell carcinoma of the bladder. J Urol 146:316–318

Lipponen PK, Eskelinen MJ, Nordling S (1991) Relationship between DNA flow cytometric data, nuclear morphometric variables and volume corrected mitotic index in transitional cell bladder tumors. Eur Urol 19:327–331

Lutzeyer W, Rubben H, Dahm H (1982) Prognostic parameters in superficial bladder cancer: an analysis of 315 cases. J Urol 127:250–252

Malmström P-U, Norlen BJ, Andersson B et al. (1989) Combination of blood group ABH antigen status and DNA ploidy as independent prognostic factors in transitional cell carcinoma of the bladder. Br J Urol 64:49–55

Mostofi FK, Sobin LH, Torloni H (1973) Histological typing of urinary bladder tumours. International histological classification of tumours, no 10. World Health Organization, Geneva

Nagy GK, Frable WJ, Murphy WM (1982) Classification of premalignant urothelial abnormalities. A Delphi study of the National Bladder Cancer Cooperative Group A. Pathol Annu 17:219–265

Nielsen K, Colstrup H, Nilsson T et al. (1986) Stereological estimate of nuclear volume correlated with histopathological grading and prognosis of bladder tumour. Virchows Arch [B] 52:41–54

Nielsen K, Örntoft T, Wolf H. (1989) Stereological estimates of nuclear volume in non-invasive bladder tumors (Ta) correlated with the recurrence pattern. Cancer 8:2269–2274

Norming U, Nyman CR, Tribukait B (1989) Comparative flow cytometric deoxyribonucleic acid studies on exophytic tumour and random mucosal biopsies in untreated carcinoma of the bladder. J Urol 142:1442–1447

Olsen PR, Wolf H, Schröder T et al. (1988) Urothelial atypia and survival rate of 500 unselected patients with primary transitional-cell tumour of the urinary bladder. Scand J Urol Nephrol 22:257–263

Ooms ECM, Essed E, Veldhuizen RW et al. (1981) The prognostic significance of morphometry in T1 bladder tumours. Histopathology 5:311–318

Ooms EMC, Anderson WAD, Alons CD et al. (1983) Analysis of performance of pathologists in the grading of bladder tumors. Hum Pathol 14:140–143

Prior JP (1973) Factors influencing the survival of patients with transitional cell tumours of the urinary bladder. Br J Urol 45:586–592

Quilty PM, Hargreave TB, Smith G, Duncan W (1987) Do abnormal mucosal biopsies predict prognosis in patients with transitional cell carcinoma of bladder treated by radical radiotherapy? Br J Urol 59:242–247

Richards B, Parmar MKB, Anderson CK et al. (1991) The interpretation of biopsies of "normal" urothelium in patients with superficial bladder cancer. Br J Urol 67:369–375

Robertson AJ, Beck JS, Burnett RA et al. (1990) Observer variability in histopathological reporting of transitional cell carcinoma and epithelial dysplasia in bladder. Clin Pathol 43:17–21

Smith G, Elton RA, Beynon LL et al. (1983) Prognostic significance of biopsy of normal-looking mucosa in cases of superficial bladder cancer. Br J Urol 55:665–669

Smith G, Elton RA, Chisholm GD et al. (1986) Superficial bladder cancer: intravesical chemotherapy and tumour progression to muscle invasion or metastases. Br J Urol 58:659–663

Tribukait B (1987) Flow cytometry in assessing clinical aggressiveness of genito-urinary neoplasms. World J Urol 5:108–122

Weinstein RS, Miller AW III, Pauli BU (1980) Carcinoma in situ: comments on the pathobiology of a paradox. Urol Clin North Am 7:523–531

Wijkström H, Nilsson B, Tribukait B (1992) DNA analysis in predicting survival of irradiated patients with transitional cell carcinoma of the bladder. Br J Urol 69:49–55

Wolf H, Höjgaard K (1983) Urothelial dysplasia concomitant with bladder tumours as a determinant factor for future new occurrences. Lancet ii:134–136

Wolf H, Olsen PR, Höjgaard K (1985) Urothelial dysplasia concomitant with bladder tumours: a determinant for future new occurrences in patients treated with full course radiotherapy. Lancet i:1005–1007

Wolf H, Kakizoe T, Smith PH et al. (1986) Bladder tumours. Treated natural history. In: Denis L, Niijima T, Prout GR et al. (eds) Development in bladder cancer. Progress in clinical and biological research, vol 221 Alan Liss, New York, pp 223–255

Wolf H, Olsen PR, Fischer A et al. (1987a) Urothelial atypia concomitant with primary bladder tumour. Incidence in a consecutive series of 500 unselected patients. Scand J Urol Nephrol 21:33–38

Wolf H, Iversen H-G, Olsen PR et al. (1987b) Transurethral surgery in the treatment of invasive bladder cancer (T1 and T2). Scand J Urol Nephrol Suppl. 104:127–132

Zincke H, Utz DC, Farrow GM (1985) Review of Mayo Clinic experience with carcinoma in situ. Urology Suppl. 24(4):39–46

Chapter 4

New Techniques in Management and Treatment of Superficial Bladder Cancer

J. Franklin and M. C. Benson

It is estimated that 51 600 new cases of bladder cancer will be diagnosed in the USA during the year 1992 (Boring et al. 1992). More than 70% of these tumours will be superficial, being stages Ta, Tis, and T1. The International Union Against Cancer defines Ta as a non-invasive papillary tumour, Tis as a flat and often diffuse malignant change of the urothelium and T1 as tumour invading the lamina propria (Witjes and Debruyne 1991). These tumours may occur as either solitary or multiple lesions, exhibit different grades (I–III) and possess different potentials for recurrence and progression. Because of this heterogeneity, therapy should be stratified according to the particular characteristics of the presenting tumour. For instance, a solitary small papillary stage Ta grade I tumour, which poses the least risk for recurrence and progression, can be managed by primary resection alone (Morrison et al. 1984). However, multifocal stage Ta, Tis or any T1 tumour will usually require adjuvant intravesical chemotherapy including thiotepa, mitomycin-C, adriamycin and epodyl. Biologic response modifiers that have been employed in the treatment of transitional cell bladder cancer consist of various strains of Bacillus Calmette–Guérin, alpha-2 interferon and keyhole limpet haemocyanin (Herr et al. 1987; Soloway 1987; Stricker et al. 1987; Herr and Landone 1988; Jurincic et al. 1988; Lum and Torti 1990). In addition to these intravesical therapies, new therapeutic modalities are under investigation for a wide range of indications.

The objective in the treatment of superficial bladder cancer is to rid the patient of existing disease and to prevent or at least retard recurrence and progression. This chapter will evaluate the various therapeutic options presently available for the treatment of superficial transitional cell carcinoma (TCC) of the bladder.

Surgery

Transurethral electrocautery resection (TUR) together with fulguration remains the most commonly used therapy for superficial TCC (Soloway

1987). Its efficacy against both solitary and multiple papillary lesions has been well established. However, approximately 50% of patients experience a recurrence, and of these up to 20% will progress to invasion (Lutzeyer et al. 1982). Carcinoma in situ (often diffuse in the bladder) presents a different problem since it is not amenable to resection and as many as 80% of patients will recur and up to 50% will invade after primary TUR (Lum and Torti 1990).

Neodymium-YAG laser therapy has been promoted for its ability to produce full thickness homogeneous coagulation necrosis of the bladder while preserving bladder wall integrity and avoiding perforations (Staehler and Hofstetter 1979; McPhee et al. 1982). This procedure, which produces less pain than TUR, is well tolerated under local anaesthesia. However, neodymium-YAG requires TUR of lesions greater than 1.5 cm in diameter prior to treatment of the tumour base in order to obtain tissue for pathological assessment. The ability to accurately stage patients may be compromised by the failure to assess pathologically the entire specimen.

In one randomised study, laser therapy has been shown to be more effective than TUR in preventing recurrence of disease at the treated site, resulting in 0/47 and 13/50 recurrences respectively (Beisland and Seland 1986). The follow-up period in this study was from three to 24 months. All recurrences in the TUR series were from large T1 tumours suggesting that laser irradiation may be destroying residual unresected tumour. No differences in recurrence rates have been observed within non-treated areas or when used to treat cis (Beisland and Seland 1986).

Intravesical Chemotherapy

The introduction of chemotherapeutic agents into the bladder subjects urothelial tumours to high concentrations of cytotoxic agents while avoiding systemic toxicity. Drugs are introduced into the bladder via a urethral catheter following the drainage of any residual urine. The drug is retained in the bladder for approximately 2 h and in order to diminish dilution and aid in retention, patients are advised to refrain from fluid intake for 4 h prior to therapy. A typical treatment course consists of six weekly instillations beginning 3 to 14 days after TUR. Repeat cystourethroscopy is usually performed at three months to assess efficacy (Witjes and Debruyne 1991).

The "ideal" antitumour agent for intravesical use is one with minimal local side effects and a high molecular weight in order to prevent absorption and systemic toxicity. The "ideal" agent should be highly effective both in its ability to eradicate existing tumours and in preventing future tumours (Mishina et al. 1986; Knuchel et al. 1989). Efficacy should be optimal at physiological urinary pH (Groos et al. 1986). Not only has the ideal agent not yet been identified, but many important questions remain about the manner in which the currently employed agents are administered. Among these questions are: (a) how long should the agents be retained in the bladder? (b) should the patient be rotated to promote total bladder coating? and (c) should the intravesical pH be adjusted with the use of buffers to improve efficacy?

Another major consideration is the ability to predict if a tumour is susceptible or has acquired resistance to a given agent, for example by utilising tumour markers, such as the expression of the multidrug resistance (MDR-1) gene (Floyd et al. 1990; Benson et al. 1991). We have preliminary data that MDR-1 expression can be induced during intravesical chemotherapy and that this may prove useful in determining a tumour's susceptibility to certain intravesical therapies.

Dalton et al. (1991) studied the pharmacokinetics of intravesical therapy. They found that:

1. There is a large intra- and intersubject variability to exposure of the drug.
2. The residual urine volume at the time of drug administration, the urine production rate and the rate of drug removal by degradation or absorption are inversely proportional to the intravesical drug exposure.
3. Urinary pH affects intracellular degradation of the drug.

Further investigation in this area is necessary and should improve our understanding of the pharmacokinetics of the various intravesical chemotherapeutic agents.

Thiotepa

Since its introduction in 1961, thiotepa (triethylene-thiophosphoramide) has been extensively utilised as an intravesical chemotherapeutic agent. Thiotepa has a molecular weight of 189 and is therefore easily absorbed from the bladder. This absorption can cause systemic toxicity, including myelosuppression (Soloway and Ford 1983). When used to treat existing superficial bladder tumours, thiotepa has been shown to have a complete response rate of 23%–47% and a partial response rate of 24%–38% (Esquivel et al. 1965; Abbassian and Wallace 1966; Veenema et al. 1969; Koonz et al. 1981). However, other investigators have demonstrated a significant benefit over controls (Herr and Landone 1988). When used as a prophylactic agent after complete TUR, Koonz et al. (1981) reported leucopenia, thrombocytopenia and urinary tract symptoms such as pyuria in 17% in the treatment group and 11% in the prophylaxis group. The toxicity, which did not appear to be affected by dose level, led to the termination of therapy in 10 patients; four patients in the treatment and six patients in the prophylaxis groups.

Adriamycin

Adriamycin (doxorubicin), a water-soluble glycoside, has a molecular weight of 580 and is therefore not absorbed (Crawford et al. 1986; Herr and Landone 1988). When used as definitive therapy, adriamycin has been reported to yield complete and partial response rates of 33% and 31%, respectively.

Prophylactically, adriamycin prevented recurrence in 69% compared with 59% after TUR alone (Herr and Landone 1988). The addition of monthly maintenance therapy resulted in no improvement in either frequency of recurrence or tumour progression (Flamm 1990). Side effects are usually local with irritative symptoms secondary to chemical cystitis predominating. These symptoms may lead to discontinuation of therapy in 5%–20% of patients (Edsmyr et al. 1980). Adriamycin can also cause fibrosis of the submucosal tissue of the bladder and potentiates the fibrotic effects of radiation. This can lead to severe contraction of the bladder (Phillips and Fu 1976).

Mitomycin-C

Mitomycin-C (Mutamycin) has a molecular weight of 329 and, as a result, myelosuppression has been only rarely reported (Witjes and Debruyne 1991). Heney (1985) reported haematological side effects in 5/76 (6.6%) of patients treated with intravesical mitomycin-C. Chemical cystitis and skin rash are the most frequent side effects and may be severe enough to limit therapy (Flanigan et al. 1986; Heney et al. 1988).

Mitomycin-C, when used as definitive therapy, exhibits a complete response rate of 39%–78% (Mishina et al. 1975; Soloway 1985; Stricker et al. 1987; Herr and Landone 1988). Although tumour recurrences developed in many of these patients, tumour free rates of 58% at an average of 21 months have been reported (Stricker et al. 1987). As prophylaxis, intravesical mitomycin-C prevented recurrence in 58% of patients compared to 46% treated with TUR only (Herr and Landone 1988). Isaka et al. (1987) observed tumour free rates of 72% at one year, 66% at three years and 66% at five years for mitomycin-C compared with 53%, 39% and 23% at the corresponding years for the untreated controls ($P < 0.01$). In another study, Tsushima et al. (1987) reported non-recurrence rates at one and two years of 76% and 63% respectively for mitomycin-C compared with to 30% and 22% in controls ($P < 0.01$).

Side effects occurred in 10%–14% of patients (Isaka et al. 1987; Tsushima et al. 1987), bladder irritability being the most common untoward event. Side effects led to the discontinuation of treatment in 4.2% of patients (Tsushima et al. 1987).

Epodyl

Ethoglucid or epodyl (triethylene glycol diglyceride ether), with a molecular weight of 262, was described by Mufti et al. (1990) as having efficacy against superficial grade I-II tumours. In several studies, this agent has exhibited combined (complete and partial) responses in 71% of patients treated definitively for papillary tumours, but only a 35% complete response against cis (Kurth et al. 1984). Although side effects, including both mild and chemical cystitis and systemic reactions, were reported as rare by Kurth et al. (1984), cystitis, severe enough to interrupt treatment, was observed by Mufti et al. (1990) in 19% of patients.

Table 4.1. Comparison among drugs

Drug	Patients	Rx	Follow-up (months)	Response	P (%)	Reference
TT vs ADR	25	P	36	75 vs 85	NS	Horn et al. (1981)
TT vs ADR	61	P	3	70 vs 68	NS	Zincke et al. (1983)
TT vs MMC	40	P	12	93 vs 84	NS	Flanigan et al. (1986)
TT vs MMC	56	T	12	27 vs 39	0.02	Heney (1985)
MMC vs ADR	81	P	12	74 vs 73	NS	Jacobi et al. (1981)
MMC vs ADR	41	P	24	85 vs 47	0.01	Jauhiainen et al. (1986)
MMC vs ADR	16	T	24	82 vs 80	NS	Jauhiainen and Alfthan, (1987)
MMC vs ADR	70	P	24	63 vs 74	NS	Tsushima et al. (1987)
Epodyl vs ADR	171	P	12	56 vs 46	NS	Kurth et al. (1984)

TT, Thiotepa; ADR, Adriamycin; MMC, Mitomycin; P, prophylactically; T, therapeutically.

Comparison of Intravesical Chemotherapy Agents

The efficacy of thiotepa, adriamycin and mitomycin-C has been compared in a number of reports (Lutzeyer et al. 1982; Herr et al. 1987; Soloway 1987; Herr and Landone 1988; Lum and Torti 1990; Herr 1991; Witjes and Debruyne 1991) in which several studies were reviewed (Table 4.1). These drugs were equally effective as prophylactic agents, but in terms of definitive therapy, mitomycin-C and adriamycin seem to be superior to thiotepa. The combination of adriamycin and mitomycin-C, explored by Ferraris (1988) has shown no advantage over single agent treatment. An in vitro study demonstrated that adriamycin and thiotepa were considered more effective in killing cells of a bladder tumour cell line compared with combined adriamycin and mitomycin-C (Serpahim et al. 1991). Definitive randomised trials with combination therapy have not been performed.

Biologic Response Modifiers

Bacillus Calmette–Guérin (BCG) was the first active biologic response modifier to gain wide acceptance as an antitumour agent against superficial bladder cancer. BCG causes a local granulomatous inflammatory reaction and a systemic immune response. These reactions may result in the eradication and/or growth inhibition of TCC (Lamm et al. 1989; Bohle et al. 1990). Although the actual mechanism of action is not known, the binding of the bacilli to fibronectin has been demonstrated to be essential for the induction of the BCG mediated response (Hudson et al. 1987a; Kavoussi et al. 1990).

A variety of BCG strains (TICE, Pasteur, Connaught, Armand Frappier, Glaxo, Moreau and RIVM) are currently in use, and others are under investigation. These strains are provided in different concentrations, reported as colony forming units (CFUs) (Table 4.2) (Reitsma et al. 1991). The activity of the BCG strains may differ from each other based on their method of preparation and the number of CFUs in the final product (Morales et al. 1976).

Since Morales et al. (1976) first reported the activity of BCG against super-ficial TCC, there have been numerous reports of this agent in the literature

Table 4.2. BCG: Strain, weight and strength

Strain	Weight/ampoule (mg)	Colony-forming units (CFUs)
TICE	50	$2{-}8 \times 10^8$
Pasteur	75	6×10^8
Connaught	40	$8{-}32 \times 10^8$
Armand Frappier	120	10^7
Glaxo	75	$8{-}26 \times 10^6$
Moreau	100	2×10^9

showing complete remission rates ranging from 20%–100% (average 61%) for superficial TCC, and remission rates of 40%–94% (average 69%) against carcinoma in situ (Reitsma et al. 1991). BCG, therefore, compares favourably with intravesical chemotherapy in its activity against Ta and T1 tumours, and demonstrates superiority over these agents in its activity against cis (Herr et al. 1987; Soloway 1987; Herr and Landone 1988; Lum and Torti 1990; Herr 1991; Witjes and Debruyne 1991) (Table 4.3). In a recent randomised study reported by Lamm et al (1991a) comparing intravesical BCG and adriamycin, the 5-year disease-free rates of Ta and T1 tumours were 37% and 17% after BCG and adriamycin respectively. The time to treatment failure as measured by persistence, recurrence or progression of disease was 10.4 months after adriamycin and 22.5 months after BCG. For cis, complete response rates were observed in 70% of patients treated with BCG, compared with 34% after adriamycin. The median time to treatment failure was shorter for adriamycin, 5.1 months as opposed to BCG, 39 months. Moreover, at 5 years, disease-free survival was 18% for adriamycin and 45% for BCG.

The relative efficacy of mitomycin-C and BCG remains unanswered. Although most studies suggest that BCG is the superior agent, Debruyne et al. (1989), in a randomised study, demonstrated no difference between intravesical mitomycin-C and BCG RIVM in their ability to prevent recurrence. A significant consideration was whether BCG RIVM was less effective than other commonly used BCG strains. To address this issue, Guttman (1992) compared the BCG RIVM and TICE strains with mitomycin-C. He reported preliminary results which demonstrated that mitomycin-C had a similar efficacy to both strains of BCG. In contrast to these results, the Southwest Oncology Group recently terminated a large randomised study because TICE BCG was significantly more effective than mitomycin-C.

The most efficacious treatment schedule for BCG therapy remains in question. The use of monthly intravesical BCG after the initial six-weekly course has not been shown to add therapeutic benefit (Badalament et al. 1987; Hudson et al. 1987b). However, Lamm et al. (1992a) recently reported improved outcome after a maintenance regimen consisting of three weekly BCG doses at three months, six months, 12 months, 18 months, 24 months, 30 months and 36 months after completion of the initial six-weekly course. This regimen differs from the monthly intravesical dosage and may in fact be repeat therapy. Repeat therapy, constituting a second six-weekly course of BCG at the time of initial recurrence, has also been shown to improve the

Table 4.3. BCG vs chemotherapy

Drug	Patients	Rx	Follow-up (months)	Response (%)	P	Reference
BCG vs TT	49	P	24	100 vs 60	0.01	Brosman (1982)
BCG vs ADR	151	P	12	74 vs 34	0.01	Mori et al. (1986)
BCG vs ADR	100	T	12	72 vs 53	0.001	Mori et al. (1986)
BCG vs ADR	131	P	60	37 vs 17	0.015	Lamm et al. (1991b)
BCG vs ADR	131	T	60	45 vs 18	0.001	Lamm et al. (1991b)
BCG vs MMC	315	P	13	71 vs 79	NS	Debruyne et al. (1989)

TT, thiotepa; ADR, adriamycin; MMC, mitomycin C; P, prophylactically; T, therapeutically.

overall response rate (Brenton et al. 1990; Melekos et al. 1990). Based on Lamm's recent data, additional treatment with three week courses as outlined above may be indicated in high risk cases. A randomised prospective study by Lamm et al. (1990) has shown that oral BCG has no effect on bladder TCC. Adjunctive percutaneous BCG with intravesical therapy has similarly been shown to add no therapeutic advantage (Lamm et al. 1991b).

Adverse reactions related to BCG therapy appear to be more frequent than with other forms of intravesical therapy and are largely localised to the bladder (Lamm et al. 1992b) (Table 4.4). Side effects include cystitis (91%), which is self-limiting and can be successfully treated with medications such as phenazopyridine, propantheline bromide or oxybutynin. The frequencies of other less common, but more serious complications are fever >37°C (2.9%), granulomatous prostatitis (0.9%), major haematuria (1.0%), pneumonitis/hepatitis (0.7%), arthritis/arthralgia (0.5%), skin rash (0.3%), ureteral obstruction (0.3%), orchitis/epididymitis (0.4%), contracted bladder (0.2%), renal abscess (0.1%) and cytopenia (0.1%). All these complications appear to be responsive to isoniazid 300 mg.

For fevers >39.5°C not attributable to other sources, it is recommended that patients be hospitalised and treated with antituberculous antibiotics. Progressive adverse reactions must be carefully managed to avoid sepsis and possible death which has been attributed to BCG sepsis in seven reported cases. Systemic BCG infections such as granulomatous pneumonitis or hepatitis, should be treated with combination therapy of isoniazid 300 mg, rifampicin 600 mg, and ethambutol 1200 mg daily for 6 months. If BCG sepsis develops or is suspected, patients should be treated with the above combination therapy plus cycloserine 500 mg twice daily for five days.

Risk factors for systemic infection include direct intralesional injection of BCG, the use of BCG immediately following TUR and its use after a traumatic catheterisation. BCG is contraindicated in patients who are severely immunocompromised, such as patients with acquired immunodeficiency syndrome (AIDS), leukaemia, Hodgkin's disease or patients who have had organ transplants. BCG should not be given to patients who are pregnant, lactating, or to patients with intractable urinary tract infection.

Table 4.4. BCG complications in 2602 patients

	Total	%
Fever	75	2.9
Granulomatous prostatitis	23	0.9
Pneumonitis/hepatitis	18	0.7
Arthralgia	12	0.5
Haematuria	24	1.0
Rash	8	0.3
Ureteral obstruction	8	0.3
Epididymitis	10	0.4
Contracted bladder	6	0.2
Renal abscess	2	0.1
Sepsis	10	0.4
Cytopenia	2	0.1

Interferon

Intravesical interferon therapy is presently being evaluated as a therapeutic agent in superficial transitional cell cancer. The interferons alpha, beta and gamma are lymphokines produced by a variety of cells in response to viral infections, bacterial endotoxins, polyanions, polynucleotides and polysaccharides and have been shown to possess antiviral, antiproliferative, immunomodulatory and surface membrane activity. Torti et al. (1988) reported the use of intravesical administration of 50 million units of recombinant alpha interferon in 53 patients, and showed that, of the 19 patients with cis, complete and partial responses occurred in six and eight patients respectively. Four complete and no partial responses occurred in the 16 patients with Ta and T1 tumours. Of the eight cis patients with a partial response, three had complete elimination of their cis but developed interval papillary tumours. Of the ten complete responders, five remained disease free at 18–37 months. In a study comparing low (10 million units) versus high (100 million units) dosage of intravesical alpha interferon for cis, the high dose was significantly more efficacious with 20/47 (43%) complete responders compared with 2/38 (5%) for low dose treatment. Only minor flu-like symptoms were observed in 15 of 55 courses of treatment (Glashan 1990). No local symptoms were seen and systemic absorption or the formation of neutralising antibodies were not detected.

Using recombinant beta interferon, Niijima (1989) observed reductions in tumour size in 14/41 (34%) of patients treated with consecutive administration of daily or twice daily dosages. Local side effects included dysuria in two patients and pollakiuria in one case. Systemic toxicity was also observed. Two patients experienced febrile reactions and one patient developed a cutaneous eruption.

These studies demonstrate that therapy with interferons has potential efficacy in TCC. However, additional studies are needed to assess their full role in prophylaxis, and to determine the most appropriate dose regimen. Randomised studies will then be required to compare their effectiveness to other accepted therapies.

New Intravesical Agents

Intravesical therapy has proved to be an extremely significant tool in the management of superficial TCC, and a continued search for new agents with improved efficacy exists. It is impossible to provide an evaluation of all these agents in this chapter; however, a discussion of 4'-epidoxorubicin and keyhole-limpet haemocyanin (KLH) is provided because of the recent attention these two agents have received in the literature. 4'-Epidoxorubicin (a derivative of doxorubicin) has been shown in two phase II studies to have efficacy against Ta and T1 tumours, with reported complete remission rates of 22.5% (Whelan et al. 1991) and 67% (Calais da Silva et al. 1988).

Complications were seen in 32.5% of patients and included chemical cystitis, haematuria and bacteriuria.

Keyhole-limpet haemocyanin was observed by Olsson et al. (1973) to have antitumour activity against TCC of the bladder. More recently, Jurincic et al. (1988), in a randomised study, showed that recurrences were significantly less frequent in 21 patients following KLH treatment than after the treatment of 23 patients with intravesical mitomycin-C (39%) ($P < 0.05$). The follow-up period was 20.7 months for KLH and 18.3 months for mitomycin-C. In the same study, a second group of 81 patients was treated with KLH with a mean follow-up of 22.8 months. In this group recurrences were observed in 21%. KLH was administered as a 1 mg intracutaneous injection followed by monthly 10 mg intravesical instillation. The only side effects noted were low-grade fevers (37.5°C–37.8°C) after intracutaneous KLH in three patients.

Photodynamic Therapy

Photodynamic therapy is a therapeutic modality which has not been approved for use in any country; however, it has been used in several series of patients to treat superficial bladder cancer with some very encouraging results (Prout et al. 1987). This therapy consists of the systemic injection of a photosensitising agent (photofrin II) which is selectively retained in tumour cells (Dougherty 1989). The in vivo stimulation of this agent by a laser light source, which can be introduced by a cystoscope, results in the release of cytotoxic singlet oxygen radicals which induce damage to the microvasculature of the tumour as well as a direct cellular injury to the tumour cells. Photofrin II (PII, dihaematoporphorin ether, DHE), a mixture of non-metalloporphyrins, is the only agent currently being utilised in phase III studies. The drug is given intravenously at a dose of 2.0 mg/kg body weight and photoactivated by laser irradiation two to three days later. Photoactivation may be either focal to broad base papillary tumours or diffuse for multifocal papillary tumours and carcinoma in situ. Several studies are presently in progress to evaluate the efficacy of photodynamic therapy. Published results, thus far, have shown varied response rates. Because of the small number of patients and short follow-up time, caution must be taken in the interpretation of these results.

One major side effect to this mode of treatment is the development of photosensitivity secondary to the systemic cutaneous retention of the photoactive agent. Patients are advised to avoid direct sunlight for six to eight weeks following therapy.

Conclusion

The practising urologist must be aware of the available therapeutic modalities and their varied therapeutic potentials to effectively treat the patient with superficial transitional cell carcinoma of the bladder. Because superficial TCC of the bladder exhibits distinctive presentations in terms of stage, grade, size and tumour number, the treatment options for this disease should be individualised. Surgical resection of the presenting lesion(s) continues to be the therapy of choice, and whereas TUR remains the gold standard, neodymium YAG laser is an alternative.

Elimination of the primary tumour is but the first task in the management of superficial bladder TCC, following which various chemotherapeutic agents and immune response modifiers may be utilised to prevent or retard tumour recurrence and progression in high-risk patients.

There is ongoing research to determine the most efficacious agent(s) as well as the best dosing regimen and form of delivery. Further work is being done to develop new agents that will improve the therapeutic outcome of superficial TCC. Carcinoma in situ although not amenable to resection, has been susceptible to the immune response modifiers with BCG being the first-line drug. The ability for photodynamic therapy to treat the whole bladder implies that a role may develop for this mode of therapy in the management of cis.

References

Abbassian A, Wallace DM (1966) Intracavitary chemotherapy of diffuse non-infiltrating papillary carcinoma of the bladder. J Urol 96:461

Badalament RA, Herr HW, Wang GY et al. (1987) A prospective randomized trial of maintenance versus non-maintenance intravesical Bacillus Calmette–Guérin therapy of superficial bladder cancer. J Clin Oncol 5:441

Beisland HO, Seland PA (1986) A prospective randomized study of neodymium-YAG laser irradiation versus TUR in the treatment of urinary bladder cancer. Scand J Urol Nephrol 20:209

Benson MC, Giella J, Whang IS et al. (1991) Flow cytometric determination of the multidrug resistant phenotype in transitional cell cancer of the bladder: implications and applications. J Urol 146:982

Bohle A, Gerdes J, Ulmer AJ et al. (1990) Effects of local Bacillus Calmette–Guérin therapy in patients with bladder carcinoma on immunocompetent cells of the bladder wall. J Urol 144:53

Boring CC, Squires TS, Tong T (1992) Cancer statistics 1992. Cancer 42:19

Brenton PR, Herr HW, Whitmore WF Jr et al. (1990) The response of patients with superficial bladder cancer to a second course of intravesical Bacillus Calmette–Guérin. J Urol 143:710

Brosman SA (1982) Experience with BCG in patients with superficial bladder carcinoma. J Urol 128:27

Calais da Silva F, Denis L, Bono A et al. (1988) Intravesical chemoresection with 4-epi-doxorubicin in patients with superficial bladder tumours. Eur Urol 14:207

Crawford ED, McKenzie D, Mansson W et al. (1986) Adverse reactions to the intravesical administration of doxorubicin hydrochloride: a report of six cases. J Urol 136:668

Dalton JT, Witjes MG, Badalament RA et al. (1991) Pharmacokinetices of intravesical mitomycin C in superficial bladder cancer patients. Cancer Res 51:5144

Debruyne FMJ, van der Meijden APM, Franssen MPH (1989) BCG-(RIVM) versus mitomycin intravesical therapy in patients with superficial bladder cancer. Prog Clin Biol Res 303:435

Dougherty TJ (1989) Photodynamic therapy: status and potential. Oncology 3:67

Edsmyr F, Bertin T, Roman J et al. (1980) Intravesical therapy with adriamycin in patients with superficial bladder tumours. Eur Urol 6:132

Esquivel EL Jr, Mackenzie AR, Whitemore WF (1965) Treatment of bladder tumours by instillation of thiotepa, actinomycin D, or 5-fluorouracil. Invest Urol 2:381

Ferraris V (1988) Doxorubicin plus mitomycin C regimen in the prophylactic treatment of superficial bladder tumours. Cancer 63:1055

Flamm J (1990) Long term versus short term doxorubicin hydrochloride instillation after transurethral resection of superficial bladder cancer. Eur Urol 17:119

Flanigan RC, Ellison MF, Butler KM et al. (1986) A trial of prophylactic thiotepa or mitomycin C intravesical therapy in patients with recurrent or multiple superficial bladder cancers. J Urol 136:35

Floyd JW, Lin C, Prout GR Jr (1990) Multidrug resistant of a doxorubicin-resistant bladder cancer cell line. J Urol 144:169

Glashan RW (1990) A randomized controlled study of intravesical alpha-2b-interferon in carcinoma in situ of the bladder. J Urol 144:658

Groos E, Walker L, Masters JRW (1986) Intravesical chemotherapy: studies on the relationship between pH and cytotoxicity. Cancer 58:1199

Guttman C (1992) BCG equals mitomycin in bladder cancer study. Urol Times 20:1

Heney NM (1985) First-line chemotherapy of superficial bladder cancer: mitomycin C vs thiotepa. Urol 26 (suppl.):27

Heney MN, Koonz WW, Barton B et al. (1988) Intravesical thiotepa versus mitomycin C in patients with Ta, Ti, and TIS transitional cell carcinoma of the bladder: a phase III prospective randomized study. J Urol 140:1390

Herr HW (1991) Transurethral resection and intravesical therapy of superficial bladder tumours. Urol Clin North Am 18:525

Herr HW, Landone VP (1988) Intravesical therapy for superficial bladder cancer. Update Cancer, vol 2: Principles and Practice of Oncology. Lippincott, Philadelphia

Herr HW, Landone VP, Whitmore WF Jr (1987) An overview of intravesical therapy for superficial bladder tumours. J Urol 138:1383

Horn Y, Eidelman A, Walach N et al (1981) Intravesical chemotherapy in controlled trial thiotepa versus doxorubicin. J Urol 125:652

Hudson MA, Brown EJ, Ritchey JK et al. (1987a) Modulation of fibronectin medicated Bacillus Calmette–Guérin attachment to murine bladder mucosa by drugs influencing the coagulation pathways. Cancer Res 51:3726

Hudson MA, Ratcliff TL, Gillen DP et al. (1987b) Single course versus maintenance Bacillus Calmette–Guérin therapy for superficial bladder tumours: a prospective randomized trial. J Urol 138:295

Isaka S, Okano T, Shimazaki J et al. (1987) Prophylaxis of superficial bladder cancer with instillation of adriamycin or mitomycin-C. Cancer Chemother Pharmacol 20 (Suppl.):S77

Jacobi GH, Jakse G, Thuroff JW et al. (1981) Intravesical chemotherapy for prophylaxis of recurrent superficial bladder tumours: a randomized trial of 122 patients. Proc Am Urol Assoc (Annual Meeting) Abstract 579, p 236

Jauhiainen K, Alfthan O (1987) Mitomycin and doxorubicin instillation as recurrence prophylaxis in superficial (Ta-1) urinary bladder carcinoma. J Urol 128:27

Jauhiainen K, Sotrauta M, Penn J (1986) Effect of mitomycin C and doxorubicin instillation of carcinoma in situ of the bladder. Eur Urol 12:32

Jurincic CD, Engelmann U, Gasch J et al. (1988) Immunotherapy in bladder cancer with keyhole-limpet hemocyanin: a randomized study. J Urol 139:723

Kavoussi LR, Brown E, Ritchey JK et al. (1990) Fibronectin-medication Calmette–Guérin Bacillus attachment to murine bladder mucosa: requirements for the expression of an anti-tumour response. J Clin Invest 85:62

Knuchel R, Hofstadter F, Jenkins WEA et al. (1989) Sensitivities of monolayers and spheroids of the human bladder cancer cell line MGH-UI to the drugs used for intravesical chemotherapy. Cancer Res 49:1397

Koonz WW Jr, Prout GR Jr, Smith W et al. (1981) The use of intravesical thiotepa in the management of non-invasive carcinoma of the bladder. J Urol 125:307

Kurth KH, Schroeder FH, Tunn U et al. (1984) Adjuvant chemotherapy of superficial transitional cell bladder carcinoma: preliminary results of a European Organization for Research on Treatment of Cancer randomized trials comparing doxorubicin hydrochloride, ethoglucid and transurethral resection alone. J Urol 132:258

Lamm DL, Thor DE, Stogdill VD et al. (1989) Bladder cancer immunotherapy. J Urol 142:719

Lamm DL, Dehaven JI, Shriver J et al. (1990) a randomized prospective comparison of oral versus intravesical and percutaneous Bacillus Calmette–Guérin for superficial bladder cancer. J Urol 144:65

Lamm DL, Dehaven JI, Shriver J et al. (1991a) Prospective randomized comparison of intravesical with percutaneous Bacillus Calmette–Guérin versus intravesical Bacillus Calmette–Guérin in superficial bladder cancer. J Urol 145:738

Lamm DL, Blumenstein BA, Crawford ED et al. (1991b) A randomized trial of intravesical doxorubicin and immunotherapy with Bacillus Calmette–Guérin for transitional-cell carcinoma of the bladder. N Engl J Med 325:1205

Lamm DL, Crawford ED, Blumenstein B et al. (1992a) Maintenance BCG immunotherapy of superficial bladder cancer: a randomized prospective Southwest Oncology Group study. (Abstract) J Urol 147(Suppl):274A

Lamm DL, van der Meijden APM, Morales A et al. (1992b) Incidence and treatment of complications of Bacillus Calmette–Guérin intravesical therapy in superficial bladder cancer. J Urol 147:596

Lum BL, Torti FM (1990) Adjuvant intravesicular pharmacotherapy for superficial bladder cancer. J Natl Cancer Inst 83:82

Lutzeyer W, Rubben H, Dahm H (1982) Prognostic parameter of superficial bladder cancer: an analysis of 315 cases. J Urol 127:250

McPhee MS, Mador DR, Tulip J et al. (1982) Segmented irradiation of the bladder with neodymium YAG laser irradiation. J Urol 128:1101

Melekos MD, Pantazakos A, Markou S et al. (1990) Intravesical Bacillus Calmette–Guérin administration of the prophylaxis of superficial bladder cancer. Int Urol Nephrol 22:433

Mishina T, Oda K, Murata S et al. (1975) Mitomycin-C bladder instillation therapy for bladder tumours. J Urol 114:217

Mishina T, Watanabe H, Kobayashi T et al. (1986) Absorption of anticancer drugs through bladder epithelium. Urology 27:148

Morales A, Eidinger D, Bruce AW (1976) Intracavitary Bacillus Calmette–Guérin in the treatment of superficial bladder tumours. J Urol 116:180

Mori K, Lamm DL, Crawford ED (1986) A trial of BCG versus adriamycin in superficial bladder cancer. Urol Int 41:L 254

Morrison DA, Murphy WM, Ford KS et al. (1984) Surveillance of stage 0, grade 1 bladder cancer by cytology alone: is it acceptable? J Urol 132:672

Mufti GR, Virdi JS, Hall MH (1990) Long term follow-up of intravesical epodyl therapy for superficial bladder cancer. Br J Urol 65:32

Niijima T (1989) Intravesical treatment of bladder cancer with recombinant human interferon-beta. Cancer Immunol Immunother 30:81

Olsson CA, Chute R, Rao CN (1973) Immunologic reduction of bladder cancer recurrence rate. Trans Am Assoc Genito-Urin Surg 65:66

Phillips TL, Fu KK (1976) Quantification of combined radiation therapy and chemotherapy effects on critical normal tissue. Cancer 37:1186

Prout GR Jr, Lin C, Benson R Jr et al. (1987) Photodynamic therapy with hematoporphyrin derivative in the treatment of superficial transitional-cell carcinoma of the bladder. N Engl J Med 317:1251

Reitsma DJ, Guinan P, Lamm DL et al. (1991) Long term effect of intravesical Bacillus Calmette–Guérin (BCG) TICE strain on flat carcinoma in situ of the bladder. Urol Times 19:17

Serpahim LA, Perapato SD, Slocum HK et al. (1991) In vitro study of the interaction of doxorubicin, thiotepa, mitomycin-C, agents used for intravesical chemotherapy of superficial bladder cancer. J Urol 145:613

Soloway MS (1985) Treatment of superficial bladder cancer with intravesicular mitomycin-C: analysis of immediate and long term response in 70 patients. J Urol 134:1107

Soloway MS (1987) Selecting initial therapy for bladder cancer. Cancer 60 (Suppl):502

Soloway MS, Ford KS (1983) Thiotepa induced myelosupression: reviews of 679 bladder instillation. J Urol 130:

Staehler G, Hofstetter A (1979) Laser, transurethral laser irradiation of urinary bladder tumours. Eur Urol 5:64

Stricker PD, Grant ABF, Hosken BM et al. (1987) Topical mitomycin-C therapy for carcinoma of the bladder. J Urol 138:1164–1166

Torti FM, Shortliffe LD, Williams RD et al. (1988) Alpha-interferon in superficial bladder cancer: a Northern California Oncology Group study. J Clin Oncol 6:476

Tsushima T, Matsumura Y, Ozaki Y et al. Urological Cancer Collaboration Group (OUCCG)

(1987) Prophylaxis intravesical instillation therapy with adriamycin and mitomycin-C in patients with superficial bladder cancer. Cancer Chemother Pharmacol 20(Suppl): S72

Veenema RJ, Dean AL Jr, Uson AC et al. (1969) Thiotepa bladder instillations: therapy and prophylaxis for superficial bladder tumours. J Urol 101:711

Whelan P, Cumming JA, Garvie WHH et al. (1991) Multi-centre phase II study of low dose intravesical epirubicin in the treatment of superficial bladder cancer. Br J Urol 67:600

Witjes JA, Debruyne FNJ (1991) Optimal management of superficial bladder cancer. Eur J Cancer 27:330

Zincke H, Utz DC, Taylor WF (1983) Influence of thiotepa and doxorubicin instillation at time of transurethral surgical treatment of bladder cancer on tumour recurrence. J Urol 129:505

Chapter 5

The Role of Chemotherapy in the Treatment of Bladder Cancer

J. T. Roberts and R. R. Hall

Introduction

This chapter will not attempt to give a detailed review of data from phase II studies of systemic chemotherapy in advanced urothelial cancer, as such information has been reviewed comprehensively elsewhere (Yagoda 1987; Seidman and Scher 1991). Rather, we will seek to place in context information on the role of systemic chemotherapy in the treatment of primary muscle invasive bladder cancers, in the management of locally extensive, recurrent tumours and metastatic disease. The role of chemotherapy in the management of primary, muscle-invasive bladder cancer will be considered as follows:

1. The use of chemotherapy as sole treatment (monotherapy), in attempts to conserve bladder function. Conventional radical treatments are reserved in such patients for the treatment of local failure of chemotherapy.
2. Chemotherapy as an adjuvant to conservative surgery (partial cystectomy or endoscopic resection of tumour) and as an adjunct to conventional radical radiotherapy. In either case, the role of chemotherapy may be seen as increasing the local control rate and thus enhancing the likelihood of bladder conservation.
3. The use of systemic chemotherapy in the conventional adjuvant or neo-adjuvant setting. That is, it is given in addition to conventional radical treatment, such as cystectomy or radiotherapy, in the hope that the destruction of occult micrometastases might improve cure rates for a disease in which conventional treatments produce only modest numbers of long term survivors.

The Development of Combination Chemotherapy Regimes For Transitional Cell Carcinoma

Metastatic transitional cell carcinoma has traditionally been regarded as a chemoresistant tumour, with low response rates to single agent chemotherapy (typically less than 30%). Very few complete responses to single agents are documented and no demonstrable impact has been discerned from single agent-, or most combination-chemotherapy regimes on the poor survival of patients with metastatic disease.

Two of the most active single agents, cisplatin and methotrexate, are potentially nephrotoxic. The understandable reluctance to combine these agents in an elderly patient population in which renal impairment is common was overcome by two groups who demonstrated higher response rates, including a number of complete responses, following the combination of these two drugs than had been recorded for single agents or for other combinations (Carmichael et al. 1985; Stoter et al. 1987). There followed reports of more aggressive combinations, adding vinblastine alone (CMV) (Harker et al. 1985) or together with adriamycin (MVAC) (Sternberg et al. 1985), to produce overall response rates of the order of 60%–70%, with significant numbers of complete responders (CRs) – and the suggestion that a worthwhile impact on the survival of patients with metastatic disease was being observed.

As is frequently the case, the high response rates of early studies and the apparently spectacular improvements in mean survival have not been replicated by multicentre studies. The initial expectation of some that metastatic transitional cell carcinoma might prove reliably chemocurable has been tempered with time (Raghavan 1990). Nevertheless, numerous non-randomised studies have been undertaken in patients with locally advanced as well as metastatic urothelial cancer, the results of which merit thoughtful consideration.

Systemic Chemotherapy as Monotherapy for Muscle-Invasive Bladder Cancer

The response of primary bladder cancers to neoadjuvant chemotherapy has been reviewed by Splinter et al. (1989) and Scher et al. (1988, 1989) have reviewed their single institution experience specifically with the use of MVAC in primary bladder tumours.

Overall response rates of 60%–70% with complete response rates of the order of 30% have been observed repeatedly. There is also the impression that response rates of primary T2–T4b tumours are better than those of

Table 5.1. Muscle invasive bladder cancer: primary chemotherapy: T3 tumours only

	Complete response	
T3 tumours – all patients	23/67	(34%)
T3 tumours $\leq$ 5 cm	15/43	(35%)
T3 patients, T0 at 3 years with chemotherapy only	10/56	(18%)

metastatic lesions (Meyers et al. 1985; Scher et al.1988; Sternberg et al. 1988; Boutan-Laroze et al. 1991).

In series that have set out to examine the local response rate of primary bladder cancers to systemic chemotherapy, the reluctance of patients to accept conventional radical therapy after the documentation of an histologically confirmed complete response, or the reluctance of some surgeons to remove an apparently normal bladder, has allowed the observation of the rates and durations of complete remissions of muscle-invasive bladder cancer following systemic chemotherapy alone (Roberts et al. 1991; Scher et al. 1989). These observations led us to explore the possibility that cisplatin-based chemotherapy might prove an effective sole treatment for invasive bladder cancer.

In a series of 103 patients with muscle-invasive bladder cancer of varying clinical stages treated with a variety of cisplatin based chemotherapy regimens, we have observed complete remissions in about 37% after two to six cycles of chemotherapy, more than half of which have been durable. However, by three years the proportion of patients remaining in complete clinical remission without further intervention had fallen to only 17% (Hall and Roberts 1991). The results for T3 tumours were similar; 34% were in clinical complete remission at the end of chemotherapy but only 18% were disease free at three years without additional alternative therapy (Table 5.1).

Reviewing the published data, it is clear that muscle-invasive bladder cancer is chemosensitive and is chemocurable in a small proportion of patients. But as monotherapy, cisplatin-based chemotherapy does not produce such good durable remission rates as radiation and must therefore be regarded as inadequate as definitive sole treatment.

Conservative Surgery Combined with Chemotherapy

Soquet (1981), using a combination of partial cystectomy and systemic high-dose methotrexate, reported local control and survival figures for muscle-invasive bladder cancer that approximated those for more conventional radical therapy in 25 patients. A collaborative North of England Group, using similar chemotherapy, but combining it with a radical endoscopic resection of tumour, rather than formal open partial cystectomy, achieved similar results

Table 5.2. TUR + C/M for muscle-invasive bladder cancer; control of primary tumour: TUR + C/M only

	6m	1y	2y	3y	4y	5y
Alive T0	40	34	25	21	15	13
Dead of TCC but T0 in bladder	0	1	1	2	3	4
Total at risk	47	46	42	34	27	23
Percentage bladder tumour free	85%	76%	62%	68%	67%	74%

(Hall et al.1984). Overall, using this approach more than 60% of patients achieved tumour free status in the bladder (Hall and Roberts 1989).

Non-cisplatin chemotherapy is less than optimal in this setting. The use of cisplatin and methotrexate following radical transurethral resection (TUR) improves the outcome (Hall and Roberts 1989). In 47 patients with T2–T3b transitional cell carcinoma treated by "complete" TUR plus three to five cycles of cisplatin 70 mg/m^2 and methotrexate 40mg/m^2 $\times$ 2, 23/34 retained their bladder, disease free with normal function at three years with no additional treatment (Table 5.2). The ability of this therapeutic approach to produce a satisfactory clinical outcome in suitably selected patients has been supported by Martinez-Pineiro et al. (1992) and by Nogueira-March et al. (1991). Amiel et al. (1988) have also achieved a significant proportion of patients free of invasive tumour in the bladder using a combination of cisplatin and 5-fluorouracil and TUR.

An alternative approach is to give chemotherapy first and then to consolidate a complete response (CR) or good partial response (PR) by using TUR or partial cystectomy to clear the site of previous tumour. It has been suggested (Sternberg et al. 1992; Nativ et al. 1991) that up to 50% of muscle-invasive bladder cancers can be managed successfully by a combination of chemotherapy and postchemotherapy surgical conservative resection, either by means of partial cystectomy or TUR.

It would thus seem reasonable to consider the option of combining bladder-sparing surgery (TUR or partial cystectomy) and systemic, cisplatin based chemotherapy for selected patients with muscle-invasive bladder cancer. In suitable patients (probably those with smaller T3 tumours, i.e. less than 6 cm) such an approach appears to offer local control rates that match or better those achieved by more conventional means. The median follow-up of Newcastle patients was 57 months (15–105 months) and as no other series has followed patients for as long it is not yet possible to state with certainty that short-term local control will translate into acceptable long-term survival rates.

Chemotherapy Combined with Radiotherapy

There are suggestions that the integration of cisplatin with radiotherapy increases the local control rate, compared with that obtained by means of radiation alone (Hall 1991). Certainly, such combinations may be given safely (Shipley 1988; Howard et al. 1991; Waxman et al. 1992) and some workers have observed response rates in the bladder that are superior to those observed in historical control series (Shipley et al. 1984; Jakse et al. 1987; Prout et al. 1990).

Since complete response of the primary tumour following radiotherapy has been shown to predict a favourable outcome for muscle-invasive bladder cancer (Shipley 1988), there is the expectation that this apparently increased local control rate with pre-emptive or synchronous chemotherapy may translate into improved survival, in addition to an improved bladder preservation rate.

Various series have reported that the use of radiotherapy alone can yield immediate complete response rates of 40%–50% and maintain bladder tumour-free survival rates of the order of 30%–40% (Oosten and Janknegt 1990). Gospodarowicz et al. (1991) reported complete response rates in the bladder after treatment with modern megavoltage radiotherapy alone which are similar to those quoted above for the combination of chemotherapy and radiotherapy. This emphasises the importance of patient selection and the role of chance in determining treatment outcome in small series of patients and highlights the need for comparisons to be made within the context of randomised trials of sufficient size to have the power to detect real differences.

The published longer-term results of non-randomised studies of combined chemotherapy and radiotherapy (Rifkin and Wajsman 1991; Wohlgenannt et al. 1991) are not encouraging, the proportion of patients remaining tumour-free in the bladder being no greater than one would expect from conventional radiotherapy. The only reported randomised trial of a combination of radiotherapy and cisplatin chemotherapy is the Canadian BL3 study (Coppin et al. 1992). No survival benefit was demonstrated but the numbers in this study were small and the trial lacked the power to detect reliably a true survival benefit of 10%–15%. There was, however, an apparent reduction in the pelvic recurrence rate of some 25%.

One current study is designed to determine the level of benefit of the addition of three cycles of combination chemotherapy (cisplatin, methotrexate and vinblastine) to full-dose radiotherapy with integrated cisplatin preceded by transurethral resection of tumour. Preliminary results confirm the feasibility of such an approach (Prout et al. 1990) and the definitive results, both in terms of bladder preservation rate and survival are awaited with interest.

This, and other studies (Farah et al. 1991; Howard et al. 1991; Waxman et al. 1992) provide reassurance that a combination of chemotherapy and radiotherapy is practical and safe. Only the results of sufficiently large, randomised, comparative studies will establish the role of such treatment in the routine management of bladder cancer.

The Role of Adjuvant Chemotherapy in T2–T4a Bladder Cancer

The high response rates for transitional cell carcinoma reported in the middle of the last decade in single-centre phase II studies raised the expectation that the adjuvant use of such regimes would produce a significant survival benefit.

Randomised trials of non-cisplatin-containing chemotherapy regimens, single agent or combination, given in addition to conventional radical treatment have failed to demonstrate an advantage for the addition of chemotherapy (Richards et al.1983; Shearer et al. 1988).

Single agent cisplatin as an adjuvant to radiotherapy has likewise proved disappointing. Two similarly designed randomised studies (in Australia and in the UK) in which single agent cisplatin was given prior to radical radiotherapy closed before the anticipated numbers of patients had been recruited. Each assessed the impact on survival of cisplatin (100 mg/m^2, two or three doses at 3 weekly intervals) preceding radical radiotherapy ($60–64$ Gy in 2 Gy fractions over $6–6.5$ weeks). A total of 250 patients in two centres were randomly allocated to radiotherapy alone or to combined treatment. Factors such as preconceived ideas of the likely impact of chemotherapy, publication of the early results of combination chemotherapy trials and changes in surgical practice, with a shift towards radical cystectomy and bladder reconstruction, led to a fall in recruitment and premature closure of both studies. An analysis of the combined data from the two studies fails to reveal any difference in the actuarial 3-year survival in the two treatment arms (approximately 40% in each arm), although the numbers of patients assessed were not sufficiently large to detect a difference of less than 15% (Wallace et al. 1991).

A Spanish multicentre, randomised comparison of radical cystectomy alone with radical cystectomy following three cycles of single agent cisplatin failed to demonstrate any impact on survival of the adjuvant chemotherapy. Again, recruitment to this study flagged after an initially encouraging start "following the report of the results of MVAC". Only 122 patients were randomised in total so that the numbers of patients assessed are inadequate to detect even quite large differences in survival (Martinez-Pineiro et al. 1992).

A Swiss collaborative study, in which patients were randomly allocated after cystectomy either to observation or three cycles of cisplatin, also closed early, in this instance because of concern that the chemotherapy may have accelerated progression of metastatic disease. Only 80 patients were randomised and no statistically significant benefit for chemotherapy could be demonstrated (Studer et al. 1991).

Despite the failure of these studies to demonstrate a benefit for the addition of adjuvant cisplatin, there remains the hope that *combination* chemotherapy may confer a worthwhile benefit, particularly since a randomised trial has confirmed the superior activity of MVAC over single agent cisplatin in metastatic disease (Loehrer et al. 1992).

Skinner et al. (1991) claim to have demonstrated an advantage for the adjuvant use of a combination of cisplatin, adriamycin and cyclophosphamide (CisCA) with cystectomy both for time to progression and for survival. However, this conclusion is seriously undermined by the statistical inadequacies of the trial, which closed prematurely after the evaluation of only 91 patients. The emphasis in the statistical analysis on median time to recurrence of small groups and the use of the Wilcoxon test both favour early differences and are unreliable tests for long-term survival. The shortcomings of the study were highlighted in the editorial comments which accompanied its publication.

Over a 3.5-year period Stockle et al. (1992) randomised 49 patients with pT3b, pT4a transitional cell carcinomas with lymph node metastases to receive either three cycles of adjuvant MVAC or MVEC chemotherapy, or no chemotherapy, following radical cystectomy. This very slowly recruiting trial was terminated prematurely because a large difference in favour of adjuvant chemotherapy was found at interim analysis. Of 18 patients who received chemotherapy, three have had tumour progression compared with 18 of 23 patients in the control group. In agreement with the study by Skinner et al. (1991) these data suggest a benefit from the addition of chemotherapy in patients with lymph node metastases, but the result is undermined by several factors and is far from conclusive. Randomisation was by means of "a locked randomisation list" and seven of 26 patients allocated to chemotherapy did not receive it. Although one sympathises with the authors who were made aware of the findings of interim analysis, to stop the trial under these circumstances will have inevitably exaggerated the apparent difference.

The Nordic trial of adjuvant cisplatin and adriamycin before combined radiotherapy and cystectomy for T1G3/T4a bladder cancer has been reported (Rintala et al. 1991). Preliminary results "show that survival is 10% better for adjuvant chemotherapy". With only 325 patients randomised and a median follow-up of only 13 months, this is an encouraging, but premature conclusion.

A collaborative, international, multicentre randomised comparison of conventional radical therapy (radiotherapy, cystectomy or a combination) alone, with or without three cycles of neoadjuvant CMV chemotherapy is in progress, coordinated by the Medical Research Council (MRC) and the EORTC GU Group. It is more than half way to its planned recruitment figure of 950 patients and should be sufficiently powerful to detect a 10% improvement in survival.

The Southwestern Oncology Group (SWOG)/Intergroup study of the effect of adjuvant MVAC on survival following radical cystectomy is also under way and the results of both are awaited with interest. The problems faced in organising such trials are well reviewed by Raghavan (1991).

There are disadvantages, potential and real, in the administration of chemotherapy prior to standard radical therapy.

The delay in starting definitive curative radiotherapy is a cause for concern but our experience and that of other authors is that few tumours progress during pre-emptive chemotherapy and that patients are unlikely to be placed at additional risk by the adoption of this approach (Howard et al. 1991; Waxman et al. 1992).

Another concern, frequently voiced, is that the administration of chemotherapy will delay the palliation of tumour-related urinary symptoms. In fact several series have demonstrated prompt, effective and frequently complete relief of urinary symptoms during systemic chemotherapy (Howard et al. 1991; Roberts et al. 1991; Fossa et al. 1992). Improvement of symptoms may be independent of tumour response (Roberts et al. 1991) and may therefore depend on the effect of diuresis induced during cisplatin chemotherapy, the use of antibiotics to treat urinary infections detected during admissions for chemotherapy or endoscopic resection of tumour during pretreatment or response assessment.

A further concern is that pretreatment with chemotherapy may enhance the toxicity of radical radiotherapy leading to an increase in morbidity or compelling a reduction in radiation dose. In 43 patients treated with radical radiotherapy at various intervals after chemotherapy, using a number of different cisplatin-containing chemotherapy regimes, including some with an anthracycline (adriamycin or epirubicin), we have observed no unexpected or undue toxicity. A similar lack of enhancement of toxicity has been observed by other authors (Farah et al. 1991; Howard et al. 1991; Prout et al. 1991). The question of cisplatin chemotherapy accelerating the progression of metastatic disease has been alluded to in the report of the Swiss collaborative study (Studer et al. 1991).

A review of the results from several neoadjuvant chemotherapy series suggests that the response of the primary bladder tumour to initial chemotherapy provides a prognostic indicator for survival (Splinter et al. 1992).

Chemotherapy for the Treatment of Recurrent and Metastatic Disease

Metastatic TCC is generally regarded as incurable, is associated with a very poor prognosis and treatment has previously been directed at the palliation of symptoms. Chemotherapy has generally been regarded as offering poor palliation because of low response rates and the associated morbidity.

The response rates of metastatic disease to cisplatin containing chemotherapy regimens (Carmichael et al. 1985; Harker et al. 1985; Stoter et al. 1987) and particularly the initial results of MVAC (Sternberg et al. 1985), encouraged the expectation that metastatic TCC might prove the first reliably chemocurable adult carcinoma, akin to germ cell neoplasms (Waxman 1990).

A large multicentre cooperative study has compared MVAC with single-agent cisplatin (70 mg/m^2) in patients with metastatic TCC, confirming the greater toxicity of the combination but also confirming a higher response rate (39% vs 12%), a greater progression-free survival (10 vs 4.3 months) and a greater overall survival (12.5 vs 8.2 months) for MVAC (Loehrer et al. 1992).

These results would seem to confirm the superior activity of cisplatin/methotrexate combinations over single-agent cisplatin alone or in combination with other agents. However, the inclusion of cisplatin adds considerably to the toxicity and necessitates inpatient treatment and its contribution to overall efficacy is doubted by some. Thus its contribution to the basic cisplatin/methotrexate combination is being examined in a multicentre cooperative study coordinated by the Medical Research Council which compares cisplatin, methotrexate and vinblastine with methotrexate and vinblastine.

The Memorial Sloan-Kettering Cancer Centre (MSKCC) continues to report durable remissions in patients with metastatic TCC treated with MVAC chemotherapy (Sternberg et al. 1989). However, their long-term survivors have had nodal, rather than visceral, metastases. Furthermore, their complete or partial remissions have been "consolidated" by aggressive surgical resection of residual or of the initial sites of disease, for example by cystectomy combined with radical pelvic and retroperitoneal lymph node dissection. In our own experience of patients with metastatic disease treated by means of a variety of cisplatin based chemotherapy regimes, including MVAC, we have seen only one patient survive for more than 2 years following diagnosis and no long-term disease-free survivors. Others, although confirming the activity of MVAC in metastatic TCC, have failed to replicate the response rates observed at MSKCC and have not observed a substantial number of long-term survivors among responders (Boutan-Laroze et al. 1991; Loehrer et al. 1992).

Despite the lack of data suggesting that cure or greatly prolonged survival is reliably consequent upon the use of aggressive cisplatin-based chemotherapy combinations, the response rates observed, the rapid onset of response and apparently increased duration of survival all lend support to the concept that such combinations may provide worthwhile palliation of the symptoms of metastatic TCC.

However, given that only 14% or so of patients with metastatic disease will achieve a CR immediately following chemotherapy and that only a third to a quarter of the CRs are likely to prove durable, only 3%–5% of patients with metastatic disease can expect to experience a survival benefit from systemic chemotherapy. Its routine use outside clinical trials cannot therefore be recommended.

TCC is a disease which affects predominantly the elderly; the median age of presentation of bladder cancer in the UK is 67. Any chemotherapy regime used must therefore be applicable to this population. We have not excluded patients from chemotherapy on the basis of age alone. Reporting on a series of 36 patients aged from 76 to 84 years (median 78), Sella et al. (1991) conclude that cisplatin combination chemotherapy can be administered safely to such patients, they observed an efficacy similar to that found in younger patients and concluded that age should not exclude patients from the benefits of such therapy. Geller et al.(1991) and Loehrer et al.(1992) have also reported that older patients with metastatic disease fared better than younger patients.

Similarly, since a significant proportion of patients with advanced urothelial carcinoma present with renal impairment due to ureteric obstruction, it is important that chemotherapy is appropriate to this group. We observed no increase in chemotherapy toxicity in such patients and saw some complete responses, although not in patients with very high creatinine levels. Some of these patients underwent percutaneous nephrostomy or ureteric stenting prior to cytotoxic treatment (MacNeil et al.1991).

Conclusions

1. The observation that durable complete remissions of muscle-invasive TCC bladder (T2–T4b) can be obtained using cisplatin-based combination chemotherapy as monotherapy is of great interest; there is certainly no other common adult carcinoma in which such a proportion of patients can be rendered disease free using chemotherapy alone. However, the relatively low proportion (17%) remaining disease-free at three years

without further intervention in the form of salvage cystectomy or salvage radiotherapy reduces this observation to the level of an intriguing clinical curiosity. Certainly, when compared with the 30% or so who will remain persistently disease-free in the bladder following conventional radiotherapy there is nothing to commend this approach as a routine method of managing bladder cancer. Its adoption as a clinical routine must await the development of cytotoxic agents which are more effective than those currently available.

2. The combination of systemic chemotherapy, using cisplatin and methotrexate (or combinations containing these drugs, such as CMV, MVAC, EpiC-M etc.) and a conservative surgical procedure such as partial cystectomy or transurethral resection can allow bladder preservation without compromising survival in selected patients with muscle-invasive transitional cell carcinomas of the bladder.

3. The integration of chemotherapy with radiotherapy may improve local tumour control rates, but evidence of a survival benefit is so far lacking.

4. The value of adjuvant chemotherapy plus cystectomy or full-dose radical radiotherapy has yet to be proven. Adjuvant chemotherapy has, however, found an established role in the management of cancers, such as breast and bowel, where durable long-term control of the primary tumour has not been observed following chemotherapy alone. This observation must therefore be seen as encouraging the pursuit of trials of adjuvant chemotherapy in urothelial cancer.

5. Systemic chemotherapy for metastatic disease provides effective relief of symptoms, but durable complete remissions are unusual.

References

Amiel J, Quintens H, Thyss A et al. (1988) Association resection trans-uretrale (RTU)-chimiotherapie systematique comme traitement initiale des tumeurs infiltrantes de vessie (pT2-pT4, Nx, M0). J Urol (Paris) 94:333–336

Boutan-Laroze A, Mahjoubi M, Droz JP et al. (1991) MVAC (methotrexate, vinblastine, doxorubicin and cisplatin) for advanced carcinoma of the bladder; the French Federation of Cancer Centers Experience. Eur J Cancer 27:1690–1694

Carmichael J, Cornbleet MA, MacDougall FH et al. (1985) Cis-platin and methotrexate in the treatment of transitional cell carcinoma of the urinary tract. Br J Urol 57:299–302

Coppin C, Gospodarowicz M, Dixon P et al. (1992). Improved local control of invasive bladder cancer by concurrent cisplatin and pre-operative or radical radiation. Proc ASCO II:198

Farah R, Chodack GW, Vogelzang NJ et al. (1991) Curative radiotherapy following chemotherapy for invasive bladder carcinoma (a preliminary report). Int J Radiat Oncol Biol Phys 20:413–417

Fossa SD, Harland SJ, Kaye SB et al. (1992) Initial combination chemotherapy with cisplatin methotrexate and vinblastine in locally advanced transitional cell carcinoma of the bladder – response rate and pitfalls. Br J Urol 70:161–168

Geller NL, Sternberg CN, Penenberg D et al. (1991) Prognostic factors for survival of patients with advanced urothelial tumours with methotrexate, vinblastine, doxorubicin and cisplatin chemotherapy. Cancer 67:1525–1531

Gospodarowicz MK, Rider WD, Keen CW et al. (1991) Bladder cancer: long-term follow-up results of patients treated with radical radiation. Clin Oncol 3:155–161

Hall RR (1991) Combination chemoradiotherapy for bladder cancer with bladder sparing. Curr Opin Urol 1:65–67

Hall RR, Roberts JT, (1989) Chemotherapy of advanced bladder cancer. Therapeutic progress in urological cancers. Liss, New York, pp 525–531

Hall RR, Roberts JT (1991) Neoadjuvant chemotherapy, a method to conserve the bladder. Eur J Cancer 27 (Suppl. 2):529 (abstract)

Hall RR, Newling DWW Ramsden PD et al. (1984) Treatment of invasive bladder cancer by local resection and high dose methotrexate. Br J Urol 56:668–672

Harker WG, Meyers FJ, Freiha FS et al. (1985) Cisplatin, methotrexate and vinblastine (CMV): an effective chemotherapy regime for metastatic transitional cell carcinoma of the urinary tract. A Northern California Oncology Group Study. J Clin Oncol 3:1463–1470

Howard GCW, Cornbleet MA, Whillis D et al. (1991) Neoadjuvant chemotherapy with methotrexate and cisplatin prior to radiotherapy for invasive transitional carcinoma of the bladder. Assessment of feasibility and toxicity. Br J Urol 68:490–494

Jakse G, Fritsch E, Frommhold H (1987) Hyperfractionated, accelerated irradiation and chemotherapy in locally advanced bladder cancer. Eur Urol 13:22–25

Loehrer PJ, Einhorn LH, Elson P et al. (1992) A randomised comparison of cisplatin alone or in combination with methotrexate, vinblastine and doxorubicin in patients with metastatic urothelial carcinoma: a cooperative group study. J Clin Oncol 7:1066–1073

MacNeil HF, Hall RR, Neal DE et al. (1991) Systemic chemotherapy for urothelial cancer in patients with ureteric obstruction. Br J Urol 67:169–172

Martinez-Pineiro JA, Martin MG, Arocena F et al. (1992) Neoadjuvant cisplatin therapy before radical cystectomy in invasive transitional cell carcinoma of the bladder: CUETO study 84005. In: Villavicenio H, Fair W R (eds) Societé Internationale d'Urologie Reports: Evaluation of chemotherapy in bladder cancer. Churchill Livingstone, Edinburgh, pp 103–108

Meyers FJ, Palmer JM, Freyha FS et al. (1985) The fate of the bladder in patients with metastatic bladder cancer treated with cisplatin, methotrexate and vinblastine: a Northern California Oncology Group study. J Urol 134:1118–1121

Nativ O, Herr HW, Scher HI et al. (1991) Neoadjuvant chemotherapy and partial cystectomy for invasive bladder tumours. J Urol 145:336A (abstract)

Nogueira-March JL, Ojea A, Figueiredo L et al. (1991) Radical TUR + MVAC in the treatment of infiltrating bladder tumours. Proceedings of 22nd Congress Societé Internationale d'Urologie, Sevilla 1991, abstract 215

Oosten JK, Janknegt RA (1990) Bladder saving procedure in invasive local bladder cancer. Results of 3 years follow up in 87 responders on radiotherapy. Eur Urol 18 Suppl 1:79 (abstract)

Prout GR, Shipley WU, Kaufman DS et al. (1990) Preliminary results in invasive bladder cancer with transurethral resection; neoadjuvant chemotherapy and combined pelvic irradiation plus cisplatin chemotherapy. J Urol 144:1128–1134

Prout GR, Shipley WV, Kaufman DS et al. (1991) Interval report of a phase I–II study utilizing multiple modalities in the treatment of invasive bladder cancer: a bladder sparing trial. Urol Clin North Am 18:547–554

Raghavan D (1990) Chemotherapy for advanced bladder cancer: "Midsummer Night's Dream" or "Much ado abouth Nothing"? Br J Cancer 62:337–340

Raghavan D (1991) Keynote address. A critical assessment of trials of neoadjuvant (pre-emptive) chemotherapy for bladder cancer: lesson for future studies of combined modality treatment. Int J Radiat Oncol Biol Phys 20:233–237

Richards B, Bastable JRG, Freedman L et al. (1983) Adjuvant chemotherapy with doxorubicin (adriamycin) and 5-fluorouracil in T3, Nx, M0 bladder cancer treated with radiotherapy. Br J Urol 55:386–391

Rifkin MN, Wajsman Z (1991) Incidence and pattern of local recurrence in patients with invasive bladder cancer treated with a bladder sparing approach. J Urol 145:336A (abstract)

Rintala E, Hannisdal E, Sander S (1991) Radiotherapy versus radiotherapy and chemotherapy as precystectomy treatment in bladder cancer. Scand J Urol Nephrol Suppl 135:50 (abstract)

Roberts JT, Fossa SD, Richards B et al. (1991) Results of a Medical Research Council phase II study of low dose cisplatin and methotrexate in the primary treatment of locally advanced (T3 and T4) transitional cell carcinoma of the bladder. Br J Urol 68:162–168

Scher HI, Yagoda A, Herr HW et al. (1988) Neoadjuvant MVAC (methotrexate, vinblastine, doxorubicin and cisplatin) effect on the primary bladder lesion. J Urol 139:470–474

Scher H, Herr H, Sternberg C et al. (1989) Neoadjuvant chemotherapy for invasive bladder cancer. Experience with the MVAC regime. Br J Urol 64:250–256

Seidman A, Scher HI (1991) The evolving role of chemotherapy for muscle-infiltrating bladder cancer. Semin Oncol 6:585–595

Sella A, Logothetis CJ, Dexeus FH et al. (1991) Cisplatin combination chemotherapy for elderly patients with urothelial tumours. Br J Urol 67:603–607

Shearer RJ, Chilvers CED, Bloom HJG et al. (1988) Adjuvant chemotherapy in carcinoma of the bladder. A prospective trial preliminary report. Br J Urol 62:558–564

Shipley WU (1988) Review of factors predicting improved tumour control and survival from invasive bladder carcinoma following external beam radiation therapy. Prog Clin Biol Res 260:437–446

Shipley WU, Coombs LJ, Einstein AB et al. (1984) Cisplatin and full dose irradiation for patients with invasive bladder carcinoma: a preliminary report of tolerance and local response. J Urol 132:899–903

Skinner DG, Daniels JR, Russell CA et al. (1991) The role of adjuvant chemotherapy following cystectomy for invasive bladder cancer: a prospective comparative trial. J Urol 145:459–467

Soquet Y (1981) Combined surgery and adjuvant chemotherapy with high dose methotrexate and folinic acid rescue (HDMTX-CF) for infiltrating tumours of the bladder. Br J Urol 53:439–443

Splinter TAW, Denis L, Scher HI et al. (1989) Neoadjuvant chemotherapy of invasive bladder cancer: the prognostic value of local tumour response. Therapeutic progress in urological cancers. Liss, New York, pp 541–547

Splinter TAW, Scher HI, Denis L et al. (1992) The prognostic value of the response to combination chemotherapy before cystectomy in patients with invasive bladder cancer. J Urol 147:606–608

Sternberg CN, Yagoda A, Scher HI et al. (1985) Preliminary results of MVAC (methotrexate, vinblastine, doxorubicin and cisplatin) for transitional carcinoma of the urothelium. J Urol 133:405–407

Sternberg CN, Yagoda A, Scher HI et al. (1988) MVAC (methotrexate, vinblastine, doxorubicin and cisplatin) for advanced transitional cell carcinoma of the urothelium. J Urol 139:461–469

Sternberg CN, Yagoda A, Scher HI et al. (1989) MVAC for advanced transitional cell carcinoma of the urothelium: efficacy and patterns of response and relapse. Cancer 64:2448–2458

Sternberg C, Pansadoro V, Cancrini A et al. (1992) Neo-adjuvant MVAC (methotrexate, vinblastine, doxorubicin and cisplatin) for infiltrating transitional cell carcinoma of the bladder. Eur Urol EVA Suppl. 113 (abstract)

Stockle M, Meyenburg W, Wellek S et al. (1992) Advanced bladder cancer (stages pT3b, pT4a, pN1 and pN2): improved survival after radical cystectomy and three adjuvant cycles of chemotherapy. Results of a controlled prospective study. J Urol 148:302–307

Stoter G, Splinter TAW, Child JA et al. (1987) Combination chemotherapy with cisplatin and methotrexate in advanced transitional cell cancer of the bladder. J Urol 137:663–667

Studer VE, Hering F, Jaeger P et al. (1991) Adjuvant cisplatin chemotherapy following cystectomy for bladder cancer (SAKK 09/84). J Urol 145:335A (abstract)

Wallace DMA, Raghavan D, Kelly KA et al. (1991) Neo-adjuvant (pre-emptive) cisplatin therapy in invasive transitional cell carcinoma of the bladder. Br J Urol 67:608–615

Waxman J (1990) Chemotherapy for metastatic bladder. Is there new hope? Br J Urol 65:1–6

Waxman J, Barton C, Biruls R et al. (1992) Bladder cancer: inter-relationships between chemotherapy and radiotherapy. Br J Urol 69:151–155

Wohlgenannt M, Eberle J, Bartsch G (1991) Combined radio-chemotherapy for invasive bladder cancer – long term results. J Urol 145:335A (abstract)

Yagoda A (1987) Chemotherapy of urothelial tract tumours. Cancer 60:574–585

Chapter 6

Cystectomy and Bladder Reconstruction for Bladder Cancer

O. Seemann and P. Alken

Indications and Selection Criteria for Radical Cystectomy

The control of muscle invasive carcinoma of the urinary bladder remains a challenge for the urological oncologist and the best management is still controversial. The treatment options include radical cystectomy, full-thickness transurethral resection (TUR), radiotherapy and chemotherapy – either alone or in combination with other treatments. Radical cystectomy has become accepted as the "gold-standard" against which other treatments are compared – even though survival rates after cystectomy in any one series can be difficult to compare with others owing to differences in patient selection and recent improvement in anaesthetic techniques.

In the past, radical cystectomy carried high rates of postoperative death, complications and side effects such as impotence. Various methods of urinary diversion were carried out including ureterosigmoidostomy, but in the 1950s the ileal conduit became the standard method of urinary diversion. Because of the high rate of complications and the inevitable presence of an incontinent abdominal stoma, many urologists preferred to control bladder cancer by repeated TUR; only patients with advanced disease were subjected to radical cystectomy. In historical studies, approximately 50% of patients surviving cystectomy eventually died of their disease (Leadbetter and Cooper 1950) with widespread dissemination of the tumour. It became clear that radical pelvic surgery could be successful in controlling the primary tumour, but many patients subsequently died of metastatic disease – presumably because of micrometastases present at the time of cystectomy (Prout et al. 1979). One question was whether a more ready application of radical cystectomy at the time of presentation would have improved the final outcome: particularly in patients with T1 or T2 disease who were often treated by means of TUR.

During the last couple of decades, the operative mortality of radical cystoprostatectomy has decreased as a result of progress in anaesthesia, monitoring, intensive care and fluid replacement. The overall operative mortality now ranges from 0.4% (Montie and Wood 1989) to 3% (Malkowicz et al. 1990). Even selected elderly patients can undergo cystectomy without undue morbidity and mortality (Skinner et al. 1984; Wood et al. 1987). In addition, recent improvements in surgical technique have reduced postoperative morbidity. As a consequence of continent urinary diversion or bladder replacement, radical cystectomy need no longer be regarded as a mutilating procedure. Nerve-sparing cystectomy can preserve erectile potency in up to 64% of men without compromising cancer control (Brendler et al. 1990b). Radical cystectomy is now more willingly accepted by patients as a curative treatment for invasive bladder cancer. Many urologists in Europe are now abandoning endoscopic treatment in favour of cystectomy in patients judged at high risk of progression; many patients undergo early radical surgery for lower stages of disease (T1/T2).

The results of one study (Stöckle et al. 1987) clearly indicate that cystectomy in patients with recurrence of invasive bladder carcinoma after previous TUR carries a lower 5-year survival rate (30%) than radical surgery performed immediately after the diagnosis of invasive tumour (60%). Moreover, only 10% of patients undergoing cystectomy after unsuccessful irradiation therapy survive 5 years (Lindell 1987; Stöckle et al. 1987). Analysis of survival after cystectomy or other treatments is difficult because the series are rarely contemporaneous, selection criteria have changed and some studies were retrospective whereas others were prospective. Another source of statistical distortion is clinical and pathological stage migration. The reporting of results comparing cystectomy and other treatments differs because accurate staging is only possible after cystectomy. A careful lymphadenectomy, as suggested by Skinner (1982), uncovers a higher number of lymph nodes, thus increasing the accuracy of pathological staging. As a consequence, today, nodal involvement

Table 6.1. Five-year survival rates after radical cystectomy alone or in combination with radiotherapy or chemotherapy

Reference; Year	No. of patients/5-year survival (%)					
	Ta/cis	T1	T2	T3a	T3b	T4/N+
Brendler et al. (1990b); 1982–1988		←———47———→ 73%		←——29——→ 52%		
Pagano et al. (1991); 1979–1987		54 75%	58 63%	←——73——→ 50%	15%	19 21%
Montie et al. (1984); 1960–1979	←——34 R[a] → 88%			←———— 32 R[a] ———→ 40%		
Skinner and Lieskovsky (1984); 1971–1982		67 75%	←———108———→ 54%			59 36%
Mameghan and Fisher (1989); 1977–1982		9 R[a] 55%	22 R[a] 33%	←——132 R[a]→ 20%		28 R[a] 5%

[a]R = Radiotherapy.

is often diagnosed in patients who would have been staged free from nodal disease 20 years ago. This particular group of patients "migrates" from the N− group to the N+ group apparently improving the statistical outcome of the N− group without any change in overall outcome (Wishnow and Tenney 1991).

The distortion of stage migration in comparative past and contemporary series could be one factor which explains the apparent improved survival of patients treated by preoperative radiotherapy. It is now felt that better patient selection, improved clinical and pathological staging, as well as advanced surgery and perioperative management are probably the reasons for improved survival rates rather than radiotherapy (Skinner and Lieskovsky 1984). Table 6.1 shows survival rates after radical cystectomy alone or in combination with chemotherapy or radiotherapy. The 5-year survival of patients with advanced stage tumours or positive lymph nodes is still poor regardless of treatment. This suggests that many patients in this group are subjected to inappropriate radical treatment. On the other hand, 70%–100% of patients with T1 tumours or carcinoma in situ (cis) survive 5 years or more. Moreover, bladder reconstruction has meant that more patients with lower stage disease are being offered earlier radical treatment. This raises the critical question of how to select patients for radical surgery and how to select those who can be successfully managed with bladder-sparing treatment.

Superficial Bladder Carcinoma (Ta, T1, cis)

Between 70% and 80% of patients with newly diagnosed bladder carcinoma initially present with superficial tumours (Ta, T1, cis). Despite the use of all available intensive treatment methods consisting of repeated TUR and intravesical chemotherapy, up to 20% develop progression or metastatic disease (Droller and Walsh 1985; Raghavan et al. 1990). Several prognostic factors are available for the identification of patients at high risk of progression.

Tumour Stage and Grade

Superficial transitional cell carcinoma is often defined as those tumours without muscle invasion (Ta/T1). Many of these tumours are well-differentiated or moderately well-differentiated. The 5-year survival rate of grade 1 or grade 2 Ta/T1 tumours is 94% (Jakse et al. 1987). The incidence of poorly differentiated grade 3 superficial bladder carcinoma ranges from 6% to 23%. These tumours have a considerable risk of progression (29% to 50%) when treated by TUR alone, 21% of patients dying within 5 years (Birch and Harland 1989; see chapter 1). Of T1 G3 tumours 66% have associated cis compared with 19% of the remaining superficial bladder carcinomas (Algabe 1987). This pattern indicates the highly aggressive nature of this tumour. Vincente et al. (1991) found a recurrence and progression rate in more than 80% and 60% respectively of T1 G3 tumours. It is now generally accepted that these tumours are a different entity from low-grade Ta superficial transitional cell carcinoma which carries an excellent prognosis. It has been suggested that cis, high-grade superficial tumours, as well as muscle-invasive bladder carcinoma are a distinct type of disease (Algabe 1987) requiring more aggressive treatment.

Recently, Malkovicz et al. (1990) demonstrated that radical cystectomy is highly effective in high-grade superficial bladder carcinoma, resulting in a 5-year survival of 80%, 78% and 85% in patients with P1, P1 with Pis and Pis only lesions respectively. All patients down-staged by their previous treatments to P0/A survived 5 years. The dilemma in patient selection is that some patients of this group probably could have been cured by means of TUR and intravesical treatment alone as shown by Herr (1987). Unfortunately, there are no reliable prognostic factors available to identify these patients accurately.

Some patients respond to full-thickness or deep TUR followed by intra-vesical Bacillus Calmette-Guérin (BCG) treatment (Herr 1991). Regardless of the initial tumour stage, 8.7% of the patients had T1 tumours 3 months after BCG treatment; this was a high risk group with an 82% risk of progression. Of patients who progressed to muscle invasion 43% finally died of the disease despite cystectomy and/or systemic chemotherapy. This group accounted for six out of 195 patients who probably would have benefited most from prompt cystectomy.

Tumour Localization and Size

The growth pattern of bladder carcinoma gives some additional information when selecting patients for radical surgery. An increased risk of metastasis or relapse can be expected in cases with cis, multifocal or solid tumour growth. Other adverse prognostic factors are tumour infiltration of the bladder neck, prostatic urethra or ureteral orifice with subsequent hydronephrosis. Random biopsies of apparently normal mucosa at the time of the first resection may detect cis. In cases with known cis, it is necessary to exclude involvement of the bladder neck, the ureteric orifices and the prostate. If invasion of the prostatic ducts or the stroma is documented, simultaneous urethrectomy is recommended to lower the high risk of urethral recurrences in these cases (Hardeman and Soloway 1990).

Other Prognostic Factors

A variety of biochemical and cytological analyses have been suggested as potential tumour markers and prognostic parameters by Schneider and Huland (1990). Ploidy, the expression of oncogenes, blood group antigens or other cell surface characteristics may provide additional screening and monitoring information. However, as yet there is no marker which is sensitive or specific enough to determine a need for cystectomy.

Muscle-Invasive Tumours and Nodal Disease

Stage T2 and T3a

In muscle-infiltrating bladder cancer of stage T2 to T3 without distant metastasis, radical cystectomy is the preferred treatment. However, half of the patients still die of metastatic disease. Involvement of lymph nodes indicates a poor prognosis. The 5-year survival of patients with tumours of stage T3a is more than 50% when lymph nodes are negative, whereas nearly all patients with T3a disease and lymph node involvement die within 5 years (Pagano et al. 1991). Treatment failure in these patients is mainly related to micrometastases which may benefit from adjuvant chemotherapy, although clinical data are still non-conclusive.

Stage T3b and T4

Advanced bladder carcinoma with invasion of the perivesical tissue, affected lymph nodes or distant metastases has an extremely poor prognosis. The indication for radical surgery as an attempt at curative treatment is debatable, for 5-year survival rates ranges from 0% to 40% (Skinner 1982; Pagano et al. 1991).

Most reports suggest that the survival of patients with nodal metastases is around 5%–10%. Studies by Skinner (1982) suggest that a meticulous pelvic lymph node dissection can improve survival in cases with metastatic spread to only a few pelvic nodes. In his series of 36 patients with nodal involvement, 14 survived 3 years or more. This denotes the possible value of lymphadenectomy in the surgical management of bladder cancer.

Although most patients die from widespread metastatic disease rather than from local recurrence, a substantial number of patients suffer considerably from severe symptoms if the primary lesion is left in place. Haematuria, hydronephrosis, bladder infection, pain or incontinence can cause significant morbidity in these patients and occasionally cystectomy may be indicated in such patients for palliation.

Operative Procedure of Cystectomy

Preoperative Care

Prior to surgery, the cardiovascular, pulmonary and nutritional status must be assessed and appropriate corrective treatment given. Patients should be familiarized with the concept of urinary diversion and stoma appliances, even if a continent diversion or bladder substitution is planned. An optimum stomal site should be determined since intraoperative circumstances may indicate the need for ileal conduit formation. Warning should also be give about erectile impotence in men and difficulty with vaginal intercourse in women after operation. Bowel preparation commences two days before surgery with a low-residue diet and patients are instructed to drink a solution of polyethylene glycol, sodium sulphate, sodium bicarbonate, sodium chloride and potassium chloride (Go-Lytely or Klean-prep) the day before surgery. Prophylactic antibiotics including metronidazole are given before induction.

Surgical Procedure

All patients being operated with curative intention should first undergo meticulous pelvic lymphadenectomy from the aortic bifurcation to the external inguinal ring. Radical cystectomy for bladder cancer in males includes removal of the bladder, the prostate and seminal vesicles with ample margins and the overlying peritoneum. Erectile impotence after cystectomy is caused by injury to the branches of the pelvic plexus that innervate the corpora cavernosa. Schlegel and Walsh (1987) demonstrated the precise relationship of the neurovascular bundle to the bladder and the seminal vesicle. The operative technique of nerve-sparing radical cystectomy was recently described by Schlegel and Walsh (1987) and Burgers and Brendler (1991) in detail. Since the major aim of the operation is complete removal of the tumour, wide excision of the neurovascular bundle is recommended if infiltration is suspected. However, Schlegel and Walsh (1987) showed that preservation of only one neurovascular bundle is sufficient to preserve potency in most patients. In a series of 25 patients undergoing cystectomy 83% remained potent.

If preoperative assessment suggests an increased risk of urethral recurrence, then urethrectomy should be performed. A modified approach (Brendler et al. 1990a) may preserve erectile potency in 50% of men undergoing urethrectomy, but clinical experience with this technique is still limited. Urinary tract reconstruction follows removal of the specimen. In female patients, radical cystectomy is performed as an anterior exenteration including the excision of bladder, urethra and a segment of the anterior vaginal wall, uterus, fallopian tubes and ovary which are removed *en bloc* with the surrounding fatty tissue. It is not possible to preserve the sphincteric mechanism in women making bladder replacement impossible.

Urinary Diversion and Bladder Replacement

In 1911, Coffey described one of the very first urinary diversion techniques – the ureterosigmoidostomy. Initially, this was considered to be a good technique because some degree of urinary continence was achieved. However, incorrect patient selection for this procedure led to severe complications; progressive deterioration of renal function was also observed in some patients, the most common type being hyperchloraemic acidosis. Urine in contact with the colon can lead to acid–base and electrolyte imbalance – mainly in patients with impaired renal function. In addition, there was an increased incidence of subsequent malignancy in the bowel. Hence, in the 1950s many surgeons abandoned this technique in favour of the ileal conduit (Bricker 1950).

The ileal conduit is a non-continent diversion necessitating an external appliance and on evaluation of initial long-term results, deterioration of renal function was found in at least 20% of patients (Neal, 1985; Svare et al. 1985). During the last 15 years, this has prompted an intensive search for new techniques of continent diversion or bladder reconstruction to achieve maximum social acceptance and minimum risk.

Today, even though the ileal conduit is still regarded as the gold standard by some urologists, new techniques offer marked advantages. First, the use of a urinary reservoir and continent stoma on the abdominal wall which is emptied by periodical self-catheterisation means that the patient can dispense with an external appliance. Second, urologists are now able to construct a neobladder which is attached to the urethra and permits voiding *per urethram*.

Criteria for Patient Selection

Preoperatively, the pros and cons of each method should be discussed with each patient to determine the best solution for that individual. Prior to surgery, a stoma therapist should counsel the patient regarding the site and management of an ileal conduit with an external appliance even if a continent technique is planned. In addition, the patient may wish to meet others who have had similar procedures carried out in order to reduce anxiety. Age, motivation and the potential compliance of the patient with intermittent catheterisation must be taken into consideration for selection of the most appropriate technique. Given that self-catheterisation requires a certain amount of manual skill and cooperation, a non-continent ileal conduit is advisable in some cases.

Understandably, many patients prefer the construction of an orthotopic neobladder allowing natural micturition. However, an important principle is that cancer cure should not be compromised; the risk of urethral or pelvic recurrence must be carefully assessed. Contraindications to reconstruction of the lower urinary tract remain controversial. Reddy et al. (1991) excluded patients with a history of significant cis, multifocal tumour growth or involvement of the prostatic urethra from bladder replacement. Skinner et al. (1991) did not consider cis, nodal disease or even involvement of the perivesical fat as a contraindication for Kock urethrostomy and only excluded patients with direct invasion of the prostate or those with positive urethral biopsies. Pagano et al. (1991) recently suggested that involved pelvic lymph nodes were a contraindication, whereas Wenderoth et al. (1990) subjected patients with bladder carcinoma stage T4 N2 to radical cystectomy and bladder replacement by the "Ulm bladder". Nevertheless, bladder replacement in patients with locally advanced tumours or nodal disease involves a major risk of pelvic recurrence with subsequent infiltration of the neobladder. The survival of such patients is poor and there is a risk of incontinence so that many of this group of patients would benefit more from a continent diversion than from an orthotopic bladder reconstruction.

The greatest risk of urethral recurrence is encountered in cases of prostatic stroma or duct involvement. Thus, preoperative deep resection biopsies of the prostate are recommended and patients with positive findings should undergo simultaneous urethrectomy and urinary diversion rather than bladder reconstruction.

Previous or concomitant gastrointestinal diseases may determine the type of bladder replacement or choice of intestinal segment to be utilized. The ileocaecal segment may be difficult to use in the case of previous tuberculosis of the ileocaecal region. Utilisation of the ileocaecal segment or ileum is not recommended for patients with malabsorption. In some cases a contrast enema should be performed to rule out diverticulosis or cancer of the colon as this would exclude utilisation of the sigmoid colon; this also reveals whether the length of the sigmoid is sufficient for reconstruction. In patients who have undergone preoperative high-dose irradiation of the pelvis, transverse colon or even stomach may be suitable for bladder replacement or continent diversion. Many types of continent urinary diversion and bladder reconstruction have been reported suggesting that an optimal method has not yet been determined. The following points outline common essential principles for all forms of urinary diversion and bladder replacement: a continence mechanism, prevention of ureterorenal reflux and a compliant reservoir.

Continence Mechanism

Nipple Valve

Intussusception of the bowel to create a continent nipple valve was described by Kock (1969) for the formation of a continent ileostomy. Later, numerous investigators successfully employed this technique for a continent urinary diversion. Initially, complications such as nipple necrosis, urinary leakage or nipple sliding with consecutive incompetence of the valve were common and the rate of reoperation for nipple revision was 50% or more. In the following years, the technique was repeatedly modified and the revision rate declined to about 10% in some hands (Skinner et al. 1987). A critical point concerning the competence of the valve is the length of the intussuscepted segment which should be at least 3 cm long. Stripping of the mesentery at the site where the bowel is intussuscepted is important and fixation of the valve with three rows of staples and polyglycolic acid mesh to the base of the nipple prevents sliding of the nipple valve. Late complications were reported in only 3% of patients in a recent series by Skinner et al. (1991). However, the nipple technique is still a time-consuming and technically demanding operation.

Tapered Efferent Loop

Plication of the efferent loop in techniques utilising the ileocaecal region as a reservoir has been described by several investigators as a reliable and safe continence mechanism (Lockhart 1987; Rowland et al. 1987; Bejany and Politano 1988). The advantage of this method is that it is easier to construct than the invaginated nipple valve. Short-term follow-up reveals similar urinary continence results, but long-term results are not yet available and difficulties with catheterisation occur. Atta (1991) described a simple technique of tapering the outlet by the formation of a double-jacket intestinal tube that can be applied to either sigmoid colon or ileum providing urinary continence with easy catheterisation. Long-term follow-up results are not yet available.

The Mitrofanoff Principle

Mitrofanoff (1980) originally used the isolated appendix to create a continent vesicocutaneostomy in patients with neurogenic bladder dysfunction or those with a severely damaged urethra. The basic objective is the use of a narrow, catheterisable outlet which is implanted into the reservoir by means of an antireflux technique. This principle was successfully utilised for construction of an effective continence mechanism for continent diversion. Barker (1991) used the detubularised ileocaecal segment for construction of the reservoir. The appendix was divided, mobilised at the mesentery and the tip re-implanted into the caecum so that a portion of 3 cm was in a mucosal gutter and the base of the appendix was brought to the skin. Continence rates have been most satisfactory, but catheterisation difficulties are a general problem. A different appendix stoma procedure was described by Riedmiller et al. (1990). In a modification of the Mainz pouch, the appendix was not divided but submucosally embedded into a 3–4 cm longitudinal incision of the caecal taenia. The tip of the appendix was placed to the lower right abdominal wall or alternatively, an umbilical stoma was designed. Continence was reported in 100% of patients, although one of 13 patients required re-operation for stomal stenosis. Another procedure was reported by Bihrle et al. (1991), who created the efferent limb from a tubularised gastric strip that was implanted into the reservoir in a tunnelled, antireflux technique.

A potential hazard of all techniques of continent diversion is urinary leakage when the pouch is full. Sustained high pressures can lead to perforation. Patients must be encouraged to empty the reservoir at intervals not exceeding 6 h.

Prevention of Ureterorenal Reflux

Deterioration of renal function due to high pressure reflux or ureteral obstruction is a complication which may be encountered subsequent to urinary diversion. For this reason, careful ureteral implantation is a crucial point.

The formation of a submucosal tunnel for reflux prevention is an effective method when the ureters are implanted into large bowel segments. In the procedure described by Thüroff et al. (1988), the ureters are pulled through a 5 cm submucosal tunnel, starting at the open end of the large bowel. This is associated with a low incidence of upper tract dilation and a 98% success rate of reflux prevention. Another technique of tunnelled implantation was used by Rowland et al. (1987) and Reddy et al. (1991). The ureteroenteric anastomosis was made into the lateral taenia from the outside of the bowel in accordance with a technique originally described by Leadbetter and Cooper (1950). A non-tunnelled ureterocolonic anastomosis was described by Bejany and Politano (1988), who implanted the ureters into a mucosal sulcus with a success rate of 95%. However, in a small series, Lockhart et al. (1990) showed that a direct, freely refluxing mucosa to mucosa technique is not necessarily associated with renal deterioration provided the

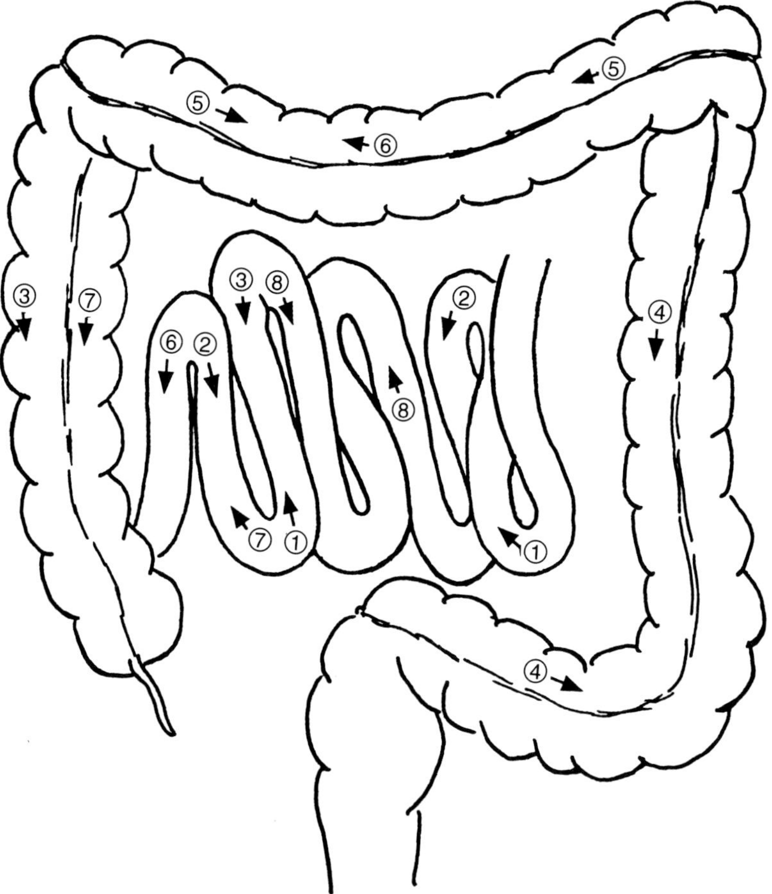

Fig. 6.1. Intestinal segments used for different techniques of urinary diversion and bladder replacement.

pouch is detubularised creating a low-pressure reservoir. Reflux only occurred in 7%, suggesting that low intrapouch pressure is an important factor in reflux prevention.

The submucosal tunnel technique is not practical in the small intestine since the mucosal layer is too thin. Kock et al. (1985) described the formation of an afferent intussuscepted nipple valve for reflux protection. The ureters were anastomosed to the proximal end of the invaginated segment. This procedure proved to be highly effective in an extensive series as reported by Skinner et al. (1989, 1991). However, this method is complicated and an additional 10 cm of ileum is required for the construction of the valve alone. An easier approach was described by Le Duc and Camey (1979). The ileal mucosa is incised over a length of 3 cm and the submucosal layer is exposed. At one end of the sulcus, the ureter is brought to the luminal side through a transmural incision and placed into the sulcus between the mucosal edges where it is fixed by interrupted absorbable sutures. This technique was also used by Wenderoth et al. (1990) in the "Ulm Bladder". In a series of 100 consecutive cases the reflux rate was less than 5%, and obstruction was reported in 8%. A modified tunnel technique similar to the Leadbetter procedure was reported by Hirdes et al. (1988). In this technique the ileal serosa and muscularis is incised creating a supple section of the intestinal wall. The ureters are anastomosed to an opening in the mucosa and buried by closing the intestinal walls over the ureters on both sides. However, reflux was reported in 19% and stenosis in 6%. It has been reported by Studer et al. (1991) that the deleterious effect of reflux can be eliminated by implantation of the ureters into an afferent, tubular, isoperistaltic ileal segment of 20 cm

Technique	Ileal segments (cm)	Colonic segments (cm)
1 Kock pouch (Kock et al. 1985)	70–80	
2 "Ulm bladder" (Hautmann et al. 1988)	70	
3 MAINZ pouch (Thüroff et al. 1988)	40–55	10–15
4 Sigmoid bladder (Reddy et al. 1991)		30–35
5 Transverse colon–gastric tube pouch[a] (Bihrle et al. 1991)		25–30
6 Florida pouch (Lockhart 1987)	15	30–40
7 Indiana pouch (Rowland et al. 1987)	30–35	20
8 Camey ileal bladder (Camey 1985)	40	

[a]Additional gastric strip from the greater curvature

length, although previous studies of ileal conduit suggest that this may not be successful (Neal 1989).

Features of the Reservoir

Almost all intestinal segments from stomach to rectum have been used for reservoir formation (Fig. 6.1). Clinical and theoretical evidence suggest that the tubular shape of the bowel is disadvantageous (Hinman 1988). Geometric considerations demonstrate that re-configuration of a given length of bowel to a spherical pouch produces the highest volume per unit length. In accordance with the Laplace relationship, the mural tension of a reservoir at constant pressure increases with the radius. Pouches with a larger radius will therefore be subjected to greater wall tension than tubular reservoirs with a smaller diameter but since the bowel wall is viscoelastic, they will accommodate more volume. Peristaltic movement of the bowel is mediated by the action of the myenteric plexus which lies between the longitudinal and the circular smooth muscle layers. The contraction of longitudinal muscle layers triggers a circular muscle contraction increasing intraluminal pressure. Detubularisation of intestinal segments does not prevent peristaltic contraction, but when the detubularised bowel is folded in a complex manner the contractile activity becomes discontinuous and disorganised. This prevents increases in intratubular pressure resulting from synchronised contraction. Indeed several investigators have pointed out that even short segments of non-detubularised bowel segments proximal to the urethral sphincter may cause incontinence in patients with a neobladder anastomosed to the urethra (Skinner et al. 1989; Thüroff et al. 1988).

It has been demonstrated that, regardless of the bowel segment used for reservoir formation, results are satisfactory as long as the bowel was detubularised and a spherical-shaped reservoir is accomplished. Thus, most surgeons have abandoned techniques using non-detubularised bowel for construction of urinary reservoirs. The anatomical and clinical condition of the patient is the deciding factor for selection of the most appropriate segment for urinary diversion. Five established techniques are described below.

Kock Pouch

Kock (1969) described a continent ileal pouch for patients undergoing proctocolectomy. The concept was soon applied to the urinary tract and finally developed into a standardised and well-documented technique for continent urinary diversion.

The technical details of the procedure were described by Skinner et al. (1987). Briefly, an 80 cm segment of ileum is isolated on its mesentery. The 44 cm middle portion is folded to a U-shape and detubularised for construction of the reservoir. The intact proximal and distal ends are then intussuscepted into the reservoir for creation of nipple valves: the afferent one prevents ileo-ureteral reflux and the efferent valve ensures stomal continence. However, nipple construction is technically demanding and possible complications include necrosis, leakage, nipple sliding or malfunction as well as stone formation. Modifications have greatly reduced complications, but reoperation is still necessary in 10%–15% of patients, even in the best hands (Skinner et al. 1987). Since 1986, Skinner et al. (1991) performed bladder replacement using a modified Kock reservoir. The pouch was constructed without an efferent nipple and directly anastomosed to the urethral stump. Day and night continence was achieved in 94% and 85% respectively.

"Ulm Bladder"

A different technique of lower urinary tract reconstruction by means of an ileal reservoir was described by Hautmann et al. (1988). A 70 cm ileal segment is mobilised 15 cm proximal to the ileocaecal valve and completely detubularised. The ileal plate is W- or M-shaped and a spherical reservoir is formed. The ureters are implanted by a non-refluxing technique as described by Le-Duc and Camey (1979) and the reservoir anastomosed to the urethra using a buttonhole in the bowel. A review of the first 100 cases (Wenderoth et al. 1990) showed no perioperative mortality, reoperation was necessary in 13 patients and day and night-time continence was achieved in 82%. However, continence was strongly dependent on patient age – 50% of patients over the age of 70 were incontinent at night.

MAINZ Pouch

Various methods have been described using the ileocaecal segment for construction of a continent urinary reservoir. The basic idea was to use the caecum as a reservoir and the terminal ileum as an efferent outlet. The continence mechanism was provided by the natural ileocaecal valve. This technique did not become common practice because continence rates were poor. When detubularisation was defined as an important principle in bladder replacement it became possible to achieve a low pressure reservoir and interest in this technique increased.

Current techniques vary with respect to the extent of colonic or ileal segment to be utilised. Thüroff et al. (1988) described a surgical procedure for construction of a urinary reservoir using 15 cm of detubularised caecum and ascending colon together with two, longitudinally split ileal loops of the same length. The pouch is fashioned by arranging the detubularised bowel in the shape of an N, a bowel plate is created by caecoileal and ileoileal side-to-side anastomosis. The ileocaecal valve is spared if a continent stoma is to be achieved. The efferent valve utilises an additional 15 cm segment of intact ileum which is left attached to create an intussuscepted nipple valve. For further stabilisation, the nipple is pulled through the ileocaecal valve and stabilised by two rows of staples. A ureterocaecal anastomosis is accomplished by a submucosal tunnel technique, the reservoir is closed and an umbilical stoma then fashioned. For bladder reconstruction, no efferent nipple is created; instead, a buttonhole incision is made into the caecal pole of the reservoir which is anastomosed to the membranous urethra. This procedure provides a low-pressure reservoir with a mean capacity of more than 600 ml and incontinence rates are 4%–7% (Thüroff et al. 1988). Alternatively, the appendix may be utilised according to the Mitrofanoff principle and anastomosed to the umbilicus (Riedmiller et al. 1990).

Sigmoid Neobladder

In the selection of bowel segments for construction of a neobladder, the sigmoid colon has significant advantages over small bowel or ileocaecal segments. The sigmoid colon is located in the pelvis so correct position of the reservoir is easily accomplished. The ileocaecal valve and the terminal ileum are not excluded from the gut and non-refluxing ureteral anastomoses are easily achieved.

A 35 cm sigmoid segment is isolated on its mesenteric pedicle. The segment is folded to a U-shape and the ureters are anastomosed into the lateral taenia in accordance with the non-refluxing technique of Leadbetter and Cooper (1950). Detubularisation is accomplished along the medial taenia and a spherical reservoir is fashioned. A small incision is made at the lowest point of the reservoir which is then anastomosed to the urethral stump. The average capacity is 600 ml and 67% of patients were continent during the day and night (Reddy et al. 1991).

Transverse Colon Pouch

Most patients undergoing salvage cystectomy after definitive radiotherapy or females previously subjected to pelvic irradiation for a gynaecological tumour undergo diversion by means of a transverse colonic conduit, since most urologists object to utilisation of potentially irradiated ileum, caecum or sigmoid colon. The transverse colon–gastric tube reservoir, as previously described by Bihrle et al. (1991), is an interesting alternative. The continent stoma is constructed from unaffected intestinal segments such as a gastric tube and the reservoir is formed from a 25–30 cm long segment of detubularised, U-shaped transverse colon. The efferent limb is constructed from a tubularised, gastric strip taken from the greater curvature. The gastric tube is implanted into the reservoir in a non-refluxing, tunnelled technique as described by Leadbetter and Cooper (1950). Adequate capacity and continence is attained by this technique, but a significant complication is skin erosion at the stomal site caused by secretion of gastric fluid from the efferent limb.

Functional Results and Urinary Continence

In general, continence after continent urinary diversion is satisfactory. Most series show an incontinence rate of less than 10%. Voiding intervals average 5 h (Table 6.2). Nipple sliding or devagination is a common cause of late leakage, but the functional length of the valve is a significant factor. Tapered

Table 6.2. Continence after continent diversion; comparison of different techniques

Reference/ Pouch	No. of Patients	Pouch volume (ml)	Daytime continence (No. Pts (%))	Night-time continence (No. Pts (%))	Continence over all (No. Pts (%))	Voiding intervals (h)	Voiding/ day	Voiding/ night
Kock et al. (1985) Kock pouch	29	700	29 (100)	29 (100)			4–5	0
Schreiter and Noll (1989) Kock pouch	46	550	41 (89)		39 (85)			
Chen et al. (1989) Kock pouch	20	320			18 (90)	2–6		
Ahlering et al. (1989) Kock pouch	12		12 (100)	12 (100)		6–8	3	1
Thüroff et al. (1988) MAINZ pouch	51	622			49 (96)			
Lockhart et al. (1990) Florida pouch	65	747			63 (97)	4–6		
Rowland et al. (1987) Indiana pouch	29	508	27 (93)	22 (76)		4		0–1
Ahlering (1989) Indiana pouch	25		25 (100)	25 (100)		5–7	3	1
Bihrle et al. (1991) Transverse colon gastric tube reservoir	4	400	3 (75)	3 (75)		4		

ileum intended for continent stoma should be approximately 10 cm long to achieve correct functioning (Bejany and Politano 1988; Lockhart et al. 1990). Chen et al. (1989) suggested that a functional nipple length of at least 3 cm is required for adequate continence of the Kock pouch urinary diversion.

The definition of continence after bladder replacement or reconstruction diverges greatly in the literature (Table 6.3). The length of time between emptying of the reservoir to ensure dryness is one critical point. Camey (1985) defined continence as an interval of more than 2 h. A more stringent definition was given by Reddy et al. (1991), who defined patients as enuretic when the reservoir was emptied more than twice per night to ensure dryness. Another criterion often included in evaluation is patient satisfaction. This value is mainly subjective and chiefly depends on the attitude taken by each individual patient, making data comparison difficult.

An adequate reservoir capacity is a precondition for convenient voiding intervals. The average reservoir capacity is 570 ml (range 320–747ml) and 480 ml (range 300–755 ml) for continent diversion and neobladder respectively (Tables 6.2 and 6.4). In the bladder replacement group, Wenderoth et al. (1990) reported a 50% rate of incontinence in men aged over 70 years compared with 11% in younger patients. Night-time incontinence is a particular problem after bladder replacement (Table 6.4). Continence in some men may only be achieved by two to three voids per night. As normal bladder filling sensation is not experienced after bladder replacement with intestinal segments, patients suffer from overflow incontinence at night. However, two other mechanisms have been proposed. Jakobsen et al. (1987) indicated that the tone of the external sphincter decreases during sleep as a result of lowered general tone of the striated muscles. Contractions of the neobladder are not, of course, accompanied by protective reflex contraction of the distal sphincter mechanism. In addition, the circadian rhythm of antidiuretic hormone (maximum excretion at midnight to 4 am) results in maximum concentration of urine at night. In patients with an intestinal reservoir, the high osmotic gradient generated by the concentrated urine leads to a fluid shift into the reservoir with subsequent increases in urine volumes at night (Koch et al. 1991).

Patients with incontinence can be treated with oral or topical anticholinergics to prevent extensive bowel contractions (Table 6.5). However, a controlled study evaluating the effect of these drugs is not yet available.

Table 6.3. Definition of continence

Reference	Definition
Allen et al. (1985) Wenderoth et al. (1990)	Day and night: no need of pads
Camey (1985)	Day: voiding no more frequent than every 2 h
Chen et al. (1989)	No wet stomal cover gauze or visible leakage in urinary diversion
Melchior et al. (1988)	Continence = no need of pads Social continence = small pads Incontinence = diapers
Reddy et al. (1991)	Night: voiding not more than twice per night to remain dry

Side Effects of Urinary Diversion

When urine is stored in a reservoir fashioned from intestinal segments, nutritional, gastrointestinal and metabolic complication may be encountered. Knowledge of the pathophysiology of urinary diversion influences patient selection and follow-up.

Metabolic Changes

The intestinal mucosa is a highly absorptive tissue. Absorption of chloride in exchange for bicarbonate takes place in ileal and colonic segments. After urinary diversion, hyperchloraemic acidosis can occur; this is caused by absorption of ammonium, chloride and hydrogen ions from the urine whilst bicarbonate and sodium undergo net secretion (Hall et al. 1991; Koch et al. 1991). However, the incidence of severe metabolic complications after bladder reconstruction is surprisingly low provided that renal functional reserve is satisfactory. Wenderoth et al. (1990) reported mild acidosis after ileal bladder replacement in more than 50% of patients. Alkalinisation therapy with bicarbonate is routinely administered to patients undergoing the formation of a Mainz pouch (Thüroff et al. 1988). However, all patients were stable after 12 months and did not require further therapy.

Gastrointestinal Complications

Gastrointestinal function and nutritional status may be severely affected after urinary diversion, depending on the bowel segment used. Bile salts as well as vitamin B12 are absorbed in the ileum. Removal of the ileal segment from intestinal continuity may lead to the passage of unabsorbed bile salts into the colon resulting in diarrhoea. On removal of more than 100 cm of ileum, loss of bile salts may exceed the capacity of the liver for resynthesis, resulting in fat malabsorption, steatorrhoea, hypovitaminosis A and D and increased reabsorption of oxalate which may result in urolithiasis. The function of the ileocaecal valve is to control the passage of ileal contents to the colon and its section results in an uncontrolled flow of bowel content, potentially overwhelming the colonic resorptive capacity and resulting in diarrhoea. Reflux of colonic content may also cause bacterial colonization of the small bowel.

Life After Cystectomy

Radical cystectomy and urinary diversion or bladder replacement can cause severe problems in all aspects of life. These include sexual problems, difficulties related to urinary diversion, postoperative incontinence and the fear of recurrence and metastasis. Questionnaire surveys reveal that social activities as well as leisure pursuits are substantially affected (Mansson et al. 1988). Surprisingly, no significant differences were found between patients with a

Table 6.4. Continence after bladder replacement; conmparison of different techniques

Reference; Pouch	No. of patients	Bladder volume (ml)	Daytime continence (No. Pts (%))	Night-time continence (No. Pts (%))	Continence overall (No. Pts (%))	Voiding intervals (h)	Voiding/ day	Voiding/ night
Camey (1985) Camey ileal bladder	150	300	143 (95)	75 (50)		2–	5–8	
Allen et al. (1985) Camey ileal bladder	11	326	5 (45)	1 (9)				several times
Roehrborn et al. (1987) Camey ileal bladder	14	362	11 (79)	1 (7)		2	7–8	
Hautmann et al. (1987) "Ulm bladder"	11	387			8 (73)	2–4		
Wenderoth et al. (1990) "Ulm bladder"	84	755	74 (84)	79 (88)			3–9	0–3
Kock et al. (1989) Hemi Kock ileal bladder	34	600	32 (94)	30 (88)			3–8	0–2
Skinner et al. (1991) Hemi Kock ileal bladder	121	709	114 (94)	102 (84)			3–5	0–3

Table 6.4. *(continued)*

Reference; Pouch	No. of patients	Bladder volume (ml)	Daytime continence (No. Pts (%))	Nighttime continence (No. Pts (%))	Continence overall (No. Pts (%))	Voiding intervals (h)	Voiding/ day	Voiding/ night
Shaaban et al. (1991) Hemi Kock ileal bladder	12	536	12 (100)	8 (70)			3–5	0–1
Schreiter and Noll (1989) Ileal S bladder	32[a]	550	30 (94)		28 (88)			
Shaaban et al. (1991) Ileal S bladder	12	500	11 (92)	7 (58)			3–5	0–1
Tscholl et al. (1987) Ileal S bladder	7	317	5 (71)	7 (100)				0–3
Melchior et al. (1988) Ileal bladder	9[b]	300	9 (100)	8 (89)		3		with alarm clock
Reddy et al. (1991) Sigmoid bladder	27	600	27 (100)	18 (67)			3–5	0–2

[a]14 patients with art. sphincter. [b]5patients social continence.

Table 6.5. Pharmacological management of incontinence in urinary diversion and bladder replacement

Reference	Pouch	No. of patients	Drug	Effect
Bihrle et al. (1991)	Colon transversum pouch	1	Phenobarbital	+
Fowler et al. (1987)	Tubular ileocaecal reservoir	6	Diphenoxylate hydrochloride and atropine sulphate	+
Goldwasser and Webster (1985)	Tubular ileocaecal reservoir	3	Oxybutinine hydrochloride	+
Ghoneim et al. (1981)	Rectal bladder		Imipramine	+
Light and Scott (1984)	Tubular sigmoid bladder	1	Oxybutinine hydrochloride, propantheline bromide, diphenoxylate hydrochloride and atropine sulphate	−
Shaaban et al. (1991)	Hemi-Kock pouch/Parks S pouch	5	Imipramine hydrochloride	+
Webster and Bertram (1986)	Tubular ileocaecal reservoir	3	Oxybutinine hydrochloride	+

normal stoma and those with continent urinary diversion. Generally, some assessment of the patient's mental constitution should be made before operation and appropriate psychological support should be given.

References

Ahlering TE, Weinberg AC, Razor B (1989) A comparative study of the ileal conduit, Kock pouch and modified Indiana pouch. J Urol 142:1193–1196

Algabe F (1987) Origin of high-grade superficial bladder cancer. Eur Urol 13:153–155

Allen TD, Peters PC, Sagalowsky AI, Roehrborn C (1985) The Camey procedure: preliminary results in 11 patients. World J Urol 3:167–71

Atta MA (1991) A new technique for continent urinary reservoir reconstruction. J Urol 145:960–962

Barker SB (1991) Continent diversion with an appendix conduit and an ileocecal bladder. J Urol 146:754–755

Bejany DE, Politano VA (1988) Stapled and nonstapled tapered distal ileum for construction of a continent colonic urinary reservoir. J Urol 140:491–494

Bihrle R, Klee LW, Adams MC, Foster RS (1991) Early clinical experience with the transverse colon-gastric tube continent urinary reservoir. J Urol 146:751–753

Birch BRP, Harland SJ (1989) The pT1G3 bladder tumour. Br J Urol 64:109–116

Brendler CB, Schlegel PN, Walsh PC (1990a) Urethrectomy with preservation of potency. J Urol 144:270–273

Brendler CB, Steinberg GD, Marshall FF, Mostwin JL, Walsh PC (1990b) Local recurrence and survival following nerve-sparing radical cystoprostatectomy. J Urol 144:1137–1141

Bricker EM (1950) Bladder substitution after pelvic evisceration. Surg Clin North Am 30:1511–1521

Burgers JK, Brendler JB (1991) Anatomic radical cystoprostatectomy. Urol Clin North Am 18:659–676

Camey M (1985) Bladder replacement by ileocystoplasty following radical cystectomy. World J Urol 3:161–166

Chen KK, Chang LS, Chen MT (1989) Urodynamic and clinical outcome of Kock pouch continent urinary diversion. J Urol 141:94–97

Coffey RC (1911) Physiologic implantation of the severed ureter or common bile-duct into the intestine. JAMA 56:397–403

Droller MJ, Walsh PC (1985) Intensive intravesical chemotherapy in the treatment of flat carcinoma in situ: is it safe? J Urol 134:1115–1117

Fowler JE, Jr, Clayton M, Mouli K, Reagan G (1987) Effect of liquid diphenoxylate hydrochloride and atropine sulfate (Lomotil) instillations on dynamics and function of continent cecal urinary reservoirs. J Urol 138:735–738

Ghoneim MA, Shehab-El-Din AB, Ashamallah AK, Haballah MA (1981) Evolution of the rectal bladder as a method for urinary diversion. J Urol 126:737–740

Goldwasser B, Webster GD (1985) Continent urinary diversion. J Urol 134:227–36

Hall MC, Koch MO, McDougal WS (1991) Metabolic consequences of urinary diversion through intestinal segments. Urol Clin North Am 18:725–735

Hardeman SW, Soloway MS (1990) Urethral recurrence following radical cystectomy. J Urol 144:666–669

Hautmann RE, Egghart G, Frohneberg D, Miller K (1987) Die Ileum Neoblase. Urologe A 26:67–73

Hautmann RE, Egghart G, Frohneberg G, Miller K (1988) The ileal neobladder. J Urol 139:39–42

Herr HW (1991) Progression of stage T1 bladder tumors after intravesical bacillus Calmette–Guérin. J Urol 145:40–44

Herr HW (1987) Conservative management of muscle-infiltrating bladder cancer: prospective experience. J Urol 138:1162–1163

Hinman F Jr (1988) Selection of intestinal segments for bladder substitution: physical and physiological characteristics. J Urol 139:519–523

Hirdes WH, Hoekstra I, Vlietstra HP (1988) Hammock anastomosis: a nonrefluxing ureteroileal anastomosis. J Urol 139:517–518

Jakobsen H, Steven K, Stigsby B, Klarskov P, Hald T (1987) Pathogenesis of nocturnal urinary incontinence after ileocaecal bladder replacement. Continuous measurement of urethral closure pressure during sleep. Br J Urol 59:148–152

Jakse G, Loidl W, Seeber G, Hofstaedter F (1987) Stage G1, Grade 3 transitional cell carcinoma of the bladder: an unfavorable tumor? J Urol 137:39–43

Koch MO, McDougal WS, Reddy PK, Lange PH (1991) Metabolic alterations following continent urinary diversion through colonic segments. J Urol 145:270–273

Kock NG (1969) Intra abdominal 'reservoir' in patients with permanent ileostomy. Preliminary observations on a procedure resulting in fecal 'continence' in five ileostomy patients. Arch Surg 99:223–231

Kock NG, Norlén LJ, Philipson BM, Akerlund S (1985) The continent ileal reservoir (Kock pouch) for urinary diversion. World J Urol 3:146–151

Kock NG, Ghoneim MA, Lycke KG, Mahran MR (1989) Replacement of the bladder by the urethral Kock pouch: functional results urodynamics and radiological features. J Urol 141:1111–1116

Leadbetter WF, Cooper JF (1950) Regional gland dissection for carcinoma of the bladder: a technique for one-stage cystectomy, gland dissection and bilateral ureteroenterostomy. J Urol 63:242

Le Duc A, Camey M (1979) Un procédé d'implantation urétéroiléale antireflux dans l'entéro-cystoplastie. J Urol Néphrol 85:449–454

Light JK, Scott FB (1984) Total reconstruction of the lower urinary tract using bowel and the artificial urinary sphincter. J Urol 1984 131:953–956

Lindell O (1987) Salvage cystectomy. Eur Urol 13:17–21

Lockhart JL (1987) Remodeled right colon: an alternative urinary reservoir. J Urol 138:730–734

Lockhart JL, Pow Sang JM, Persky L, Kahn P, Helal M, Sanford E (1990) A continent colonic urinary reservoir: the Florida pouch. J Urol 144:864–867

Malkowicz SB, Nichols P, Lieskovsky G, Boyd SD, Huffmann J, Skinner DG (1990) The role of radical cystectomy in the management of high grade superficial bladder cancer (PA, P1, Pis and P2). J Urol 144:641–645

Mansson A, Johnson G, Mansson W (1988) Quality of life after cystectomy. Comparison between patients with conduit and those with continent caecal reservoir urinary diversion. Br J Urol 62:240–245

Melchior H, Spehr C, Knop Wagemann I, Persson MC, Juenemann KP (1988) The continent ileal bladder for urinary tract reconstruction after cystectomy: a survey of 44 patients. J Urol 139:714–718

Mitrofanoff P (1980) Cystostomie continente trans-apendiculaire dans le traitment des vessies neurologiques. Chir Pediatr 21:297–304

Montie JE, Wood DP Jr (1989) The risk of radical cystectomy. Br J Urol 63:483–486

Montie JE, Straffon RA, Steward BH (1984) Radical cystectomy without radiation therapy for carcinoma of the bladder. J Urol 131:477–482

Neal DE (1985) Complications of ileal conduit urinary diversion in adults with cancer followed up for at least 5 years. Br Med J 290:1695–1697

Neal DE (1989) Urodynamic investigation of the ileal conduit: upper tract dilatation and the effects of revision of the conduit. J Urol 142:97–100

Pagano F, Bassi P, Galetti TP et al. (1991) Results of contemporary radical cystectomy for invasive bladder cancer: a clinicopathological study with an emphasis on the inadequacy of the tumor, nodes and metastases classification. J Urol 145:45–50

Prout GR Jr, Griffin PP, Sipley WU (1979) Bladder carcinoma as a systemic disease. Cancer 43:2532–2539

Raghavan D, Shipley WU, Garnick MB, Russel PJ, Richie JP (1990) Biology and management of bladder cancer. N Engl J Med 322:1129–1138

Reddy PK, Lange PH, Fraley EE (1991) Total bladder replacement using detubularized sigmoid colon: technique and results. J Urol 145:51–55

Riedmiller H, Bürger R, Müller S, Thüroff J, Hohenfellner R (1990) Continent appendix stoma: A modification of the MAINZ pouch technique J Urol 143:1115–1117

Roehrborn CG, Teigland CM, Sagalowsky AI (1987) Functional characteristics of the Camey ileal bladder. J Urol 138:739–742

Rowland RG, Mitchell ME, Bihrle R, Kahnoski RJ, Piser JE (1987) Indiana continent urinary reservoir. J Urol 137:1136–1139

Schlegel PN, Walsh PC (1987) Neuroanatomical approach to radical cystoprostatectomy with preservation of sexual function. J Urol 138:1402–1406

Schneider AW, Huland H (1990) Tumormarker und prognostische Parameter beim Harnblasen-karzinom. Urologe A 29:71–76

Schreiter F, Noll F (1989) Kock pouch and S bladder: 2 different ways of lower urinary tract reconstruction. J Urol 142:1197–1200

Shaaban AA, Dawaba MS, Gaballah MA, Ghoneim MA (1991) Urethral controlled bladder substitution: a comparison between Parks S pouch and hemi-Kock pouch. J Urol 146:973–976

Skinner DG (1982) Management of invasive bladder cancer: a meticulous pelvic node dissection can make a difference. J Urol 128:34–36

Skinner DG, Lieskovsky G (1984) Contemporary cystectomy with pelvic node dissection compared to preoperative radiation therapy plus cystectomy in management of invasive bladder cancer. J Urol 131:1069–1072

Skinner EC, Lieskovsky G, Skinner DG (1984) Radical cystectomy in the elderly patient. J Urol 131:1065–1068

Skinner DG, Boyd SD, Lieskovsky G (1987) An update on the Kock pouch for continent urinary diversion. Urol Clin North Am 14:789–795

Skinner DG, Lieskovsky G, Boyd S (1989) Continent urinary diversion. J Urol 141:1323–1327

Skinner DG, Boyd SD, Lieskovsky G, Bennett C, Hopwood B (1991) Lower urinary tract reconstruction following cystectomy: experience and results in 126 patients using the Kock ileal reservoir with bilateral ureteroileal urethrostomy. J Urol 146:756–760

Stöckle M, Alken P, Engelmann U, Jacobi GH, Riedmiller H, Hohenfellner R (1987) Radical cystectomy – often too late? Eur Urol 13:361–367

Studer UE, Spiegel T, Casanova GA et al. (1991) Ileal bladder substitute: antireflux nipple or afferent tubular segment? Eur Urol 20:315–326

Svare J, Walter S, Kristensen JK, Lund F (1985) Ileal conduit urinary diversion – early and late complications. Eur Urol 11:83–86

Thüroff JW, Alken P, Riedmiller H, Jacobi GH, Hohenfellner R (1988) 100 cases of Mainz pouch: continuing experience and evolution. J Urol 140:283–288

Tscholl R, Leisinger HJ, Hauri D (1987) The ileal S-pouch for bladder replacement after cystectomy: preliminary report of 7 cases. J Urol 138:344–347

Vincente J, Laguna MP, Duarte D, Algabe F, Chéchile G (1991) Carcinoma in situ as a prognostic factor for G3pT1 bladder tumours. Br J Urol 68:380–382

Webster GD, Bertram RA (1986) Continent catheterizable urinary diversion using the ileocecal segment with stapled intussusception of the ileocecal valve. J Urol 135:465–469

Wenderoth UK, Bachor R, Egghart G, Frohneberg D, Miller K, Hautmann RE (1990) The ileal neobladder: experience and results of more than 100 consecutive cases. J Urol 143:492–496

Wishnow KI, Tenney DM (1991) Will Rogers and the results of radical cystectomy for invasive bladder cancer. Urol Clin North Am 18:530–537

Wood DP Jr, Montie JE, Maatman TJ, Beck GJ (1987) Radical cystectomy for carcinoma of the bladder in the elderly patient. J Urol 138:46–48

Chapter 7

Prostate Cancer: More Questions Than Answers?

W. B. Peeling and K. Griffiths

Overview

A great deal of information has been gathered together during the past 50 years about the pathology of prostate cancer, its endocrinology, cell biology and particularly its clinical features and behaviour. Despite this, there is uncertainty about its causes and natural history, and as there is still considerable debate about methods of treatment it is probably not surprising that mortality from the disease remains much as it was 30 to 40 years ago. It would appear, therefore, that there has been limited forward progress in the clinical management of this disease so what should we be examining in the last decade of the twentieth century, to find some answers, particularly to reduce mortality?

Detection and successful treatment of early stage prostate cancer, perhaps by screening men at risk from the disease, might lead to better chances of a real cure for some patients. This has recently been shown to be possible after screening for breast cancer which in England and Wales is now expected to save 1250 deaths each year by the turn of the century (Reece 1991). Is it likely that screening programmes for prostate cancer can achieve likewise? Some urologists think so (Walsh 1992) whereas others strongly disagree with the concept of screening for prostate cancer because, among other reasons, it has never been proved that treatment after early diagnosis has had a beneficial effect on mortality (Blandy 1991). A solution must be found soon to this important debate for it is becoming increasingly recognised that, as a potential health care problem, prostate cancer could overwhelm the resources of health services in the western world towards the end of the century (Boyle, personal communication). However, the greatest problem at the present time is our ignorance of the natural history of this disease. For instance, it is well known that the incidence of prostate cancer, whether of clinical or microscopic proportions, increases with age ranging from about 30% in men under 50 years of age to 100% in the ninth decade (Franks 1954). Data from the USA estimated that in 1987 10 000 000 men could be expected to harbour microscopic or "latent" prostate cancer (Carter and Coffey 1988) which in general, can be expected to be a well-differentiated focal tumour (McNeal et al. 1986). And yet, it is known that only a small fraction of men with "latent" cancer will die from clinical cancer which Stamey (1982) calculated to be only one prostate cancer death out of every 1300 men with histological evidence of the disease. We do not know what switches on "latent" cancers to become clinically active, but of those that undergo this change, in the 1987 cohort in the USA, it is expected that 26 000 will die of the disease (Carter and Coffey 1988). Will it ever be possible to identify those men at risk of developing prostatic cancer before they acquire clinically active disease?

When established as a clinical entity, it is generally understood that only those patients with tumours that are completely confined within the prostate are likely have them successfully removed or destroyed and so achieve a cure. However, early diagnosis through screening to detect such patients would benefit only those with cancers that are likely to progress and become lethal if untreated. How can these be identified to enable us to select those patients who would benefit from radical treatment?

But, which treatment is best – radical prostatectomy, irradiation or is a surveillance policy safe? We do not yet know the answer to this problem.

Further along the clinical spectrum of prostate cancer is advanced disease. It could be argued that little progress has been made with endocrine methods of treatment since Huggins and Hodges (1941) showed the role of orchidectomy and diethylstilboestrol (DES) as excellent palliation for patients with advanced prostate cancer. Since then, DES has been largely discredited by the work of the Veterans Administration Co-operative Urological Research Group (VACURG) who revealed its dangerous side effects (Arduino et al. 1967). Therefore, many urologists have since favoured orchidectomy as the most direct, swift and safe treatment for advanced prostate cancer, but others quite rightly searched for new non-oestrogens as a medical alternative to surgical castration for there are occasions when orchidectomy may, for medical, cultural or psychological reasons, be contraindicated. Progestogenic derivatives were never entirely ideal and interest shifted away from these when it was recognised that chronic administration of LHRH agonists can produce an effective medical castration. Drugs such as goserelin (Zoladex) were demonstrated to be as effective clinically and as safe as orchidectomy (Peeling 1987).

However, orchidectomy and LHRH agonists share a major drawback – loss of sexual potency. Therefore, the discovery of non-steroidal antiandrogens such as nilutamide, flutamide and casodex, and more recently 5α-reductase inhibitors, was of extreme interest to clinicians for these drugs possessed the logistic advantage over orchidectomy and LHRH drugs in that they act directly on prostatic cells without suppressing the hypothalamic–pituitary–testicular axis and so avoid loss of potency. Moreover, by acting at the target prostate cell, they also block the action of androgens of adrenocortical origin that remain in serum after surgical or medical castration which, according to Labrie et al. (1988), could be sufficient to stimulate growth of prostate cancer. Thus, combination therapy of antiandrogens added to orchidectomy or LH drugs achieved the concept of "total androgen blockade" and was considered to be a major step forward in the treatment of men with advanced prostate cancer (Labrie et al, 1983). Others are not so sure and the question remains:

which treatment is best for advanced disease – castration or total androgen blockade? Furthermore, is there still a role for oestrogens?

Meanwhile, uncertainty developed about the optimal timing for hormonal treatment by orchidectomy or LHRH analogues. At the moment we have no clear guide about the safety of treatment that is deferred until patients develop symptoms from advanced prostate cancer or whether it is better to start hormonal treatment without delay when a diagnosis is made. Some experimental evidence suggests that incomplete androgen deprivation may hinder clonal changes towards hormone-refractory disease which raises the possibility that intermittent hormonal treatment might be an alternative palliative procedure (Bruchovsky, personal communication). Should this be examined in more detail?

These many questions focus, therefore, on two main issues about prostate cancer that are of great concern to urologists at the present time. First, as the only chance of cure from this disease is detection and treatment when early stage cancer is totally confined within the prostate, can screening for early prostate cancer be justified clinically, economically or ethically? Second, as endocrine treatment of advanced prostate cancer by whatever method is well known to result in only about a 70% response rate, with relapse to hormone-refractory disease and death of over 50% of these patients within 18–24 months, hormone therapy can only be regarded as a palliative process. One wonders whether endocrine therapy has reached its limit, in which case we must accept that for advanced disease, improvement in quality of life is all we can offer our patients. Or are there new treatments for advanced disease that might improve mortality rate and reduce morbidity?

The purpose of this review is to search for a balanced practical way forward with these two contentious but difficult topics: (a) is screening for early prostate cancer justifiable? and (b) can endocrine therapy be improved?

Is Screening for Early Prostate Cancer Justifiable?

Screening for any cancer must conform with two cardinal principles. First, the ultimate goal of any cancer screening programme can only be a reduction of disease-specific mortality and second, screened patients must not be harmed by the screening process either physically or psychologically. It must be emphasised that screening for prostate cancer implies that only asymptomatic, apparently healthy men who have complained of no symptoms related to prostate cancer will be investigated by screening. Some of these will become screen-positive and will be advised to undergo a sequence of diagnostic/staging investigations, possibly treatment (which could give rise to complications) and follow-up for which they may be ill prepared in their minds when they enter the screening process. Screening for asymptomatic disease should, therefore, not be undertaken lightly. It is now generally accepted that the principles for early detection of disease by screening should be according to those set out by Wilson and Jungner (1968). These are as follows.

1. The condition sought should be an important health problem.
2. There should be an accepted treatment for patients with recognisable disease.

3. Facilities for diagnosis and treatment should be available.
4. There should be a recognisable latent or early symptomatic stage.
5. There should be a suitable test or examination.
6. The test should be acceptable to the population.
7. The natural history of the condition, including development from latent to declared disease, should be adequately understood.
8. There should be an agreed policy on whom to treat as patients.
9. The cost of case-finding (including diagnosis and treatment of patients diagnosed) should be economically balanced in relation to possible expenditure on medical care as a whole.
10. Case-finding should be a continuing process and not a "once and for all" project.

The concept of screening is therefore complex and for a prostate cancer screening programme based upon Wilson and Jungner's (1968) principles, the following sequence of questions needs to be considered:

1. Which men should be screened?
2. Is prostate cancer an important health problem?
3. What should be the target for screening?
4. How reliable are current methods to detect early prostate cancer?

Table 7.1. Clinical staging of primary prostate carcinoma

DRE findings	Modified Whitmore–Jewett system	TNM system		
		UICC 1978		UICC 1989
Primary tumour				
Not assessed			Tx	
No evidence of tumour			T0	
No palpable tumour (incidental histological finding)	A	T0	T1	
Volume < 5% well differentiated	A1	T0a		T1a (< 3 foci)
Volume > 5% or not well differentiated	A2	T0b	T1b	(> foci)
Confined tumour	B	T1	T2	
< 1.5 cm nodule	B1	T1		T2a
> 1.5 cm in one lobe	B2	T1/T2		T2b
Bilateral lobar disease	B2	T2		T2b
Extracapsular spread	C	T3	T3	
Lateral sulci	C1			
Seminal vesicles	C2			
Seminal vesicles and bladder	C3	T4	T4	
Tumour fixed	C3	T4	T4	

Whitmore (1956); Jewett (1975); Cantrell et al. (1981).

5. Which prostatic biopsy technique is most appropriate in a screening programme?
6. What is the best treatment for screen-positive men?
7. Do the benefits of screening outweigh its disadvantages?
8. How much will screening cost? Can it be afforded?

Note: Staging categories in this review will be according to the 4th revised TNM system (UICC 1987) and the modified Whitmore–Jewett system (Whitmore 1956; Jewett 1975) (Table 7.1).

Which Men Should be Screened?

Few urologists would dispute the principle that men screened for prostate cancer should have an expectation of life of 10 years at least. This would exclude those with restricted life-expectancy due to pulmonary disease, cardiac conditions, other malignancies or debilitating conditions. The lower age limit for prostate cancer screening is easily determined as prostate cancer is rarely encountered under the age of 50 years (Thompson et al. 1984).

The upper cut off age limit is more difficult to decide but basing this upon an expectation of life of at least 10 years, data from England and Wales in 1992 indicate that for men aged 50 life expectation is 25.6 years, for those aged 70 it is 10.9 years whereas in 80 year olds it is 6.3 years (OPCS 1992). Data from the USA for life expectation of white men between 50 and 70 years are similar. Therefore, on the basis of such information it is reasonable to screen men aged between 50 and 70 years for prostate cancer.

Is Prostate Cancer a Major Health Problem?

"Latent" prostate cancers are unlikely to be a major health problem for they are considered to have little aggressive potential. In practical terms, "latent" prostate cancers are more likely to be encountered at autopsy or in cystoprostatectomy specimens when they may be found in as many as 30% to 50% (Walsh, 1992). These lesions would not be palpable by digital rectal examination (DRE), and give no characteristic ultrasound pattern so are not detectable by transrectal ultrasound (Peeling and Griffiths 1984). Nevertheless they can be detected by random prostatic biopsy (Dyke et al. 1990).

Whereas "latent" prostate cancers are autopsy or pathological specimen findings, "incidental" prostate cancers (stage T1a/stage A) are diagnosed in life as an unexpected finding in tissue removed at prostatectomy. These cancers are not rare and may be reported in tissue after prostatectomy in as many as 23% of patients (Chisholm 1981). In the USA in 1987, of 96 000 new cases of prostate cancer registered, 22 000 (23.4%) were classified as stage A tumours (Carter and Coffey 1988). These are considerable numbers of patients and in fact for prostate cancer as a whole, it has now been shown that it is the commonest male malignancy in the USA (Boring et al. 1991) and in England and Wales it is second to lung cancer (OPCS 1991b).

Not only is prostate cancer a common condition, there is evidence that its incidence is increasing. For instance, in the USA in 1973 the incidence of prostate cancers per 100 000 white males was 62.1, whereas in 1984 it was 79.4 (Horm et al. 1984). More recent data recorded in 1987 reported 96 000 prostate cancers in the USA (Carter and Coffey 1988) and in 1992 the expected number of new cases was 122 000 (Boring et al. 1991). In England and Wales, in 1971 there were 5819 registrations for prostate cancer whereas in 1986 this number had risen to 10 180 (OPCS 1991a).

As a cause of death from malignancy among males, prostate cancer is the second commonest cause in the USA and in England and Wales (Boring et al. 1991; OPCS 1991b). As with incidence, the projected number of disease-specific deaths from prostate cancer is expected to rise; in the USA, from the 1987 cohort 27 000 (28%) men are expected to die from the disease (Carter and Coffey 1988) and from those registered in 1992, 32 000 (26%) are expected to die. In England and Wales, in 1974 there were 4605 deaths from prostate cancer recorded (OPCS 1976) whereas in 1990, 8098 men were reported to have died from prostate cancer (OPCS 1991b).

These data indicate that prostate cancer is a major health problem in terms of incidence and mortality, but it is also a health problem of increasing magnitude.

What Should be the Target for Screening and Early Diagnosis?

For curability of prostate cancer to be feasible, the disease must still be confined within the prostate at the time of treatment, whether this is excision by radical prostatectomy or ablation by irradiation or other means. If this condition is met, survival should be no different from normal life expectation. It has been known for many years that actuarial survival of patients with only microscopic involvement with prostate cancer deviates little from the expected survival of a population of equivalent age, but that with increased staging of primary tumours from B1 tumours (palpable nodule) to B3 cancers (palpably diffuse but localised tumour) survival is progressively less (Jewett 1975). More precisely, small cancers of less than 2 cm^2 in area on DRE (or 1.4 cm diameter) can be expected to be non-aggressive in terms of survival whereas 5-year survival of tumours measuring over 2 cm^2 has been reported to be 45% (Byar 1977).

McNeal et al. (1986) linked volume with tumour differentiation by showing that prostate cancers of over 3–5 ml in volume (or about 1.5 cm diameter) tended to dedifferentiate and acquire invasive tendencies.

Based on this evidence, the target for early detection of prostate cancer in a screening programme would be a tumour of 1.5 cm or less, for, according to the evidence available, these are most likely to be non-invasive and well differentiated and therefore have the highest chance of curability

How Reliable are Current Methods to Detect Early Prostate Cancer?

Tests for screening of small volume prostate cancers must have a high sensitivity (i.e. ability to detect curable cancers), and high specificity (i.e. should avoid giving false-positive results) so that men with potentially curable prostate cancers are not overlooked and those without disease are not subjected to unnecessary investigations.

Three screening techniques are in current use; digital rectal examination (DRE), transrectal ultrasound (TRUS) and assay of serum prostate specific antigen (PSA).

Screening using DRE

The traditional method of detecting prostate cancer has been DRE to palpate the prostate for abnormalities of contour or consistency that might indicate a cancer. DRE must, therefore, be regarded as the most common screening process in clinical practice.

The reported effectiveness of DRE when used to screen for prostate cancer varies widely. Detection rates by DRE have varied from 0.1% to 7.6% (av. 1.54%) and positive predictive values (PPV) have varied from 6% to 39% (Gerber and Chodak 1990). DRE has, therefore, a low PPV to detect prostate cancer in a screening programme and becomes less effective in detecting prostate cancer as the tumours become smaller. In fact, over 50% of cancers under 1.5 cm in size may not be detected or diagnosed by DRE (Lee et al. 1987). DRE has a further disadvantage when used in screening, for over 50% of patients judged clinically to be stage B tumours may be proved surgically to be stage C or D1 disease (Chodak et al. 1989).

DRE clearly has a limited role in screening not only for diagnosis and detection, but also for staging.

Screening Using TRUS

Although TRUS has emerged as the best imaging process for the prostate, its role as a diagnostic procedure in clinical practice can only be justified if its performance is better than DRE, or can supplement DRE to improve sensitivity and PPV.

With locally invasive prostate cancers (stage T3/T4) TRUS gives no added diagnostic information to DRE for the sensitivity and specificity of both modalities is about 96% (Peeling and Griffiths 1984). However, for stage T2a prostate cancers, it has been reported that sensitivity of both DRE and TRUS were of the order of 97% whereas for DRE specificity was only 53% but for TRUS was 94% (Clements et al. 1988).

For cancers of less than 1.5 cm diameter TRUS has been shown to have twice the sensitivity of DRE and in one study TRUS detected 100% of tumours of this size whereas DRE detected only 41% (Lee et al. 1988). Impalpable cancers can also be detected by TRUS (Lee et al. 1988; Drago and Badalament 1990).

TRUS would appear to have considerable advantages over DRE for detection of early prostate cancers, but there are, nevertheless, two important limitations with TRUS. First, many hypoechoic lesions under 1.5 cm in size may not be malignant – in one study only 21% of such lesions were proved by biopsy to be cancer (Rifkin and Choi 1988). Second, 24%–30% of small prostate cancers are not demonstrable by TRUS because they are isoechoic, which means that they exhibit no characteristic ultrasonic features to distinguish them from adjacent non-malignant prostatic tissue (Dahnert et al. 1986; Salo et al. 1987).

When used as a purely screening process for prostate cancer, reported sensitivities of TRUS have varied from 100% to 48% with specificities varying from 94% to 60% (Optenberg and Thompson 1990).

Screening with TRUS alone is therefore likely to have variable results probably depending on operator skills and experience but it undoubtedly improves upon DRE to detect cancers of 1.5 cm in size or less, especially non-palpable tumours.

Screening with Prostate Specific Antigen (PSA)

PSA has mostly replaced prostatic acid phosphatase (PAP) as a front-line tumour marker for prostate cancer. In fact, there is no role for PAP in screening for it is rarely, if ever, elevated when prostate cancer is truly localised to the prostate (Vikho et al. 1985)

PSA is a highly immunogenic glycoprotein that originates only from prostate epithelium and is produced by benign as well as malignant prostate tissue. There are a number of assays available for measurement of PSA in serum of which Tandem-R (Hybritech Inc., San Diego, California) and Pros-Check (Yang Laboratories, Bellevue, Washington) are the most widely available. The Tandem-R assay employs monoclonal antibodies in a two-site immunometric assay (m-PSA) whereas Pros-Check is a radioimmunoassay employing polyclonal antibodies (p-PSA). The manufacturer's upper limit of normality for m-PSA is 4.0 ng/ml, and that for p-PSA is 2.5 ng/ml, so it is important to clarify the assay used in any statements about serum PSA levels, particularly when these are low as in screening exercises.

It is thought that prostate cancers produce more PSA per gram of tissue than BPH so that the total serum PSA level in any patient with prostate cancer should be a volumetrically related function of the combined contributions of PSA from the malignant and benign moieties of the gland. In BPH, Stamey et al. (1987) have reported that serum PSA increased by 0.3 ng/ml/g of hyperplastic tissue.

Although there have been many excellent studies to examine the role of PSA for diagnosis of prostate cancer only two investigations have specifically considered using PSA as the initial test in the early detection of the disease (Catalona et al. 1991; Brawer et al. 1992). Both studies had similar protocols and similar results. Men aged over 50 were recruited by press release or publicity to take part in a study of serum PSA measurement as a screening test for prostate cancer. Those with m-PSA less than 4 ng/ml were not investigated further. Those with m-PSA greater than 4 ng/ml were invited to undergo DRE and TRUS with biopsy of any suspect areas of the prostate. However, in Catalona's study no biopsy was taken from patients with no abnormality on DRE or TRUS if m-PSA was between 4.0 and 9.9 ng/ml.

Catalona et al. (1991) also compared in a similar way 300 men who were of similar age to the screened group (1653 men). These were being investigated for a variety of abnormal urological symptoms, signs or investigations suggesting prostatic disease and were therefore a clinical rather than a screened group.

The detection rate for prostate cancers was 2.2% in the screened group whereas in the comparison (clinical) group it was 24%. However, it was

Table 7.2.

m-PSA (ng/ml)	Screened group		Comparative (clinical) group	
	No.	Cancers (%)	No.	Cancers (%)
< 4.0			116	13 (11)
> 4.0–9.9	107	19 (18)	74	19 (26)
>10.0	30	18 (60)	45	29 (64)

From Catalona et al. (1991).

evident that m-PSA lacked sensitivity as a screening test because 11% of clinical patients with serum m-PSA less than 4 ng/ml had prostate cancer (Table 7.2). Brawer et al. (1992) reported that 23.3% of men with m-PSA less than 4 ng/ml but with a palpable prostatic abnormality had prostate cancer. When m-PSA exceeded 4 ng/ml, the yield of prostate cancer increased, particularly when over 10 ng/ml for at that level 60%–64% of men were shown to have malignancy (Table 7.2).

The credibility of PSA as an aid to early diagnosis could be increased if its sensitivity could be improved to detect prostate cancers more reliably, particularly for smaller tumours. As already mentioned, serum PSA levels are a sum of the contributions of the malignant tissue and benign tissue in the prostate so in theory subtraction of the PSA contribution by the non-malignant moiety from total PSA might expose the extent of PSA originating from prostate cancer cells.

Therefore two studies of PSA levels in men without evidence of prostate cancer are of interest. These have demonstrated a statistically significant relation between the log of the serum PSA concentration and total prostatic volume measured by TRUS (Babaian et al. 1992; Clements et al. 1992). Babaian et al. (1992) related levels of m-PSA to prostate volume and found that it was most unusual (2.2% incidence) for serum m-PSA to exceed 4 ng/ml when prostate volumes were less than or equal to 25 cm^3 and m-PSA never exceeded 10 ng/ml in these subjects (Table 7.3). As prostate volume increased so did m-PSA which in prostates greater than 50 cm^3 in volume was greater than 4 ng/ml in 65.4% of patients (Table 7.3).

Clements et al. (1992) related log m-PSA to prostatic volumes (UPV) measured by TRUS in 50 men with no clinical or other evidence of prostate

Table 7.3.

Prostate volume (cm^3)		m-PSA (ng/ml)					
		<4		>4 to <10		>10	
	(n)	n	(%)	n	(%)	n	(%)
<25	(139)	136	(97.8)	3	(2.2)	–	–
>25 to<50	(217)	177	(81.6)	32	(14.7)	8	(3.7)
>50	(52)	18	(34.6)	29	(55.8)	5	(9.6)
Totals	(408)	331	(81.1)	64	(15.7)	13	(3.2)

From Babaian et al. (1992).

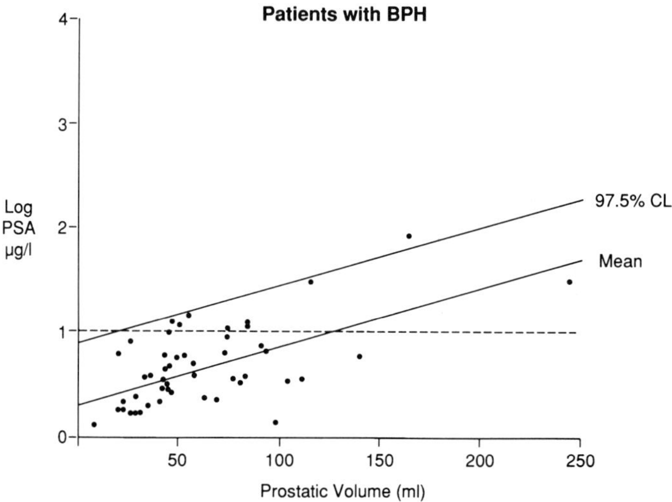

Fig. 7.1. Correlation between prostate volume (ml) and log serum prostate specific antigen (m-PSA) in patients with benign prostatic hyperplasia. (From Clements et al. 1992; with kind permission of Wiley–Liss Inc., New York.)

cancer although most had benign prostatic hyperplasia. They employed the Deming regression equation

$$\log \text{m-PSA} = 5.62 \times 10^3 \text{ (UPV)} + 0.32$$

(SD residual error of regression about $Y = 0.30$) and found a highly significant correlation between log m-PSA and prostate volume (Fig. 7.1). Using these results as a reference grid for the benign moiety, log m-PSA/volume plots for 23 men with M0 prostate cancer were superimposed on the mean regression line and 97.5% confidence limits of the non-malignant patients (Fig. 7.2). All but four values (83%) fell outside the 97.5% confidence limits of men with benign prostatic conditions.

It can therefore be argued that 83% of these patients with M0 prostate cancer had been discriminated from BPH by this process especially as the UPV of most of them was less than 100 ml.

The concept of volume-adjusted PSA for early diagnosis of prostate cancer is also being examined elsewhere (Littrup et al. 1991) but it is becoming increasingly evident that interpretation of serum PSA values, particularly when at low levels, must take prostate volume into account.

Use of DRE, PSA, TRUS in Early Diagnosis

It is clear, therefore, that measurement of serum PSA is a key but not infallible element to detect early prostate cancer but it is not the only parameter that should be used. For instance, in Catalona et al.'s (1991) study, DRE alone would have overlooked 12 of 37 cancers (32%) in the screened group of whom five had serum m-PSA greater than 4.0 ng/ml as the only suspicious finding.

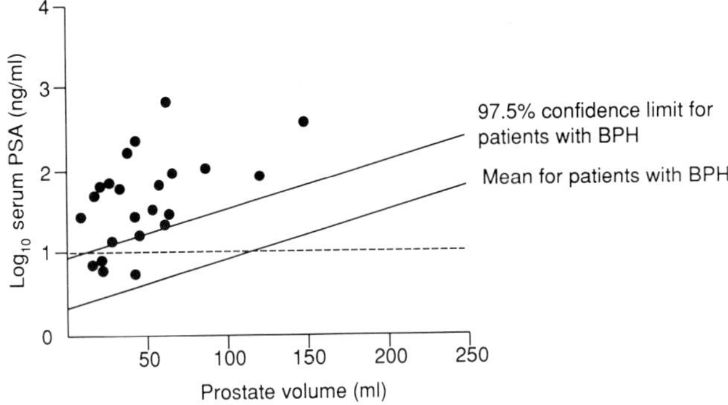

Fig. 7.2. Prostate volume (ml) and log serum m-PSA in patients with non-metastatic carcinoma of the prostate, compared with a mean correlation of 97.5% confidence limits of volume/log m-PSA for patients with BPH. (From Clements et al. 1992; with kind permission of Wiley–Liss Inc., New York.)

If TRUS had been the only screening modality, 16 of 37 cancers (43%) would have been overlooked. When DRE, PSA and TRUS were used in various combinations, the most profitable yield of cancers came from serum m-PSA linked with DRE, followed by TRUS in patients with abnormal m-PSA or DRE.

It would seem, therefore, that for screening purposes, the initial process should be serum PSA measurement with DRE, and, for those men with palpably abnormal DRE and serum PSA greater or equal to 4.0 ng/ml, second line TRUS examination should be undertaken with biopsy where indicated. The PPV for such a policy to detect cancers under 1.5 cm in diameter has been shown to be (Lee et al. 1989):

TRUS with DRE+/PSA+	71%
TRUS with DRE+/PSA−	26%
TRUS with DRE−/PSA+	34%
TRUS with DRE−/PSA−	5%

Nevertheless, from the evidence so far available m-PSA values of 10 ng/ml would appear to be an important watershed for this was the demarkation line of curability for early prostate cancers in Catalona's study. All men with m-PSA less than or equal to 9.9 ng/ml had organ confined cancer, whereas all but one whose m-PSA was greater than or equal to 10.0 ng/ml had either clinical or pathological evidence of extra prostatic spread.

Which Prostate Biopsy Technique is Best for Screening?

The usual primary indications for prostate biopsy are:

1. A palpable prostatic abnormality

2. A hypoechoic prostate lesion demonstrated by TRUS
3. Serum m-PSA equal to or greater than 4.0 ng/ml when DRE has revealed
    no abnormality of the prostate.

Traditionally, prostatic biopsy was carried out by digitally guided 14 gauge Vim
Silverman or Tru-cut needles either transrectally or transperineally which in
experienced hands would have an accuracy of about 80% for palpable lesions
(Kaufman and Schultz 1962). For a while, the transperineal route of biopsy
was preferred because it reduced the septic complications of transrectal biopsy
(Hillyard 1987). Other urologists preferred fine needle aspiration cytology
which even when carried out transrectally not only had a complication rate of
less than 1% (Esposti and Franzen 1980) but was also inexpensive and did not
require anaesthesia. However, cytological aspiration carries a false negative
rate of 5%–30% depending largely upon the experience of the cytopathologist
(Fornage 1988).

The situation has changed dramatically during the past few years with
two developments. First, spring-loaded biopsy guns which can use finer
needles (18 gauge) have been shown to produce prostatic tissue specimens
suitable for histological examination but with very low infective complications
(0.8%) when used transrectally with prophylactic antibiotics (Hodge et al.
1989). Second, the immense technical advances of transrectal ultrasound
probes, particularly of multiplanar probes which can image the prostate
transversely or sagittally to produce a 3-dimensional appreciation of the
prostate, have now provided technology in which biopsy can be carried
out extremely accurately (Torp-Pederson et al. 1989). With this technique,
biopsy of prostate lesions even as small as 0.4 cm can be achieved with few
complications (Bertermann 1990)

For antibiotic prophylaxis, ciprofloxacin 500 mg given 1h before biopsy and
a further 500 mg taken the following morning has proved most effective
(Clements and Peeling, unpublished data).

For screening to detect early "curable" prostate cancer, reliable biopsy
of tumours of less than 1.5 cm in size must be achieved. Lee et al. (1987)
compared the performance of aspiration biopsy and core biopsy under TRUS
guidance and achieved a rate of cancer diagnosis of 53% for cytological
examination and 54% by core biopsy. This included cancers of less than
1.0 cm in size and 56% of cancers measuring 1.0–1.5 cm. Of the lesions
examined 13 (57%) were non-palpable on DRE.

However, the problem of the localisation of small isoechoic cancers has to
be solved. This is particularly relevant as prostate cancer is often multifocal
so that its true extent may be underestimated when biopsying only a solitary
palpable lesion. Many urologists, particularly in the USA, carry out six sector
random prostatic biopsies with up to three cores from each lobe in addition to
biopsy of any palpable lesion. This can result in diagnostic yields of up to 14%
of unsuspected possibly focal cancers but often does not significantly alter the
patients' management (Dyke et al. 1990). However, TRUS guided biopsy of
small hypoechoic prostatic lesions is irrelevant when both DRE and serum
PSA are normal because the PPV for these patients was only about 5% (Lee
et al. 1989).

In a screening context, therefore, when small tumours of 1.5 cm diameter
or less are being sought TRUS-guided biopsy is most appropriate. The value

of random sector biopsies is doubtful as a practical procedure as this could result in overdiagnosis of "latent" or focal cancers that may not be a biological threat to the patient.

How Should Screen-positives be Managed?

Which Patients Should be Treated?

Any discussion about screening for prostate cancer has to focus on the treatment and management of patients in whom prostate cancer is revealed. These will be mostly stage T1/T2 tumours but a few T3/M1 cancers will also come to light. Men who consent to screening are usually fit people without urological symptoms and as these have voluntarily consented to undergo examination they will therefore expect clear sympathetic guidance about the way forward if a prostate cancer is detected. How can they be properly advised?

The options for management are well known but are a constant source of debate, particularly between North American and British urologists. These are:

1. A surveillance policy
2. Radical retropubic prostatectomy
3. External beam irradiation

The case for a surveillance policy of localised prostate cancer has been admirably presented by Smith (1990) who argued that neither radical prostatectomy nor irradiation has been shown to influence beneficially patients with poorly differentiated cancers localised to the prostate, and that more patients with well-differentiated tumours die of causes other than prostate cancer and so could be treated when symptoms arise.

This policy would seem to be reasonable for men with stage T1a/A1 focal "incidental" prostate cancer but a closer examination of the literature is confusing. In general, it has been thought that these tumours imply low volume, low grade cancers which are clinically insignificant and unlikely to progress within the lifetime of the patient. For instance, it was observed that men with untreated stage A1 disease had a life expectancy similar to that of age-matched controls (Hanash et al. 1972; Jewett 1975) and that disease-specific deaths occurred in only 1% of these patients (Lowe and Listrom 1988). However, reports that 2%–9% of men with untreated stage T1a/A1 disease develop progressive disease are disturbing (Cantrell et al. 1981; Lowe and Listrom, 1988) but of extreme concern is the report that, if stage T1a/A1 prostate cancer is left untreated for 10 years, there is a 12% chance of death from the disease (Epstein et al. 1986).

Would a surveillance policy be reasonable for men with infiltrating "incidental" prostate cancer (stage T1b/A2) for this is generally recognised as a more serious condition. Many of these lesions are less differentiated than stage T1a cancers and approximately 25% of patients with stage T1b/A2 tumours have pelvic node metastases at the time of diagnosis (Smith et al. 1983). If left untreated there is a high rate of progressive disease and nearly 20% of men with this type of prostate cancer die from the malignancy whatever the treatment.

Is surveillance of palpable prostatic malignancy (stage T2/B) safe? If these cancers are not treated, it was reported that only 19% of patients survived for 5 years (Hanash et al. 1972). However, the outlook of patients with such palpable tumours when clinically confined to the prostate depends largely upon their grading and volume. For instance, with low grade (Gleason 2–4) stage B cancers, pelvic lymph nodes may be involved in only 4%–9%; but with high grade (Gleason 8–10) tumours, nodal involvement of stage B cancers can increase from 33% to 43% (Smith et al. 1983).

Therefore, which patients should be actively treated in a programme designed to screen or establish early diagnosis of prostate cancer? From the preceding data, it would be reasonable to keep under surveillance, patients with stage T1a/A prostate cancer unless PSA increases or its tumour becomes palpable (stage T2/B). Active treatment of those with stage T1b/T2 (stage A2/B) prostate cancer should be a balancing act that takes into account:

1. The volume of the cancer, (preferably it should be no larger than 1.5 cm diameter)
2. The histological or Gleason grade of the cancer
3. The potential years of life that the patient has to lose if he remains untreated

Which Active Treatment – Radical Prostatectomy or Irradiation?

Extensive debates have been reported over many years between proponents of radical prostatectomy who claim to cure prostate cancer (which is undoubtedly true for some patients) and advocates of radiotherapy (whom some urologists say do not cure many of their patients).

Direct comparison of the effectiveness of surgery versus radiotherapy is always complicated by variables between different studies, such as grade and staging of the tumour, age and activity of patients, and even changing technology and diagnostic procedures. A comparison of a major series from Stanford University Hospital after irradiation showed no significant difference from surgical series from Johns Hopkins Hospital and the Virginia Mason Medical Centre; the 15-year survival of all series was just over 50% (Hanks 1989). However, a trial of 97 men with stage A2/B prostate cancer when randomised to radical prostatectomy or irradiation suggested better local disease control after surgery (Paulson et al. 1982) but it has been pointed out that as the treatment failures of the irradiated group behaved like stage C disease, the irradiated arm of the trial must have been biased by inadvertent inclusion of patients with stage C cancer (Hanks 1989). Other studies have shown similar disease-specific death rates after radical prostatectomy or irradiation. Middleton and Larsen (1990) reported a disease-specific death rate of 13% for B1 and 23% for B2 prostate cancers 10 years after radical prostatectomy in patients with negative lymph nodes. The overall survival rate of these patients was 71% and 51% respectively of whom none of the survivors had evidence of recurrent disease. After radiotherapy, Kaplan et al. (1992) reported that the actuarial survival for a series of patients with Stanford stage 1 prostate cancer (which is equivalent to UICC stage 2) was 84.2% ± 2.6% at 10 years.

Superficially, there seems to be little to choose between surgery or irradiation, even the loss of potency after nerve sparing prostatectomy or external beam radiotherapy being similar at about 25% (Hanks 1989). Therefore, most British and even some American urologists would consider that a randomised clinical trial to compare the two treatment modalities is the only way to establish firmly and finally the answer to this debate.

Do the Benefits of Screening Outweight the Disadvantages?

Early diagnosis by screening would benefit only those men with the type of prostate cancer that would progress and kill them if untreated and that at the time of treatment could be completely eradicated. Curability is the target for prostate screening but protection of those men with clinically insignificant disease who do not need aggressive treatment is an equally prime issue.

Therefore, is it possible to select out those patients with potentially aggressive cancers so that they can be specifically recommended for treatment? Tumour size is important, particularly as larger tumours become heterogenous (McNeal et al. 1986). On the other hand, sampling by needle-biopsy of small, apparently low-grade prostate cancers may overlook high-grade parts of the same tumour (Epstein and Steinberg 1990) and give a false impression of the oncological potential of the tumour. DNA ploidy analysis by flow cytometry may be useful as a predictor of biological potential and as a prognostic indicator, but this does not have adequate sensitivity or specificity to be useful for screening (Mitchell et al. 1990). Examination of cell proliferation characteristics could indicate the potentialities of small cancers. Nucleolar organiser region (NOR) activity is a sign of cellular proliferation, and it has been claimed that high NOR activity in small prostate cancers predicts potentially aggressive disease (Lardennois et al. 1990). Patients with low proliferating cell nuclear antigen (PCNA) scores survived significantly longer than those with high PCNA scores (Harper et al. 1992a). Studies of the proliferative cell fraction defined by the monoclonal antibody Ki-67 have indicated that decreasing differentiation of prostate carcinoma was associated with higher Ki-67 values; there was also an association with metastases at the time of diagnosis, for patients with M1 disease had higher Ki-67 scores than those known to be M0 category (Harper et al. 1992b). To be of practical value, such investigations for oncological potential of early prostate cancer should ideally be capable of using needle biopsy material taken at the time of histological or cytological biopsy. It is clear, therefore, that at the moment there are few means of selecting men at risk from aggressive disease but studies towards this principle surely must be top of the agenda of scientific priorities for the 1990s.

What harm could come to patients from a screening programme? It is unlikely that DRE, PSA and TRUS would give rise to any serious injury to patients although TRUS-guided biopsy can cause minor complications. The major damage from screening would be of emotional and psychological trauma of false-positive tests and the costs associated with them. However, the greatest threat to patients undergoing screening is unnecessary treatment. The urologist can be a greater threat to the patient than his prostate cancer. For instance radical prostatectomy has a 1%–2% mortality (Walsh 1986) and it has been suggested that if 30% of all men in the USA aged over 50 had an early stage prostate cancer excised and removed by radical retropubic prostatectomy, with a 1% mortality rate, 75 000 deaths could be expected. This would be 45 000 more deaths than the number of men expected to die from prostate cancer itself (Chodak and Schoenberg 1989).

How Expensive is Screening for Prostate Cancer?

Screening by TRUS in the USA has been quoted to be six times as expensive as screening by DRE with a yield of only a 3%–5% detection rate (Hinman 1991). If all 25 million American males aged over 50 were screened by TRUS, of whom 30% might be biopsied, it has been estimated that the cost would be $7 million annually (Chodak and Schoenberg 1989). Furthermore, if all 5000 urologists in the USA spent 15 min per patient carrying out TRUS for screening, they would spend 6 months per year doing nothing else (Chodak and Schoenberg 1989).

Most British urologists agree that no prostate cancer screening programme in the United Kingdom can be based upon TRUS as a primary screening process. It is likely that in England and Wales any early diagnosis or screening programme should be set up at a community level and the only experience of this was the pilot study carried out in Bristol (Chadwick et al. 1991b). This study invited asymptomatic men aged 55–70 years for a health check that included DRE and PSA. Those with a palpably suspicious prostate or m-PSA >4.0 ng/ml were referred for TRUS of whom 29 patients underwent biopsy. Cancer was detected in seven out of 331 men who responded to the invitation (2.1% detection rate). The cost of detecting one treatable prostate cancer in this programme was £1654.10.

A screening programme for prostate cancer has many pitfalls. First, there is "lead time bias" which is the interval that elapses between detection – diagnosis by a screening process and diagnosis by standard means (Love and Camilli 1981). Second, there is "length time bias" in which tumours detected in asymptomatic men will tend to be less aggressive and more indolent than those diagnosed by conventional means in symptomatic patients (Love and Camilli 1981). Third, there is the possibility of over-detection of prostate cancer which is known to have a high prevalance in men aged over 50 years as was demonstrated by the classical autopsy study by Franks (1954). The biggest pitfall of all is to overlook the consequences of a screening programme on screen-positive patients and society in general. The effects of the whole sequence of screening, followed by investigation, followed by treatment and eventual follow-up is frequently overlooked and those embarking towards screening for prostate cancer would do well to read the review by Optenberg and Thompson (1990) concerning the economics of prostate screening on a national basis in the USA. They estimated that a national screening programme would change spending allocation for prostate cancer from 0.06% of the total health care budget of $458.2 billion annually to a slice of over 5% of that figure. Comparatively, in the United Kingdom, expense on such a scale is beyond the national purse. However, the epidemiological warning signs of an impending health care overload of prostatic cancer cannot be swept under the carpet and ignored. Therefore, the immediate priorities should focus on (a) recognition of those men at risk of developing prostatic cancer, (b) developing improved techniques of early detection and diagnosis, (c) methods to select those who should be treated and who might die if left alone and (d) lowering the morbidity of aggressive treatments such as radical prostatectomy and radiotherapy by searching for ways of in situ surgical or medical eradication of early prostatic cancers. Although screening on a national scale may be unaffordable, new insight into the natural history of prostate cancer can only emerge if controlled early diagnosis programmes are accepted in principle and carried out properly.

Can Endocrine Therapy be Improved?

Advanced-stage prostate cancer is generally accepted to mean locally invasive, apparently non-metastatic cancers (stage T3 N0 M0; stage C), those with involved pelvic lymph nodes, or disseminated spread of the disease. In numerical terms, it is a significant health problem because untreated, advanced-stage prostate cancer – particularly disseminated disease – will almost invariably progress within 5 years and those with M1 disease (stage D2) have a median survival of about 30 months with an expected 5-year survival rate of about 20%. Consequently, most of these patients will develop symptoms and will seek treatment to alleviate these, but only about 70% will respond objectively and subjectively to any form of "androgen deprivation". Duration of response may vary from several months to several years, with the majority of patients with initial disseminated disease relapsing into a hormone-refractory state within 6–18 months.

There is no doubting the effectiveness and the role of androgen-deprivation treatment as effective management for advanced stage prostate cancer, but as it is a purely palliative process, not achieving cure, in recent years increasing attention has been directed towards the quality of life of men undergoing this form of treatment rather than length of survival. Consequently, several controversies have arisen particularly relating to the best form of treatment to be used, and the timing of treatment, when the debate is usually directed not only at the effectiveness of symptomatic relief but also at such issues as improved times to progression, increased activity and well-being.

Which Treatment?

Orchidectomy, Oestrogen or LHRH Agonist?

For half a century bilateral total orchidectomy has been the gold standard as the best primary endocrine therapy for advanced prostate cancer. It has been pointed out repeatedly that this is the quickest way to reduce plasma testosterone as a castrate state may be reached in 2.5 h. Furthermore, orchidectomy involves a single procedure, rather than a lifetime commitment for regular medication. Nevertheless, in some individuals, and particularly in some parts of Europe and elsewhere, there is profound distaste for an empty scrotum which for psychological and cultural reasons can be a humiliation incompatible with self-respect.

As an alternative to total orchidectomy, bilateral subcapsular orchidectomy leaves the shell of the testis in the scrotum and has been demonstrated to be as effective as total orchidectomy in achieving a castrate state (Burge et al. 1976). DES 1 mg tds will also reduce plasma testosterone concentrations to castrate levels but side effects of DES, such as gynaecomastia, nausea and particularly cardiovascular toxicity which were exposed by VACURG (Arduino et al. 1967) have discredited this drug. Despite these drawbacks, it is still widely used in some places. Nevertheless, although DES given in conventional doses is no longer considered to be safe, there is a very attractive argument for its use at 1 mg/day. At that dose there is little chance of cardiovascular complications but its clinical effectiveness is as good as DES taken at 5 mg/day (Byar 1973). This is surprising because plasma testosterone levels will not be fully suppressed to castrate range (Shearer et al. 1973). "Minidose DES" (0.1 mg/day) when combined with megestrol acetate (120 mg/day) has been claimed to give clinical results equal to DES (3 mg/day) for patients with M1 (stage D2) disease but with much less toxicity than DES at conventional dosage (Venner et al. 1988).

In Scandinavia, oestrogens still hold favour. Unlike DES 1 mg tds, the long-acting intramuscular oestrogen polyoestradiol phosphate (Estradurin), only suppresses LH secretion weakly (Jonsson et al. 1975) but when combined with oral ethinyloestradiol, the combination was shown to be more effective in delaying progression of advanced prostate cancer than orchidectomy alone, particularly in patients with M1 disease (Haapiainen et al. 1991). Perhaps this benefit for the oestrogen-treated group was due to a cytotoxic effect of oestrogens, but the mortality was not different from patients treated by orchidectomy. This combination of oestrogens was associated with less toxicity than that expected from DES.

In the 1970s various progestational steroids were investigated as alternative treatment to oestrogens. These included medroxyprogesterone acetate (Provera), hydroxyprogesterone acetate (Delalutin) and chlormadinone acetate but their clinical effectiveness was never evaluated by randomised clinical trials. Furthermore, their role in the treatment of prostate cancer was overshadowed by the development of LHRH agonists such as goserelin (Zoladex) as primary treatment for advanced stage disease. It was established, for instance, from phase I and phase II clinical studies that the slow-release (depot) formulation of goserelin injected subcutaneously as a 3.6 mg pellet every 28 days effectively reduced serum testosterone to castrate levels after about 15 days (Walker et al. 1984). Phase III studies indicated that long-term treatment of the depot formulation of goserelin (3.6 mg monthly) was clinically no different from orchidectomy and that side effects were, if anything, slightly less than after orchidectomy (Peeling 1987). Phase III studies have also clearly demonstrated the safety of goserelin over DES (Waymont et al. 1992). Studies with other LHRH analogues such as buserelin and leuprorelin have indicated a similar role to goserelin in the treatment of advanced prostate cancer. The current trend is towards development of longer-acting depot formulations such as a 3-monthly preparation of goserelin (10.8 mg) which, in a preliminary report, has been shown to be comparable with the monthly 3.6 mg formulation of the drug (Dijkman et al. 1990).

Rather surprisingly, considerable debate has developed on two counts since depot LHRH analogues have proved their place as alternatives to orchidectomy. First, there has been the question "which do patients prefer – surgical or medical orchidectomy?" That gives rise to the ethical rights of patients to be involved in their choice of treatment. In Austria, 86% of patients when offered a choice, selected medical castration with goserelin (Lunglmayr and Girsch 1987); in the USA, 78% chose goserelin (Cassileth et al. 1989) whereas in Bristol 23 of 50 patients (46%) chose orchidectomy because they preferred a single short stay in hospital rather than a commitment for monthly visits to hospital or a local health centre for LHRH injections (Chadwick et al. 1991a). Those patients in the USA who chose orchidectomy did so for similar reasons, whereas those who chose LHRH depot wished to avoid an operation (Cassileth et al. 1989; Chadwick et al. 1991a). When questioned after 3 months in the Austrian and American surveys, over 90% of patients and their wives were satisfied with their original choice of treatment.

Few would disagree that the patient's preference is important but there are urologists who point out that the relative costs of LHRH agonists and orchidectomy, and the time taken to see patients in clinics for their monthly injections, have to be important factors in favour of orchidectomy or even DES over LHRH analogues. No treatment is less expensive than DES which at a dose of 3 mg/day costs £60 per year for each patient. The cost of goserelin is about £1200 for 12 months treatment but there is considerable disagreement about the cost of orchidectomy. According to McClinton et al. (1989), this was up to £287.59p but other estimates made in 1987 from 51 hospitals in the United Kingdom varied from an average of £113 to £525 for NHS hospitals, to £660 for private hospitals in the NHS, and to £815 in private hospitals (Peeling 1991). In that survey it was pointed out that the break-even point for the cost of goserelin with the cost of orchidectomy in NHS hospitals was 5 months but in private hospitals it was 8 months. Consequently if drug costs remain unchanged or fall, and hospital costs continue to rise each year as at the present time, there might come a time when it will be surgical castration that will be uneconomical and not medical castration with LHRH analogues.

When Should Total Androgen Blockade be Used?

There has always been considerable unease that no endocrine treatment of advanced stage prostate cancer has achieved more than a 60%–70% response rate, so the claim by Labrie et al. (1983) that combination therapy of an LHRH agonist with an antiandrogen achieved a positive objective response rate of 97% was startling. These observations were not based on a randomised clinical trial and subsequent properly controlled trials have not substantiated the extent of Labrie's claims. Nevertheless, some have given limited support to the concept of total androgen blockade reporting, for instance, that combination therapy (leuprorelin and the antiandrogen flutamide) showed significant advantages for median time to progression and median time to survival (by 2.6 months and 7.3 months respectively) when compared with monotherapy by leuprorelin (Crawford et al, 1989).

A significantly delayed time to progression was also observed when a combination of goserelin and flutamide was used (Denis et al. 1991) whereas in two other trials with this combination there was no benefit at all (Iversen et al. 1990; Tyrrell et al. 1991). Nor was there any apparent advantage for combination therapy by means of surgical castration plus antiandrogen (Beland et al. 1991).

The concept of total androgen blockade presupposes that androgens of adrenocortical origin are sufficient to maintain and stimulate the activity and growth of hormone-sensitive prostate cancer cells that have previously been suppressed by orchidectomy or LHRH agonists. Proponents of the hypothesis base their views on in vitro studies of androgen sensitivity (Labrie et al. 1988), but other evidence based upon the human situation suggests that normal adrenal glands do not have a significant stimulating effect on human prostatic tissue and are not capable of maintaining prostatic growth (Oesterling et al. 1986). Is there yet a case for total androgen blockade? Clinical studies do not show clear cut support for such a policy, and therefore total androgen blockade would hardly be justified for routine use particularly as it is extremely expensive. Alternatively, there could be a case for routine combination therapy by castration and an antiandrogen specifically for patients with "minimal disease" for it was this group that had significantly better progression-free survival after combination therapy when compared with patients with more advanced metastatic disease (Crawford and Nabors 1991).

When to Treat?: Early, Deferred or Intermittent Endocrine Therapy?

For 25 years after the work of Huggins and Hodges (1941) prompt androgen-deprivation treatment for men with advanced-stage prostate cancer was recommended because analysis of the clinical effect of orchidectomy, DES or both treatments combined had shown a survival benefit (Nesbit and Baum 1950). These studies were retrospective, non-randomised and used historical controls, but were nevertheless highly influential in clinical urology until the results of the first VACURG study were published (Arduino et al. 1967). In this trial, 1764 men with stage C or D prostate cancers were randomised into four treatment groups: (a) placebo, (b) bilateral orchidectomy, (c) DES 5 mg/day, (d) orchidectomy with DES 5 mg/day. For placebo patients, as soon as progression of disease was recorded, hormone therapy was commenced. Consequently, the placebo group could be regarded as having received deferred endocrine treatment. Analysis of the data showed, however, that "deferred hormone treatment" had not affected survival of these patients adversely and was not inferior to any of the other active treatment arms.

A second VACURG study randomised patients of similar clinical status to: (a) placebo, (b) DES 0.2 mg/day, (c) DES 1 mg/day, (d) DES 5 mg/day (Byar 1973, 1977). This work also indicated that there was no difference of overall survival between the treatment arms, and in particular placebo was no worse than active treatment with DES. Other studies also suggested that hormonal treatment does not increase survival in men with advanced prostate cancer (Lepor et al. 1982).

Consequently, a view has developed that, if timing of treatment in the VACURG studies had no significant influence on survival, it would be reasonable to defer initiation of endocrine treatment until patients develop symptoms; at the same time side effects from treatment such as impotence would also be deferred. The arguments in favour have been reviewed by Kirk (1987) but he pointed out that in the VACURG protocols, conversion of placebo-designated patients onto active endocrine treatment was ill-defined and that in reality these studies suggested the option of deferred treatment. Nevertheless, uncertainty about the clinical merits of this issue may not even be resolved when the findings of the Medical Research Council trial has been made known, in which patients with advanced prostate cancer have been randomised to undergo either immediate orchidectomy or orchidectomy deferred until symptoms occur (Kirk 1987). In this trial, survival is unlikely to be affected by either of these policies and time to progression may be difficult to pin-point. The absence of obvious symptoms in patients with advanced prostate cancer such as bone pain may hide more subtle effects due to anaemia, weight loss, loss of energy and well-being, all of which are difficult to measure but are so important to patients and their families. Theoretically, it could be argued that early treatment with a smaller tumour burden is more likely to be effective than later treatment when tumour burden is greater with an increased chance of dedifferentiation. Furthermore, can a deferred treatment policy be justified to patients some of whom may develop urinary retention from growth of the primary cancer requiring transurethral resection, ureteric obstruction, or pathological fractures or paraplegia? In other words, what is the chance of harm coming to men with advanced prostate cancer whose treatment is deferred until they complain of pain or other symptoms? In the placebo arm of the VACURG study, 70% of men with stage C prostate cancer and 100% of those with stage D disease required hormonal treatment. More recently, it was reported that 49% of 278 patients managed by a deferred treatment policy, required eventual treatment because of progressive disease. It was of particular concern that 17% of patients who died from prostate cancer in this study had done so without receiving treatment (Handley et al. 1988).

What are the risks of immediate hormone treatment? Side effects from orchidectomy, LHRH agonists, and even DES 1 mg/day frequently occur but may be of more nuisance value to some patients than real harm. Antiandrogens such as flutamide are usually well tolerated although they may cause gastrointestinal upsets and gynaecomastia (like DES). There are theoretical arguments that early androgen deprivation can disrupt the clonal balance between androgen-dependent, androgen-sensitive and androgen-independent cell populations (Bruchovsky et al. 1990).

What benefits could result from early hormonal intervention? The VACURG studies demonstrated that untreated stage C disease progressed to stage D at a rate of 30% at 24 months and 50% at 52 months, whereas progression from stage C to stage D disease was reduced from 50% to 10% when DES 1 mg/day or 5 mg/day was given (Byar 1973; Blackard 1975). Recently, it was observed that in patients with D1 prostate cancer there were advantages for both time to progression to stage D2 disease and also survival for those undergoing immediate endocrine treatment (Kramolovsky 1988). In laboratory studies on Dunning R3327 rat prostate adenocarcinoma, androgen ablation (with or without chemotherapy) was most effective and increased survival when given early (Isaacs, 1984).

Therefore the evidence supporting either side of the debate about the timing of hormone treatment for advanced prostate cancer gives little help to urologists, but it is of considerable interest that a recent review of VACURG data using a covariate analysis has suggested that certain patients may benefit from immediate treatment (Byar and Corle 1988). Younger patients with more aggressive stage D prostate cancers (Gleason score 7–10) had a survival benefit when hormonal treatment was commenced at the time of diagnosis but at least 3 years follow-up was needed to show differences between the early and deferred treatment groups.

A third approach to management of patients with advanced prostate cancer requiring hormonal treatment could be by intermittent administration of drugs. This has received little attention and is controversial. In experiments involving a hormone-dependent breast cancer in the Noble rat, it was found that moderate reduction of hormone levels diminished tumour growth while progression to a hormone-independent state was delayed. On the other hand, castration accelerated progression towards hormone-independent autonomy and death of the animal (Noble 1977). Also of great interest are studies of the progression of androgen-dependent Shionogi mouse mammary carcinoma to an androgen-independent condition (Bruchovsky et al. 1990). It was observed that androgen withdrawal by castration altered the ratio of stem cells in the tumour cell population, and that with progression and recurrence of the carcinoma there was a 20-fold increase in the proportion of stem cells and a 500-fold increase in the number of androgen-independent stem cells over the proportions measured in the parent tumour. These results suggested that development of androgen-independent stem cells in the recurrent Shionogi carcinoma was linked to discontinuation of androgen-induced differentiation of stem cells in the parent tumour. It was suggested that if androgens are replaced before progression begins, the surviving stem cells should give rise to an androgen-dependent tumour which is amenable to retreatment by androgen withdrawal.

These experimental observations, albeit in rodents, suggest that incomplete, or intermittent, androgen withdrawal in patients with prostate cancer might influence the development of hormone-refractory disease. However, clinical experience with intermittent endocrine treatment for advanced stage prostate cancer has been anecdotal and has shown no survival benefit whatsoever although there was satisfactory symptomatic palliation with improved quality of life because of preservation of sexual function (Klotz et al. 1986; Bruchovsky, unpublished data). It would be unreasonable to expect intermittent endocrine treatment for such patients to give better survival than standard endocrine regimes for it has to be presumed that hormone refractory clones of prostate cancer cells would already have been established before treatment had commenced. Nevertheless, it has already been noted in this review that screening for prostate cancer should search for tumours of ≤ 1.5 cm in diameter because these are most likely to be well differentiated. Therefore, if experimental data from Noble and Bruchovsky are to have an area of application to prostate cancer, it should be for treatment of early tumours before they tend towards dedifferentiation. It is most unlikely that conventional endocrine therapy can be improved dramatically for all reasonable combinations of treatment modalities have already been tried and none has proved to be markedly superior to orchidectomy. It is arguable that the only new concept in recent years about endocrine therapy arises from the experimental observations of Noble and Bruchovsky but if there is an area of clinical application from these, it should be towards treatment of early prostate cancer with either intermittent or incomplete androgen depression but, as with all other studies of treatment in early stage prostate cancer, a ten or even 15 year follow-up period would need to be undertaken to assess its worth.

References

Arduino LJ et al. (Veterans Administration Co-operative Urological Research Group) (1967) Carcinoma of the prostate: treatment comparisons. J Urol 98:516–522

Babaian RJ, Miyashita H, Evans RB, Ramirez EJ (1992) The distribution of prostate specific antigen in men without clinical or pathological evidence of prostate cancer: relationship to gland volume and age. J Urol 147:837–840

Beland G, Elhilali M, Fradet Y et al. (1991) Total androgen ablation: Canadian experience. Urol Clin North Am 18:75–82

Bertermann H (1990) Ultrasound-guided prostatic biopsy. In: Peeling WB (ed.) The role of imaging in prostatic cancer. Medical Group (UK) Limited, Abingdon, Oxon. pp 51–57

Blackard CE (1975) The Veterans Administrative Co-operative Urological Research Group studies of carcinoma of the prostate: a review. Cancer Chemother Rep 59:225–227

Blandy JP (1991) The rationale for screening for cancer of the prostate. The arguments against. Urol Top 4:40–41

Boring CC, Squires TS, Tong T (1991) Cancer statistics, 1991. Cancer 41:19–36

Brawer MK, Chetner MP, Beatie J, Buchner DM, Vessella RL, Lange PH (1992) Screening for prostatic cancer with prostate specific antigen. J Urol 147:841–845

Bruchovsky N, Rennie PS, Coldman AJ, Goldenberg SL, To M, Lawson D (1990) The effects of androgen withdrawal on the stem cell composition of the Shionogi carcinoma. Cancer Res 50:2275–2282

Burge PD, Harper ME, Hartog M, Gingell JC (1976) Subcapsular orchidectomy – an effective operation? Proc R Soc Med 69:663–664

Byar DP (1973) The Veterans Administrative Co-operative Urological Research Group studies of cancer of the prostate. Cancer 32:1126–1130

Byar DP (1977) VACURG studies on prostatic cancer and its treatment. In: Tannenbaum M (ed.) Urologic pathology: the prostate. Lea and Febiger, Philadelphia, pp 241–267

Byar DP, Corle DK (1988) Hormone therapy for prostate cancer: results of the Veterans Administrative Co-operative Urological Research Group studies. In: Consensus Development Conference in the management of clinically localized prostate cancer. NCI Monogr 7:165–170

Cantrell BB, de Klerk DP, Eggleston JC, Botnott JK, Walsh PC (1981) Pathological factors that influence prognosis in stage A prostate cancer. The influence of extent versus grade. J Urol 125:516–520

Carter HB, Coffey DS (1988) Prostate cancer: the magnitude of the problem in the United States. In: Coffey DS, Resnick MI, Dorr FA et al. (eds) A multidisciplinary analysis of controversies in the management of prostatic cancer. Plenum Press, New York, pp 1–7

Cassileth BR, Soloway MS, Vogelzang NJ et al. (1989) Patients' choice of treatment in stage D prostate cancer. Urology 33 (suppl):57–62

Catalona WJ, Smith DS, Ratliff TL et al. (1991) Measurement of prostate-specific antigen in serum as a screening test for prostate cancer. N Engl J Med 324:1156–1161

Chadwick DJ, Gillatt DA, Gingell JC (1991a) Medical or surgical orchidectomy: the patients' choice. Br Med J 302:572

Chadwick DJ, Kemple T, Astley JP et al. (1991b) Pilot study of screening for prostate cancer in general practice. Lancet 338:613–615

Chisholm GD (1981) Carcinoma of the prostate: perspectives and prospects. In: Duncan W (ed) Prostate cancer – Recent results in cancer research. Volume 78. Springer-Verlag, Heidelberg, pp 173–184

Chodak GW, Schoenberg HW (1989) Progress and problems in screening for carcinoma of the prostate. World J Surg 13:60–64

Chodak GW, Keller P, Schoenberg HW (1989) Assessment of screening for prostate cancer using the digital rectal examination. J Urol 141:1136–1138

Clements R, Griffiths GJ, Peeling WB, Roberts EE, Evans KT (1988) How accurate is the index finger? A comparison of digital and ultrasound examination of the prostatic nodule. Clin Radiol 39:87–89

Clements R, Penney MD, Etherington RJ, Griffiths GJ, Hughes H, Peeling WB (1992) Volume of normal prostate, of prostate cancer and benign prostatic hyperplasia: are correlations with prostate specific antigen clinically useful? Prostate (Suppl 4):51–57

Crawford ED, Nabors WL (1991) Total androgen ablation: American experience. Urol Clin North Am 18:55–63

Crawford ED, Eisenberger MA, McLeod DG et al. (1989) A controlled trial of leuprolide with and without flutamide in prostatic carcinoma. N Engl J Med 321:419–424

Dahnert WF, Hamper UM, Eggleston JC, Walsh PC, Sanders RC (1986) Prostatic evaluation by transrectal sonography with histopathologic correlation: the echopenic appearance of early carcinoma. Radiology 158:97–102

Denis L, Smith P, Carneiro de Moura JL et al. (1991) Total androgen ablation: European experience. Urol Clin North Am 18:65–73

Dijkman GA, Fernandez del Moral P, Plasman JWMH et al. (1990) A new longer-acting LHRH analog depot: preliminary results of a Dutch open phase II clinical study on a 10.8 mg Zoladex 3-monthly depot. Eur Urol 18 (suppl 3):22–25

Drago JR, Badalament RA (1990) Prostate cancer: early detection and screening. In: Resnick MI (ed) Prostatic ultrasonography. B C Decker Inc, Philadelphia, pp 103–112

Dyke CH, Toi A, Sweet JM (1990) Value of random ultrasound-guided transrectal prostate biopsy. Radiology 176:345–349

Epstein JI, Steinberg GD (1990) The significance of low-grade prostate cancer on needle biopsy. Cancer 66:1927–1932

Epstein JI, Paull G, Eggleston JC, Walsh PC (1986) Prognosis of untreated stage A1 prostatic carcinoma: a study of 94 cases with extended follow-up. J Urol 136:837–839

Esposti PL, Franzen S (1980) Transrectal aspiration biopsy of the prostate. A re-evaluation of the method in the diagnosis of prostatic carcinoma. Scand J Urol Nephrol (Suppl 55):49–52

Fornage BD (1988) Ultrasound guided biopsy. In: Fornage BD (ed) Ultrasound of the prostate. Wiley, Chichester, pp 239–269

Franks LM (1954) Latent carcinoma of the prostate. J Pathol Bacteriol 68:603–616

Gerber GS, Chodak GW (1990) Digital rectal examination in the early detection of prostate cancer. Urol Clin North Am 17:739–744

Haapiainen R, Rannikko S, Ruutu M et al. (1991) Orchiectomy versus oestrogen in the treatment of advanced prostatic cancer. Br J Urol 67:184–187

Hanash KA, Utz DC, Cook EN, Taylor WF, Titus JL (1972) Carcinoma of the prostate – a 15 year follow-up. J Urol 107:450–453

Handley R, Carr TW, Travis D, Powell PH, Hall RR (1988) Deferred treatment for prostate cancer. Br J Urol 62:249–253

Hanks GE (1989) External beam radiation therapy for prostate cancer clinically confined to the gland. Urology 33 (suppl):21–26

Harper ME, Glynne-Jones E, Goddard L et al. (1992a) Relationship of proliferating cell nuclear antigen (PCNA) in prostatic carcinomas to various clinical parameters. Prostate 20:243–253

Harper ME, Goddard L, Wilson DW et al. (1992b) Pathological and clinical associations of Ki-67 defined growth fractions in human prostatic carcinoma. Prostate 20:371–376

Hillyard JW (1987) Bacteraemia following perineal prostatic biopsy. Br J Urol 60:252–254

Hinman H Jr (1991) Screening for prostatic carcinoma. J Urol 145:126–130

Hodge KK, McNeal JE, Stamey TA (1989) Ultrasound guided transrectal core biopsies of the palpably abnormal prostate. J Urol 142:66–70

Horm JW, Asire AJ, Young JL, Pollack ES (1984) Cancer incidence and mortality in the United States: 1973–81. NIH Publication No 85–1837, National Cancer Institute, November 1984

Huggins C, Hodges CV (1941) Studies on prostate cancer I: The effect of castration, of estrogen and of androgen injection on serum phosphatases in metastatic carcinoma of the prostate. Cancer Res 1:293–297

Isaacs JT (1984) The timing of androgen ablation therapy and/or chemotherapy in the treatment of prostatic cancer. Prostate 5:1–17

Iversen P, Suciu S, Sylvester R, Christensen I, Denis L (1990) Zoladex and flutamide versus orchiectomy in the treatment of advanced prostatic cancer. Cancer 66:1067–1073

Jewett HJ (1975) The present status of radical prostatectomy for stages A & B prostatic cancer. Urol Clin North Am 2:105–124

Jonsson G, Olsson AM, Luttrop W, Cekan Z, Purvis K, Diczfalusy E (1975) Treatment of prostatic carcinoma with various types of oestrogen derivatives. Vitam Horm 33:351–376

Kaplan ID, Prestidge BR, Bagshaw MA, Cox RS (1992) The importance of local control in the treatment of prostatic cancer. J Urol 147:917–921

Kaufman JJ, Schultz JI (1962) Needle biopsy of the prostate: a re-evaluation. J Urol 87:164–168

Kirk D (1987) Trials & Tribulations in prostatic cancer. Br J Urol 59:375–379

Klotz LH, Herr HW, Morse MJ, Whitmore WF Jr (1986) Intermittent endocrine therapy for advanced prostate cancer. Cancer 58:2546–2550

Kramolovsky EV (1988) The value of testosterone deprivation in stage D1 carcinoma of the prostate. J Urol 139:1242–1244

Labrie F, Dupont A, Belanger A et al. (1983) New approaches in the treatment of prostate cancer: complete instead of partial withdrawal of androgens. Prostate 4:579–594

Labrie F, Veilleux R, Fournier A (1988) Low androgen levels induce the development of androgen-hypersensitive cell clones in Shionogi mouse mammary carcinoma cells in culture. J Natl Cancer Inst 80:1138–1147

Lardennois B, Vazeux H, Visseaux-Coletto B, Adnet JJ, Ploton D (1990) The value of nucleolar organizer regions (NORs) with the histo-prognosis determination of prostatic cancer. Eur Urol 18(suppl 1):68

Lee F, Littrup PJ, McLeary RD et al. (1987) Needle aspiration and core biopsy of prostate cancer: comparative evaluation with biplanar transrectal US guidance. Radiology 163:515–520

Lee F, Littrup PJ, Torp-Pedersen ST et al. (1988) Prostate cancer: comparison of transrectal ultrasound and digital rectal examination for screening. Radiology 168:389–394

Lee F, Torp-Pedersen ST, Littrup PJ et al. (1989) Hypoechoic lesions of the prostate: clinical relevance of tumor size, digital rectal examination and prostate-specific antigen. Radiology 170:29–32

Lepor H, Ross A, Walsh PC (1982) The influence of hormonal therapy on survival of men with advanced prostatic cancer. J Urol 128:335–340

Littrup PJ, Kane RA, Williams CR et al. (1991) Determination of prostate volume with transrectal ultrasound for cancer screening. Part I: comparison with prostate specific antigen assays. Radiology 178:537–542

Love RR, Camilli AE (1981) The value of screening. Cancer 48:489–494

Lowe BA, Listrom MB (1988) Incidental carcinoma of the prostate: an analysis of the predictors of progression. J Urol 140:1340–1344

Lunglmayr G, Girsch E (1987) Patient choice in the treatment of advanced prostate cancer. In: Chisholm GD (ed) Zoladex, a new treatment for prostatic cancer. Alden Press, Oxford (Royal Society of Medicine Services International Congress & Symposium Series, No. 125) pp 47–51

McClinton S, Moffat LEF, Ludbrook A (1989) The cost of bilateral orchidectomy as a treatment for prostatic carcinoma. Br J Urol 63:309–312

McNeal JE, Bostwick DG, Kindrachuk RA, Redwine EA, Freiha FS, Stamey TA (1986) Patterns of progression in prostate cancer. Lancet i:60–63

Middleton RG, Larsen RH (1990) Radical prostatectomy for Stage B disease. Urol Clin North Am 17:779–785

Mitchell CB, Ring K, Giella J (1990) Flow cytometry in carcinoma of the prostate. Urol Clin North Am 17:885–891

Nesbit RM, Baum WC (1950) Endocrine control of prostatic carcinoma: clinical and statistical survey of 1818 cases. JAMA 143:1317–1320

Noble RL (1977) Hormonal control of growth and progression in tumors of Nb rats and a theory of action. Cancer Res 37:82–94

Oesterling JE, Epstein JI, Walsh PC (1986) The viability of adrenal androgens to stimulate the adult human prostate: an autopsy evaluation of men with gonadotrophic hypogonadism and panhypopituitarism. J Urol 136:1030–1034

Office of Population Censuses and Surveys (1976) In: Series DH2 No.1. Cancer statistics: mortality in England and Wales, 1974. HMSO, London

Office of Population Censuses and Surveys (1991a) In: Series MB1 No. 19. Cancer statistics: registrations: cases of diagnosed cancer registered in England & Wales, 1986. HMSO, London

Office of Population Censuses and Surveys (1991b) In: Series DH2 No. 17. Cancer statistics: mortality in England and Wales, 1990. HMSO, London

Office of Population Censuses and Surveys (1992) England and Wales: Population Estimate Unit. HMSO, London

Optenberg SA, Thompson IM (1990) Economics of screening for carcinoma of the prostate. Urol Clin North Am 17:719–737

Paulson DF, Lin GH, Hinshaw W, Stephani S and the Uro-Oncology Research Group (1982) Radical surgery versus radiotherapy for adenocarcinoma of the prostate. J Urol 128:502–504

Peeling WB (1987) A phase III trial comparing ICI 118630 (Zoladex) with orchidectomy in the management of advanced prostatic cancer. In: Chisholm GD (ed) Zoladex, a new treatment for prostatic cancer. Alden press, Oxford, (Royal Society of Medicine Services International Congress and Symposium Series, No 125) pp 27–44

Peeling WB (1991) Are stilboestrol and orchidectomy outmoded? In: Alderson AR, Oliver RTD, Hanham IWF, Bloom HJG (eds) Urological oncology. Dilemmas and developments. Wiley, Chichester, pp 203–210

Peeling WB, Griffiths GJ (1984) Imaging of the prostate by ultrasound J Urol 132:217–224

Reece D (1991) Breast cancer screening is doing well. Br Med J 302:311

Rifkin MD, Choi H (1988) Implications of small, peripheral hypoechoic lesions in endorectal ultrasound of the prostate. Radiology 166:619–622

Salo JO, Rannikko S, Makinen J, Lehtonen T (1987) Echogenic structure of prostatic cancer imaged on radical prostatectomy specimens. Prostate 10:1–9

Shearer RJ, Hendry WF, Sommerville IF, Fergusson JD (1973) Plasma testosterone: an accurate monitor of hormone treatment in prostatic cancer. Br J Urol 45:668–677

Smith JA Jr, Seaman JP, Gleidman JB, Middleton RG (1983) Pelvic lymph node metastasis from prostatic cancer: influence of tumor grade and stage in 452 consecutive patients. J Urol 130:290–292

Smith PH (1990) The case for no initial treatment of localized prostate cancer. Urol Clin North Am 17:827–834

Stamey TA (1982) Cancer of the prostate. An analysis of some important contributions and dilemmas. Monogr Urol 3:67–94

Stamey TA, Yang N, Hay AR, McNeal JE, Freiha FS, Redwine E (1987) Prostate specific antigen as a serum marker for adenocarcinoma of the prostate. N Engl J Med 317:909–916

Thompson IM, Ernst JJ, Gangai MP, Spence CR (1984) Adenocarcinoma of the prostate: results of routine urological screening. J Urol 132:690–692

Torp-Pedersen S, Lee F, Littrup PJ et al. (1989) Transrectal biopsy of the prostate guided with transrectal ultrasound: longitudinal and planar scanning. Radiology 170:23–27

Tyrrell CJ, Altwein JE, Klippel F et al. (1991) A multicenter randomized trial comparing the luteinizing hormone-releasing hormone analogue goserelin acetate alone and with flutamide in the treatment of advanced prostate cancer. J Urol 146:1321–1326

Union Internationale Contre le Cancer (1978) In: Harmer MH (ed) TNM Classification of malignant tumours, 3rd edn. G. de Buren SA, Geneva, pp 118–121

Union Internationale Contre le Cancer (1987) In: Hermanek P, Sobin LH (eds) TNM classification of malignant tumours, 4th edn. Springer-Verlag, Berlin, pp. 121–126

Venner PM, Klotz G, Klotz LH et al. (1988) Megestrol acetate plus minidose diethylstilbestrol in the treatment of carcinoma of the prostate. Semin Oncol 15 (suppl 1):62–67

Vikho P, Kontturi M, Lukkarinen O, Ervasti J, Vikho R (1985) Screening for carcinoma of the prostate. Rectal examination, and enzymatic and radio-immunologic measurements of serum acid phosphatase compared. Cancer 56:173–177

Walker KJ, Turkes AO, Turkes A et al. (1984) Treatment of patients with advanced cancer of the prostate using a slow release (depot) formulation of the LHRH agonist ICI 118630 (Zoladex). J Endocrinol 103:R1–R4

Walsh PC (1986) Radical retropubic prostatectomy. In: Walsh PC, Gittes RF, Perlmutter AD,

Stamey TA (eds) Campbell's urology, Vol 2, 5th edn. W B Saunders Co, Philadelphia, pp 2772–2775
Walsh PC (1992) Why make an early diagnosis of prostate cancer. J Urol 147:853–854
Waymont B, Lynch TH, Dunn JA et al. (1992) Phase III randomised study of Zoladex versus stilboestrol in the treatment of advanced prostate cancer. Br J Urol 69:614–620
Whitmore WF Jr (1956) Hormone therapy in prostatic cancer. Am J Med 21:697–713
Wilson JMG, Jungner G (1968) Principles and practice of screening for disease. In: Public Health Paper No 4, World Health Organization, Geneva, pp 26–27

Chapter 8

Biochemistry of Prostate Cancer

F. K. Habib

Introduction

Research on the prostate and other male accessory sexual organs is producing new insights into the regulatory mechanisms responsible for the normal and abnormal growth of the prostate. This chapter is an attempt to review some of the most recent developments in both fundamental and clinical research on the endocrinology of the human prostate and to highlight the significance of the findings on the long-term management of prostate cancer.

For many years there was a prevailing consensus that the prostate was regulated only by androgens. However, it now appears that androgens are not directly implicated in the initiation of DNA synthesis but that other regulatory factors may also be involved. Some of these non-steroidal factors act in synergy with androgens to ensure the normal growth of the prostate whereas others bypass steroid hormones and imprint their own characteristics on the gland thus rendering the prostate cell androgen independent. Much of our understanding of these alternative processes has been made possible due in part to the powerful tools of recombinant DNA technology combined with a refined understanding of the biological processes in the cell.

The body of the literature relating to the mechanisms of metabolism in the prostate is vast and still growing. This chapter is by no means a survey of the advances in the field but merely an attempt to identify target areas with particular relevance to future management of cancer of the prostate.

Androgen Regulation

Since the pioneering work of Huggins and Hodges (1941), androgen deprivation has become the primary therapy for patients with metastatic prostate cancer. Even so, 20% of tumours do not respond to endocrine manipulation. Furthermore, remission is transient and, following a variable period of response, the tumours become refractory to endocrine treatment and a hormone-unresponsive tumour develops. Many attempts have been made to identify the cellular and molecular factors associated with this transition. The key to our understanding lies in the mechanism(s) that are interspersed between the entry of the steroid hormone into the cell and the activation of transcription of androgen responsive genes.

The fundamental model for the mechanism of action of androgens in the prostate follows an integrated sequence of events described by Habib (1990). Initially, the entering testosterone molecule is metabolised to dihydrotestosterone (DHT) in a reaction catalysed by the nuclear membrane-bound steroid 5α-reductase enzyme. DHT, in turn, binds to nuclear protein receptors which exhibit a high affinity and a selective preference for this steroid. The formation of DHT–androgen receptor complexes is crucial to the biological pathways concerned with both growth regulation and the synthesis and secretion of secretory proteins (Montgomery et al. 1992). The binding of DHT to androgen receptors releases the DNA binding domain of the receptor protein allowing it to associate with hormone responsive elements (HRE) of the genome thereby modulating the transcription of specific genes and the regulation of particular biological responses (Tsai et al. 1991). Therefore, both androgen receptors acting as transcription factors and 5α-reductase, modulating intracellular DHT concentrations, are essential to the normal growth, function and differentiation of the human prostate gland. Additionally, a functionally active receptor is essential for the growth of androgen-dependent prostate cells. Whether a modification in the structure of either the androgen-metabolising enzyme or indeed the receptor would lead to the development of androgen-insensitive tumours has not been satisfactorily resolved. Part of the problem stems from an incomplete knowledge of the molecular structure of the genes for both 5α-reductase and androgen receptor. However, over the last few years considerable advances have been made in this area and this is enhancing our knowledge of the mechanisms regulating the expression of both the 5α-reductase and androgen receptor in healthy and diseased prostates.

Steroid 5α-reductase

The incidence of prostate cancer varies widely between countries and ethnic groups. To account for these perplexing patterns, a study was undertaken to investigate whether differences in serum androgen and androgen conjugates might explain the low risk of prostate cancer amongst native Japanese (Ross et al. 1992). This study demonstrated that Japanese men had significantly lower serum concentrations of 3α,7β-androstanediol glucuronide and androsterone glucuronide – an indirect measure of 5α-reductase activity – than either their black or white counterparts in the USA (Ross et al. 1992). These findings combined with the earlier data on tissue testosterone 5α-reductase patterns in normal and diseased prostate (Habib et al. 1985) highlight the unique feature of prostate cancer, among major cancers, being driven by the action of an androgen-metabolising enzyme.

Very little is known about the physicochemical properties of testosterone 5α-reductase since the enzyme has not yet been purified (Sargent and Habib 1991). However, the conversion of testosterone into DHT is essential for both the formation of the complete male phenotype during embryogenesis and for androgen-mediated growth of secondary sex organs such as the prostate (Griffin and Wilson 1992).

Single gene defects that impair this conversion lead to pseudohermaphroditism in which 46 X,Y males have male internal urogenital tracts but female external genitalia (Thigpen et al. 1992). In man, two separate genes encoding two steroid 5α-reductase isoenzymes with 50% sequence homology, designated type I and type II have been cloned (Andersson and Russell, 1990; Jenkins et al. 1992). The type I enzyme which maps to chromosome 5, has a neutral pH optimum and is expressed mainly in non-genital skin and liver. Type II enzyme is located on chromosome 2, is predominantly associated with the prostate and genital skin and has an acidic pH optimum. Unlike type I, 5α-reductase type II is mutated in male pseudohermaphroditism (Andersson et al. 1991). The mechanism regulating 5α-reductase gene expression is unusual. In rat prostate DHT induces expression of its own steroid 5α-reductase which is secondary to enhancement of 5α-reductase messenger RNA levels (George et al. 1991). This in turn increases DHT synthesis thereby triggering a positive developmental cascade resulting in a feed-forward control of prostatic growth. There is a possibility that a similar mechanism is found in human prostate tissue. Treatment of a group of benign prostatic hypertrophy (BPH) patients with 5α-reductase inhibitors not only inhibited the 5α-reductase activity of the gland but also appeared to reduce the expression of the enzyme itself (Tate and Habib, unpublished). It is, therefore, conceivable that the loss of 5α-reductase activity in prostate cancer (Habib et al. 1985) may be directly related to a down-regulation in 5α-reductase mRNA level which is secondary to mutational changes in the gene of the type II 5α-reductase isoenzyme. We have not investigated the impact of the "feed-forward" mechanism on the expression of androgen receptors but it is conceivable that the mechanism which underlies the 5α-reductase mRNA response also controls androgen receptors.

Androgen Receptors

The mechanism responsible for the progression of prostate cancer from androgen-dependent to androgen-insensitive growth has recently been the subject of extensive research. Studies on animal models particularly the Dunning rat prostatic adenocarcinoma have suggested that relapse following androgen ablation is due to the outgrowth of a population of androgen-independent carcinoma cells (Isaacs and Coffey 1981). There are also reports demonstrating that the transition to a hormone refractory state is related to a change in the level of expression of the androgen receptor caused by diminished androgen receptor mRNA levels (Tilley et al. 1990).

There was, however, no evidence to suggest that the down-regulation of androgen receptor mRNA was induced by major alterations in the structure of the androgen receptor gene. This does not exclude the possibility of subtle mutations such as point mutations present within the androgen receptor gene which could account for its inactivity in the receptor negative prostate cancer. The identification of the genes encoding the androgen receptor (Chang et al. 1988; Lubahn et al. 1988) together with the description of specific sequences of DNA termed hormone responsive elements (HREs) that bind the hormone receptor(s) and control the efficiency of transcription, has allowed the application of molecular techniques to this problem.

By comparison with other steroid receptors (Kumar et al. 1986) it is now possible to define three functionally important domains in the androgen receptor. Each receptor has a centrally located DNA binding domain which shows a high degree of sequence homology across receptor classes, a less well conserved carboxy-terminal ligand binding domain and an amino-terminal domain widely variant in size and sequence between receptors (Fig. 8.1). The gene encoding the human androgen receptor is located on the X chromosome in the Xq11-12 region and has a size >90 kb (Brinkmann and Trapman 1992) and the information for the protein coding region is separated over 8 exons (Fig. 8.1). The sequence encoding the amino-terminal domain is present in exon 1 whereas the DNA-binding domain is encoded by exons 2 and 3. The information for the steroid binding domain is distributed over five exons (exons 4–8) (Brinkmann and Trapman 1992). In an attempt to understand further the genetic basis of androgen escape in advanced prostate cancer, the molecular structure of human androgen receptors was examined initially in hormone-sensitive (LNCaP) but also in hormone-insensitive (DU-145, PC-3) cell lines. mRNA and genomic DNA were extracted and analysed after amplification by polymerase chain reaction (PCR) and the sequencing of the individual exons of the androgen receptor gene was carried out (Veldscholte et al. 1990; Yong et al. 1990). The presence of androgen receptor mRNA was demonstrated in all three cell lines though with higher levels of expression in LNCaP cells. However, the sequencing of the putative steroid binding domain of the androgen receptor mRNA from LNCaP cells demonstrated a point mutation which changed amino acid 876 Thr (ACT) to Ala (GCT). This might account for the shift in specificity by the androgen receptor in LNCaP with an increased preference for progestogens and oestradiol, a characteristic not associated with androgen receptors in normal cells

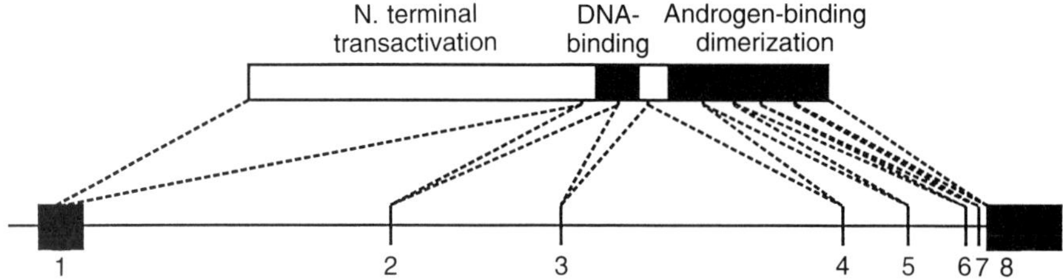

Fig.8.1. Diagram of the structure of the androgen receptor. Numbers denote exons (1–8) corresponding to the different functional domains. (Adapted from Brinkmann and Trapman 1992.)

(Brinkmann et al. 1991). To determine whether this substitution affects the functional properties of the LNCaP androgen receptor, the mutant cDNA was cloned in an expression vector and transiently expressed in COS-1 cells. The mutant receptor displayed increased binding affinity for progestogens and oestradiol confirming that the observed point mutation in the LNCaP androgen receptors is the cause of the broad steroid binding specificity found in these cells (Brinkmann et al. 1991). Whether this point mutation is a first step in the progressive growth of tumours in the prostate remains to be established. We are also uncertain whether it is possible to reverse the hormonal status of androgen insensitive prostate cancer by introducing the androgen receptor gene to the cell. To test this possibility, an expression vector carrying androgen receptor cDNA was transfected into DU-145 cells to determine the growth characteristics of this cell line in response to androgen and antiandrogen treatment. Surprisingly, exposure of these transfected cells to androgen resulted in a decreased cell proliferation and a marked decrease in characteristics associated with the malignant state (Grant and Habib, unpublished). Similarly, in a parallel set of experiments in PC-3 cells, a mild decrease in characteristics associated with the malignant phenotype and the ability to form colonies was noted following exposure to exogenous androgens (Yuan et al. 1993). These findings might have important implications for new directions in the future treatment of both androgen-dependent and -independent prostate cancer.

Through the years, wide interest in steroid hormone receptors in human prostate had developed because of their potential use as markers for predicting responsiveness to hormone therapy in cancer patients. An earlier review of the literature (Habib 1990) considered the previously reported studies and highlighted the problems inherent in the measurement of steroid hormone binding to specific receptors by biochemical and autoradiographic methods. The results were disappointing and this was attributed to the heterogeneity of the prostate cell and the difficulties in localising the receptor sites. However, with the advent of monoclonal and polyclonal antibodies for androgen receptors more refined techniques such as immunohistochemistry and flow cytometry were introduced. It has now been possible to pinpoint the site of the androgen receptor to the nucleus of the prostate epithelium and to demonstrate that androgen receptor content was significantly higher in well-differentiated adenocarcinoma compared to moderately and poorly differentiated cancers (Chodak et al. 1992). But whether it will be possible to employ these techniques for quantifying receptor concentrations and correlating these measurements with hormone responsiveness still remains to be established. It is worth noting that high androgen receptor measurements had been obtained on patients with metastasis who had escaped hormonal therapy (Habib et al. 1986). There is a distinct possibility that the receptors are non-functional but this will not prevent their recognition by the antibodies to androgen receptors if the relevant epitope is present.

Stromal Epithelial Interactions

The control of prostate growth is a very complex process dependent in part on the balance between the stromal and epithelial components of the gland (Cunha et al. 1987). Based on epithelial-mesenchymal recombination studies, it now appears that during development, epithelial cells are directed by mesenchymal signalling towards specific pathways of differentiated function. These signals may involve the production of soluble growth factors, either stimulatory or inhibitory, which exercise a paracrine influence on the adjacent epithelial tissue. Although both stromal and epithelial cells of the prostate are potential target sites for androgen action, both possess 5α-reductase activity as well as androgen receptors; prostatic growth in situ has been observed only when urogenital mesenchyme was grafted on to the mature rat prostate (Cunha et al. 1987). This would account for the failure of epithelial cells in primary cultures to respond to androgens in the absence of stroma (Chaproniere and McKeehan 1986) and lend further support to the concept for the presence of diffusible trophic growth factors in the human prostate. It is also worth noting that the environment in which the prostate cells live also influences their growth and their ability to proliferate. Interaction of cells with basement membrane components including collagen IV, laminin, fibronectin and heparan sulphate proteoglycans via specific cell surface receptors (Hay 1987) are found in the epithelial cells from which the cancer is derived. Even so, stromal/epithelial interactions continue to be of fundamental importance to the growth of the prostate from the fetal period into adulthood and it is becoming increasingly apparent that these interactions could also play a significant role in the carcinogenic process. In support of this concept are the co-inoculation studies in athymic mice demonstrating a fibroblast-mediated acceleration of epithelial tumours in vivo (Gleave et al. 1991). By employing cell to cell recombination techniques, Gleave et al. (1991) found that non-tumorigenic fibroblast accelerated the growth of solid tumours derived from non-tumorigenic human epithelial cells in vivo by at least three orders of magnitude. This highlights the importance of fibroblasts as the critical cell type within the fibromuscular stroma that supports epithelial proliferation via paracrine mechanisms at both the primary and metastatic sites. Studies to identify the type of growth factors involved are in progress and it is hoped that these may lead to a better understanding of the nature of this interaction and provide new opportunities in our quest to contain and reverse cancer growth.

Growth Factors

Growth factors differ from peptide hormones not only in the response elicited but also in their mode of delivery from the secretory to the responding cell.

Growth factors do not usually act in an endocrine manner, the consensus of opinion is that they diffuse over a short distance through intra/intercellular spaces and act locally, in either a paracrine or autocrine manner (James and Bradshaw 1984). Unlike classical endocrine hormones each growth factor may be synthesised by a variety of tissues, both adult and embryonic, and is thought to be released by many, if not all cells, in culture. Growth factors have a wide range of biological activities and are considered to be multifunctional agents (Sporn and Roberts 1988).

The role of growth factors and their receptors as mediators of prostate cancer cell growth has in recent years come under intense investigation. Many workers are now coming to recognise that growth factors play a major role in the progression of androgen-dependent to androgen-independent prostate cancer cell growth, though the evidence in the literature remains contradictory and no clear pattern is emerging (Habib and Chisholm 1991). In this section brief consideration will be given to growth factors which have been associated with the prostate gland.

Epidermal Growth Factor

Epidermal growth factor (EGF) is produced by rodent and human prostates and has been detected in large concentrations in the prostate fluid with the fluid titre being significantly lower in BPH patients than in normal controls (Gregory et al. 1986). EGF is mitogenic for primary cultures of prostate epithelium and its biological effects are mediated by the interaction with specific plasma membrane receptors (Chaproniere and McKeehan 1986). High affinity receptors for EGF (EGFr) have been found in normal prostate tissue and human BPH. The receptors were predominantly located along the basal layers of the epithelial cells with no apparent receptors in the stromal component (Maddy et al. 1987). Although EGFr are also expressed in human prostate cancer, their levels diminish as the tumour gradually progresses to a poorly differentiated state (Maddy et al. 1989). Significantly, this reduced sensitivity to EGF coincides with the development of a hormone-refractory tumour, a phenomenon which has been observed in some other systems and may be linked to the autologous production of other growth factors. In support of these observations are the experiments which showed that androgen-responsive prostate cancer (LNCaP) cell lines had relatively low numbers of EGF receptors whereas androgen unresponsive (DU-145) cells expressed higher EGF receptor numbers (MacDonald and Habib 1992). The correlation between EGF receptor expression and endocrine status suggests that steroid hormones do influence the response to growth factors, by altering growth factor receptor expression. However, this response may also reflect the species from which the prostate cells were derived. Studies on normal rat prostate demonstrated that the receptors for EGF were down-regulated following treatment of rats with exogenous androgens (Traish and Wotiz 1987). It is not clear, therefore, whether the loss of hormone sensitivity in prostate cancer and the development of hormone insensitive tumours are in any way interrelated. It would seem that the progression to an androgen-independent state may, in part, be due to a reduced need for exogenous mitogens because of the autologous production of other growth factors. Indeed, earlier studies in our laboratory and by others on a number of human prostate cell lines, demonstrated that the prostate can produce its own growth factor-like molecules which reduce the cells' needs for exogenous mitogens and thereby render these cells autostimulatory (MacDonald et al. 1990; Story 1991); one of these growth factors is transforming growth factor α.

Transforming Growth Factor α.

The EGF receptor serves as a binding site not only for EGF but also for transforming growth factor α (TGFα) which is structurally and functionally related. TGFα is a 5.6 kDa polypeptide with some sequence structure homology similar to EGF. The peptide shows a variety of biological activities similar to those of EGF although in some cases TGFα is more potent.

A lot of interest has focused on TGFα as they are a family of peptides which confer upon non-transformed cells several properties associated with the transformed phenotype, including anchorage – independent growth in semisolid medium. Some studies have revealed that prostate cancer cell lines contain high levels of TGFα mRNA, proliferate in response to TGFα and maintain a capacity to produce their own TGFαs (Wilding et al. 1989a; MacDonald et al. 1990; Hofer et al. 1991). This reduces the need by the cancerous cells for exogenous factors while at the same time promoting an autoregulatory mechanism for enhancing further growth of the tumours (MacDonald et al. 1990). TGFα may also exhibit a paracrine function and stimulate physiological activities such as angiogenesis which impart a selective advantage towards malignancies. In recent studies with transgenic mice, TGFα cDNA under the transcriptional control of inducible metallothionein-1 enhancer/promoter sequences produced significant epithelial hyperplasia and focal dysplastic changes that resembled carcinoma in situ in the anterior prostate (Sandgran et al. 1990). It is noteworthy that these phenotypic alterations correlated with high levels of the transgene mRNA.

Transforming Growth Factor β

The transforming growth factor β (TGFβ) family of polypeptides are stable, multifunctional factors with a wide variety of effects on the growth and differentiation of virtually all cell types (Massague 1990). The actions of TGFβ may be stimulatory or inhibitory, depending on the cell type, growth conditions, state of differentiation and on the presence of other growth factors. This family of growth factors consists of a number of polypeptides, some distantly related and others more closely related, designated TGFβ-1, TGFβ-2, TGFβ-1.2, TGFβ-3, TGFβ-4 and TGFβ-5. Although the full range of the biological activities of the different TGFβ isoforms have not been explored, there are reports on in vitro models showing differences in potencies, which suggest differential receptor affinities for some cell types (Massague 1992). Three classes of binding sites have been characterised from various cells and tissues: type 1 binding sites of 60–70 kDa are the most common and have an affinity for TGFβ-1 and a lower affinity for TGFβ-2; type 2 sites of 85–110 kDa vary between species and cell types; type 3 binding sites with an apparent mass of 250–350 kDa have high affinity for at least three members of the family, TGFβ-1, TGFβ-2 and TGFβ-1.2 (Massague 1990, 1992). Rat prostate cancer cells contain functional receptors for TGFβ. These receptors are up-regulated during the active phase of prostatic regression, implicating the potential role of TGFβ in prostate cell death following androgen withdrawal (Kyprianou and Isaacs 1988). Although TGFβ is predominantly inhibitory towards the growth of prostate cells, it also exhibits bifunctional properties on the basis of its ability to act as a growth promoting agent. The hormone-insensitive human prostate cancer cell lines, DU-145 and PC-3, were inhibited by TGFβ in a dose–response fashion whereas the hormone-sensitive cell line, LNCaP, did not respond (Wilding et al. 1989b). The androgen-independent cells also exhibited a capacity to produce and secrete TGFβ suggesting a possible autoinhibitory role in prostate cancer (Wilding et al. 1989b). However, in experiments undertaken in our laboratories, TGFβ stimulated the growth of fibroblasts derived from human benign prostatic hyperplasia and this pattern was also observed in immortalised but non-tumorigenic neonatal prostate epithelial cells (Kaighn et al. 1989). Additionally TGFβ is known to modulate the cellular responses to other growth factors since stimulation of LNCaP cells by EGF and the synergistic action with androgens were inhibited by TGFβ (Schuurmans et al. 1988), even though TGFβ receptors were not found on these cells (Wilding et al. 1989b).

The mechanism responsible for the control of TGFβ expression in prostate tissue is poorly understood. Although TGFβ mRNA levels were found to be elevated in poorly differentiated mouse prostate adenocarcinomas induced by the overexpression of the *ras* and *myc* oncogenes (Thomson 1990), it is not known how the *ras* oncogene affects the expression of growth factors in human prostate cancer cell lines. Clearly the mitogenic effects of EGF and other growth factors are counterbalanced by the inhibitory effects of TGFβ and this raises the possibility that an imbalance in the activities of these opposing factors might, in some way, contribute to the abnormal development of the prostate. Of relevance to this hypothesis are the elevated TGFβ concentrations reported in BPH samples when compared to normal tissues (Mori et al. 1990). However there is no evidence, so far, to suggest that a further elevation in TGFβ expression might be instrumental in the development of prostate cancer but this obviously is worth exploring.

Heparin Binding (Fibroblast) Growth Factors

In 1988, Mydlo et al. discovered a growth factor in prostate extracts which they named "prostate growth factor". Subsequent investigations revealed that this peptide exhibited a 100% homology with basic fibroblast growth factor (b-FGF) both at the transcribed and translated levels. Fibroblast growth factors (FGF) are a family of polypeptides which share an affinity to heparin. To date seven members of the FGF family have been identified of which only b-FGF and acidic-FGF (a-FGF) have been implicated in prostate growth (Mansson et al. 1989; Gelmann 1991). There are also reports from Dr Leder's laboratory at Harvard University suggesting that a third member, heparin binding growth factor-3 (HBGF-3), might also be involved in prostate growth: a new DNA construct was engineered into a mouse genome. This construct contained the int-2 gene which is associated with HBGF-3 production and was found to enlarge the prostate gland of the animal in a manner similar to human BPH (Muller et al. 1990). Interestingly substantial amounts of b-FGF mRNA and protein were detected in BPH tissues and these were significantly higher than in normal prostate, suggesting that this growth factor might be involved in the pathogenesis of BPH (Mori et al. 1990).

There are also reports showing that a-FGF mRNA is abundant in the prostate epithelium of immature rats but those peptides disappear as the animal matures (Mansson et al. 1989). However, the expression of a-FGF mRNA in the slow growing androgen-responsive Dunning R3327PAP prostate carcinoma appears to be specific to the mesenchymal cells of the tumour, leading to speculation that the mesenchyme-derived a-FGF supports the growth of the malignant epithelium in a paracrine fashion (Thomson 1990). Differences in the expression and binding kinetics of a-FGF receptor with respect to the mesenchymal and epithelial compartments were also observed, indicating the true complexity of a-FGF induced growth (Thomson 1990). The production of a-FGF in the prostate was also found to be under hormonal control since castration reduced the levels of this growth factor; these were subsequently increased to baseline levels after the administration of exogenous testosterone (Mydlo and Macchia 1992). Thus there may be a role for FGF intervention in BPH and cancer as an adjunct to hormonal therapy but more studies are needed to clarify the nature of these interactions with the prostate in health and disease.

Osteoblastic Factors

Prostate carcinomas frequently metastasise to bone and induce bone formation at specific sites. These so called osteoblastic metastases result from an imbalance in the rate of bone resorption and formation, with osteoblast depositing bone at sites independent of osteoclast resorption. The mechanisms by which prostate tumour cells induce new bone formation have yet to be determined. One possibility is that the tumour cells secrete growth factors or cytokines which act locally to stimulate the proliferation and differentiation of osteoblasts. As indicated above, human prostate cancer cells produce a variety of known growth factors, some of which stimulate new bone formation whereas others induce breakdown of bone. It should be emphasised, however, that in most situations bone resorption is a pre-requisite for new bone formation and so growth factors may be viewed as modulators of bone remodelling. Thus certain factors stimulate or inhibit bone resorbing cells (osteoclasts), whereas others act mainly on bone forming cells (osteoblasts). Koutsilieris et al. (1987) have demonstrated the presence of potent osteoblast stimulating activity in hyperplastic and cancerous prostatic tissue. Unfortunately the identity of the active mitogen has so far not been resolved.

Whereas metastasising prostate cells possess the capacity to produce growth factors which enhance their growth, the environment in which the tumour cells live also influences the growth and the ability of these cells to metastasise. In support of this theory are experiments which demonstrate that bone marrow stromal cell conditioned medium stimulates proliferation of two prostatic cell lines, PC-3 and DU-145, whereas none of the other tumour cell lines tested showed a similar response (Chackal-Roy et al. 1989). Since this activity had not been attributed to any of the growth factors so far discussed, our group investigated the possibility that other haemopoietic growth factors might be involved. We have, in particular, concentrated on granulocyte macrophage colony stimulating factor (GM-CSF) and erythropoietin (EPO) which are found in very large concentrations in bone marrow and in response to which PC-3 and DU-145 are significantly stimulated (Lang et al. 1994). Analysis of the bone marrow conditioned media identified GM-CSF as one of the active ingredients (Lang and Habib unpublished) which was also found to be secreted by these cells. Significantly, the hormone sensitive LNCaP, which did not respond to the bone cell conditioned media, was also found not to produce GM-CSF. We now suspect that the production of GM-CSF is an important step in the transition of the malignant prostate cell from hormone-sensitive to a hormone-insensitive status but this will have to be verified.

Other Considerations Relating to Prostate Cancer

Various factors, other than steroid hormones and growth factor polypeptides may well have a particular function in the maintenance of prostate growth and an implication in the aetiology of prostate diseases. Recently, attention has been directed at the effectors potentiating the trophic characteristics of androgens in the human prostate. The majority of these effectors are peptide hormones, many of which have attracted the interest and attention of researchers not least because of their potential role in prostate cancer.

Prolactin

Evidence accumulated over the last 30 years suggests that the pituitary hormone, prolactin, maintains a direct effect on the prostate. Prolactin acts both independently and in synergy with testicular adrenal androgens (Farnsworth 1990). Simultaneous injections of either testosterone or dihydrotestosterone and prolactin to mature castrated rats stimulates an increase in mRNA, DNA and protein synthesis. Furthermore prolactin accelerates the uptake of testosterone in human prostate that is 5α-reduced to dihydrotestosterone both in vivo and in vitro (Farnsworth 1990). By contrast treatment of prostate cancer patients with bromocriptine, a dopamine agonist suppressing prolactin secretion, reduced androgen uptake into the prostate (Jacobi et al. 1978). This leaves the question of how exactly prolactin promotes the uptake of testosterone. Studies in our own laboratory have established a presence of prolactin receptors in the human prostate membrane (Leake et al. 1984). It is conceivable that the presence of these receptors might facilitate the entry of androgens into the prostate gland by inducing the lipolysis of membrane phosphatides (Dave and Witorsch 1985). This in turn enhances fluidisation of the plasma membrane which should increase the permeability of the steroid (Farnsworth 1990); this may well account for the high correlation found between blood prolactin and androgen receptors in BPH (Odoma et al. 1985). Although a loose association between raised prolactin levels and poor prognosis in patients with prostate cancer has been reported in cross-sectional studies (Mee et al. 1984), no longitudinal studies of plasma prolactin and its relation to adrenal and testicular androgens have so far been reported. If the findings on the interrelationship between blood prolactin levels and androgen receptors in BPH can be confirmed in patients with cancer of the prostate then the measurement of blood prolactin concentrations on all patients might be useful since those with high prolactin and positive androgen receptors could benefit from treatment with adjuvant prolactin suppressants. This should ensure that the "oestrogen escape phenomenon" observed in some cancer patients because of the probable rise in prolactin levels will no longer occur.

Growth Hormone

Interest in growth hormone (GH) in prostate disease was prompted by the observation that patients with metastatic disease had elevated plasma GH compared to patients without metastasis (British Prostate Group Study 1979); whether this is a cause/effect in the spread of the tumour is not clear. The presence of endogenous GH in prostate tissue has been established following the immunohistochemical staining of prostate sections (Sibley et al. 1984) and GH binding sites have been detected in the stromal and epithelial components of both benign and malignant human prostate. However, the functional significance of these binding sites or indeed their importance in relation to the androgenic activity of the gland has not yet been elucidated.

Thyrotropin-releasing Hormone

Equally interesting is the role of the thyrotropin-releasing hormone (TRH) in the prostate. TRH is a tripeptide secreted primarily by the hypothalamus but recent reports revealed the presence of these peptides in both rat and human prostate in concentrations even greater than those present in the hypothalamus; it is now believed that the prostate gland might be actively involved in the synthesis of this peptide hormone (Sheth et al. 1987). Additionally, new experimental evidence suggests that TRH might also be associated with the autocrine/paracrine regulation of stromal and epithelial cells within the prostate gland. Although TRH biosynthesis is stimulated by testosterone, the peptide inhibits the 5α-reductase activity of the prostate and regulates pituitary prolactin secretion (Sheth et al. 1987). Many of these observations underline a probable role for TRH in the function and well being of the prostate. Although the bulk of the earlier experiments has been on animal models, this work provides a new and fresh outlook into the physiology of the human prostate and may well form the basis for a better understanding of the mechanisms involved.

Conclusions and Prospects

The development of the prostate is very much influenced by androgens. But the prostate also maintains a capacity to produce a number of polypeptide growth factors which act either in synergy with androgens or independently to regulate cell growth and differentiation and may play a crucial role in cancer and other diseases of the prostate.

Growth factors are secreted by both the stromal and epithelial components of the gland, exercise autocrine as well as paracrine effects and induce a diversity of responses. The mode of action of these growth factors and the nature of the stimulatory and inhibitory responses will vary depending on the cell type, growth conditions, state of differentiation and on the presence of other growth factors. The full range of these biological activities in the prostate has not yet been totally explored. Furthermore, many of the established pathways appear to undergo changes as the cell is gradually transformed to the neoplastic state and becomes hormone refractive. Some of these changes occur at an early stage in the development of the cancer long before neoplasia becomes histologically evident, others are manifested at later stages in the disease highlighting the nature of tumorigenesis as a multistep process.

The molecular events that underly the initiation and progression of cancer have been identified (Weinberg 1989) and an elegant model for the genetic basis of colorectal tumours formulated (Fearon and Vogelstein 1990). The general features of this model have been adapted to a number of other cancers. The suggested pathway through which prostate cancer may develop is outlined in Fig. 8.2 (Sandberg 1992). This is based on the genetic alterations observed by a number of workers which involve known mutational activation of oncogenes combined with mutational inactivation of tumour suppressor

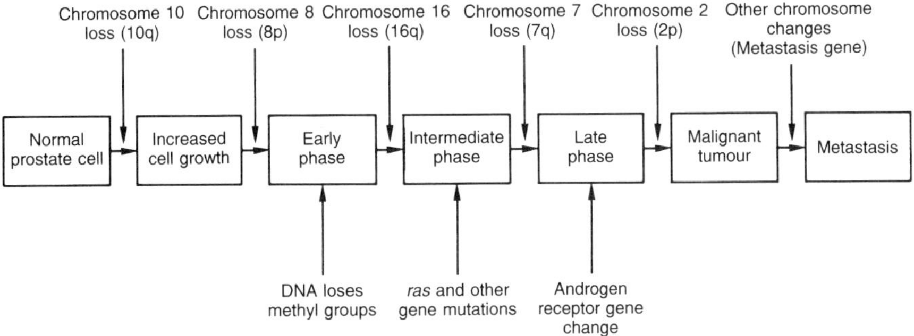

Fig.8.2. Chromosomes in prostate cancer. (From Sandberg 1992.)

genes (Bookstein et al. 1990; Isaacs et al. 1991; Mellon et al. 1992; Visakorpi et al. 1992). Genetic alterations of other genes such as those for the androgen receptor and 5α-reductase are very much implicated in this process and it is the accumulation of these changes which give rise to the sequence of events leading ultimately to the development of metastases. Scientists have put together a few pieces in the genetic jigsaw but it will take a few more years before we can obtain a complete picture of the prostate puzzle.

References

Andersson S, Russell DW (1990) Structural and biochemical properties of cloned and expressed human *ras* steroid 5α-reductases Proc Natl Acad Sci USA 87:3640–3644

Andersson S, Birman DM, Jenkins EP, Russell DW (1991) A deletion of steroid 5α-reductase 2 gene in male pseudohermaphroditism. Nature 354:159–161

Bookstein R, Shew JY, Chen PL et al. (1990) Suppression of tumorigenicity of human prostate carcinoma cells by replacing a mutated RB gene. Science 247:712–715

Brinkmann AO, Trapman J (1992) Androgen receptor mutants that affect normal growth and development. Cancer Surv 14:95–111

Brinkmann AO, Kuiper GGJM, Ris-Stalpers C et al. (1991) Androgen receptor abnormalities Steroid Biochem Mol Biol 40:349–352

British Prostate Group Study (1979) Evaluation of plasma hormone concentrations in relation to clinical staging in patients with prostate cancer. Br J Cancer 51:382–389

Chackal-Roy M, Niemeyer C, Moore M et al. (1989) Stimulation of human prostatic carcinoma cell growth by factors present in human bone marrow. J Clin Invest 84:43–50

Chang C, Kokontis J, Liao S (1988) Molecular cloning of human and rat complementary DNA encoding androgen receptors. Science 240:324–326

Chaproniere DM, McKeehan WL (1986) Serial culture of single adult prostatic epithelial cells in serum free medium containing low calcium and a new growth factor from bovine brain. Cancer Res 46:819–824

Chodak GW, Cranc DM, Libertad AP et al. (1992) A nuclear localisation of androgen receptor in heterogenous samples of normal, hyperplastic and neoplastic human prostate. J Urol 147:798–803

Cunha JR, Dontjacour AA, Cooke PS et al. (1987). The endocrinology and developmental biology of the prostate. Endocrinol Rev 8:338–363

Dave JR, Witorsch RJ (1985) Prolactin increases lipid fluidity and prolactin binding of rat prostatic membranes. Am J Physiol 248:E687

Farnsworth WE (1990) Prolactin. In: Farnsworth WE, Ablin RG (eds) The prostate as an endocrine gland. CRC Press, Boca Raton, FL, pp 177–185

Fearon ER, Vogelstein B (1990) A genetic model for colorectal tumorigenesis. Cell 61:759–767

Gelmann EP (1991) Oncogenes and growth factors in prostate cancer. J NIH Res 3:62–64

George FW, Russell DW, Wolfson JD (1991) Feed-forward control of prostate growth: dihydrotestosterone induces expression of its own biosynthetic enzyme, steriod 5α-reductase. Proc Nat Acad Sci USA 88:8044–8047

Gleave ME, Hsieh JT, Gao C et al. (1991) Acceleration of human prostate cancer growth in vivo by factors produced by prostate and bone fibroblast. Cancer Res 51:3753–3761

Gregory H, Wilshire IR, Cavanagh JP et al. (1986) Urogastrone – epidermal growth factor concentration prostatic fluid of normal individuals and patients with benign prostatic hypertrophy. Clin Sci 70:359–363

Griffin JE, Wilson JD (1992) Disorders of the testis and the male reproductive tract. In: Wilson JD, Foster DW (eds) Williams textbook of endocrinology 8th edn, W.B. Saunders, Philadelphia, pp 799–851

Habib FK, (1990) Prostate mechanisms of normal and abnormal metabolism. In: Chisholm

GD, Fair WR (eds) Scientific foundations of urology, 3rd edn. Heinemann Medical, London, pp 358–365

Habib FK, Chisholm GD (1991) The role of growth factors in the human prostate. Scand J Nephrol 126:53–58

Habib FK, Busuttil A, Robinson RA, Chisholm GD (1985) 5α-reductase activity in human prostate cancer is related to the histological differentiation of the tumour. Clin Endocrinol 23:431–438

Habib FK, Odoma S, Busuttil A, Chisholm GD (1986) Androgen receptors in cancer of the prostate: correlation with the stage and grade of the tumour on receptor content. Cancer 57:2351–2356

Hay ED (1987) Cell matrix interaction in the embryo: cell shape, cell surface and their role in differentiation. In: Trelstad RL (ed) The role of extra cellular matrix in development. Alan R Liss, New York, pp 1–31

Hofer DR, Sherwood ER, Bromberg WD et al. (1991) Autonomous growth of androgen-independent human prostatic carcinoma cells: role of transforming growth factor α. Cancer Res 51:2780–2785

Huggins C, Hodges CV (1941) Studies on prostate cancer I. Effect of castration, of oestrogen and of androgen injection on serum phosphatase in the metastatic carcinoma of the prostate. Cancer Res 1:293–297

Isaacs JT, Coffey DS (1981) Adaptation versus selection on the mechanism responsible for the relapse of prostatic cancer to androgen ablation therapy as studied in the R-3327-H adenocarcinoma. Cancer Res 41:5070–5075

Isaacs WB, Carter BS, Ewing CM (1991) While type p53 suppresses growth of human prostate cancer cells containing mutant p53 alleles. Cancer Res 51:4716–4720

Jacobi GH, Interhauf K, Kurth KH et al. (1978) Bromocriptine and prostatic carcinoma: the plasmid kinetics, production and tissue uptake of radiolabelled testosterone in vivo. J Urol 119:240–243

James R, Bradshaw RA (1984) Polypeptide growth factors. Annu Rev Biochem 53:259–292

Jenkins EP, Andersson S, Imperato-McGinley J, Wilson JD, Russell DW (1992) Genetic and pharmacological evidence for more than one human steroid 5α-reductase. J Clin Invest 89:293–300

Kaighn ME, Reddel RR, Lechnar JF et al. (1989) Transformation of human neonatal prostate epithelial cells by strontium phosphate transfection with a plasmid containing SV40 earlier lesion genes. Cancer Res 49: 3050–3057

Koutsilieris M, Robbani SA, Goltzman D (1987) The effects of human prostatic mitogens on rat bone cells and fibroblast. J Endocrinol 115:447–454

Kumar V, Green S, Staub A, Chambon P (1986) Localisation of the oestradiol binding and putative DNA binding domains of the human oestrogen receptor. EMBO J 5:2231–2236

Kyprianou N, Isaacs JT (1988) Identification of a cellular receptor for transforming growth factor β in rat ventral prostates and its negative regulation by androgens. Endocrinology 123:2124–2131

Lang SH, Miller WR, Duncan W, Habib FK (1994) The role of granulocyte macrophage-colony stimulating factor and erythropoietin in prostate cancer. Cancer Res (in press)

Leake A, Chisholm GD, Habib FK 1984) Interaction between prolactin and zinc in the human prostate gland. J Endocrinol 102:73–76

Lubahn DB, Joesph DR, Sullivan PM, Willard HF, French FS, Wilson EM (1988) Cloning of human androgen receptor complementary cDNA and localisation on the X chromosome. Science 240:327–330

MacDonald A, Habib FK (1992) Divergent responses to epidermal growth factor in hormone sensitive and insensitive human prostate cancer cell lines. Br J Cancer 65:177–182

MacDonald A, Chisholm GD, Habib FK (1990) Production and response of a human prostatic cancer line to transforming growth factor-like molecules. Br J Cancer 62:579–584

Maddy SQ, Chisholm GD, Hawkins RA, Habib FK (1987) Localization of epidermal growth factor receptors in the human prostate by biochemical and immunocytochemical methods. J Endocrinol 113:147–153

Maddy SQ, Chisholm GD, Busuttil A, Habib FK (1989) Epidermal growth factor receptors in human prostate cancer: correlation with histological differentiation of the tumour. Br J Cancer 60:41–44

Mansson PE, Adams P, Kan M et al. (1989) Heparin-binding growth factor gene expression and receptor characteristics in normal rat prostate and two transplantable rat prostate tumours. Cancer Res 49:2485–2494

Massague J (1990) Transforming growth factor β family. Annu Rev Cell Biol 6:597–641

Massague J (1992) Receptors for TGFβ family. Cell 69:1067–1070

Mee ED, Khan O, Mashiti K (1984) High serum prolactin associated with poor prognosis in carcinoma of the prostate. Br J Urol 56:698–701

Mellon K, Thomson S, Charlton RG et al. (1992) p53, c-erbB-2 and the epidermal growth facor receptor in the benign and malignant prostate. J Urol 147:496–499

Montgomery BJ, Young CWF, Bilhartz DL et al. (1992) Hormonal regulation of prostate specific antigen (PSA) glycoprotein in the human prostate adenocarcinoma cell line, LNCaP. Prostate 21:63–73

Mori HM, Maki K, Oishi M et al. (1990) Increased expression of genes for basic fibroblast growth factor and transforming growth factor type β-2 in human benign prostatic hyperplasia. Prostate 16:71–80

Muller WJ, Lee FS, Dickson C, Peters G, Pattingale P, Leder P (1990) The int-2 gene product acts as an epithelial growth factor in transgenic mice. EMBO J 9:907–913

Mydlo JH, Macchia RJ (1992) Growth factors in urologic tissues: detection, characterization, and clinical applications. Urology 40:491–498

Mydlo JH, Bulbul MA, Richon VM et al. (1988) Heparin binding growth factor isolated from human prostate extracts. Prostate 12:343–355

Odoma S, Chisholm GD, Nicol K, Habib FK (1985) Evidence for the association between blood prolactin and androgen receptors in BPH. J Urol 133:717–720

Ross RK, Bernstein L, Lobo RA et al. (1992) 5α-reductase activity and risk of prostate cancer among Japanese and US white and black males. Lancet 339:887–889

Sandberg AA (1992) Chromosomal abnormalities and related events in prostate cancer. Hum Pathol 23:368–380

Sandgran EP, Luetteke NC, Palmitar RD et al. (1990) Over expression of TGFα in transgenic mice: induction of epithelial hyperplasia, pancreatic metaplasia and carcinoma of the breast. Cell 61:1211–1235

Sargent NSE, Habib FK (1991) Partial purification of human prostatic 5α-reductase (3-oxo-5α-steroid: NADP$^+$ 4-ene-oxido-reductase; EC 1.3.1.22) in a stable and active form. J Steroid Biochem Mol Biol 38:73–77

Schuurmans ALG, Bolt J, Mulder E (1988) Androgens in transforming growth factor β modulate the growth response to epidermal growth factor in human prostate tumour cells (LNCaP). Mol Cell Endocrinol 60:101–104

Sheth NA, Vanaga GR, Hurkadly KS et al. (1987) The prostate – an extra gonadal source of inhibin: demonstration of inhibin in normal, benign, malignant human prostate and rat prostate by bioassay, immunoassay, immunocytochemical localisation and biosynthesis. In: Sheth AR (ed) Inhibins, chemistry, measurement and physiology CRC Press, Boca Raton, FL, pp 109–132

Sibley PEC, Harper ME, Peeling WB et al. (1984) Growth hormone and prostatic tumour localisation using a monoclonal human growth hormone antibody. J Endocrinol 103:311–315

Sporn MB, Roberts AB (1988) Peptide growth factors are multifunctional. Nature 332:217–219

Story MT (1991) Polypeptide modulators of prostatic growth and development. Cancer Surv 11:123–145

Thigpen AE, Davis DL, Milatovich A et al. (1992) Molecular genetics of steroid 5α-reductase to deficiency. J Clin Invest 90:799–809

Thomson TC (1990) Growth factors and oncogenes in prostate cancer. Cancer Cells 2:345–354

Tilley WD, Wilson CM, Marcelli M, McPhaul MJ (1990) Androgen receptor gene expression in human prostate carcinoma cell lines. Cancer Res 50:5382–5386

Traish AM, Wotiz HH (1987) Prostatic epidermal growth factor receptors and irregulation by androgens. Endocrinology 121:1461–1467

Tsai SY, Tsai MY, O'Malley BW (1991) The steroid receptor super family: transactivators of gene expression. In: Parker MG (ed) Nuclear hormone receptors. Academic Press, London, pp 103–124

Veldscholte J, Ris Stalpars C, Kuiper JG et al. (1990) Invitation to ligand binding domain of the androgen receptor human LNCaP cells affects steroid binding characteristic and responses to anti androgens. Biochem Biophys Res Commun 173:534–540

Visakorpi T, Kallioniemi P, Heikkinen A et al. (1992) Small sub-group of aggressive, highly proliferative prostatic carcinomas defined by p53 accumulation. J Natl Cancer Inst 84:883–887

Weinberg RA (1989) Oncogenes, anti-oncogenes and the molecular basis of multi-step carcinogenesis. Cancer Res 49:3713–3721
Wilding GE, Valverius E, Knabbe C, Gelmann EP (1989a) The role of transforming growth factor α in human prostate cancer cell growth. Prostate 15:1–12
Wilding G, Zugmeier G, Knabbe C (1989b) Differential effects of transforming growth factor β on human prostate cancer cells in vitro. Mol Cell Endocrinol 62:79–87
Yong CYF, Qiu SD, Prescott JL, Tindall DJ (1990) Over expression of a partial human androgen receptor in *E coli:* characterisation of steroid binding, DNA binding and immunological properties. Mol Endocrinol 4:1841–1849
Yuan S, Trachtenberg J, Mills GB et al. (1993) Androgen induced inhibition of cell proliferation in an androgen-insensitive prostate cancer cell line (PC-3) transfected with a human androgen receptor complementary DNA. Cancer Res 53:1304–1311

Chapter 9

The Endocrinology of Prostate Cancer

H. Wasan and J. Waxman

Introduction

In the West over recent years, there has been a virtually exponential increase in the incidence of prostate cancer. In the United Kingdom, it is now the second most common cancer of men and in 1990, caused 8098 deaths (OPCS Monitor 1991). This increased incidence is reflected worldwide, and is disproportionately greater in areas such as Japan where the disease was once rare (Waterhouse et al. 1982). Prostatic cancer is a tumour that increases in incidence with age but the increased longevity of our populace and improved detection of the disease only partially explain this change and suggest a true epidemic.

It is almost a century since the androgen dependency of the human prostate was first shown by White (1893), who treated patients with benign and malignant prostatic enlargement by orchidectomy. Medical treatments for prostatic cancer were widely introduced 50 years later (Huggins and Hodges 1941) but despite five decades of experimentation with medical therapies, no evidence of improved survival with any treatment has been demonstrated. This is remarkable in the context of subjective improvements with androgen deprivation in 85% of patients.

All current treatments of advanced prostatic cancer are therefore to be regarded as palliative, aiming for an improvement in life quality. In this context, we review current treatments for carcinoma of the prostate and prostate cancer biology.

Hormonal Treatment for Early Stage Disease

The use of hormonal manipulation cannot currently be recommended for early stage prostate cancer (T0–2 N0 M0) because of the disadvantages of therapy – flushes and impotence and the probable lack of a survival advantage to such therapies. Indeed questions regarding the benefit of any local therapies in early disease are still to be answered. In this clinical situation, there have been only limited randomised trials comparing local therapy with radiation or surgery. These studies have involved small numbers of patients with limited follow-up. Contrasts have been made between the results of treatment with single modality therapy. In one study, 97 patients with T1–2 N0 M0 prostatic cancer were randomised after staging, which included pelvic lymphadenectomy to either radical prostatectomy or to radiotherapy. The true pelvis was irradiated to between 4500 and 5000 cGy in 40 days, with a 2000 cGy boost to the prostate. Follow-up ranged up to 5 years. It is not clear what the median follow-up was of these patients, but, in the course of the study, four in the radical surgery arm and 17 in the radiation arm had disease progression. This difference was significant (Paulson et al. 1982). In a limited meta-analysis Whitmore described an 84%–92% 10-year survival for patients followed by observation alone, 92%–97% for patients treated by radical surgery and 62%–86% for patients treated by radiotherapy (Adolfsson et al. 1993). Since no adjustment was made for deaths from other causes, and because of the obvious bias in selection for surgery, no significant conclusion can be made as to the "best" therapy for early stage prostatic cancer.

Hormonal Treatment for Advanced Disease: Immediate or Deferred?

Hormonal treatments were prescribed in the confident belief that their use prolonged patients' lives. This misconception was confirmed by a study comparing hormone-treated patients to historical untreated controls where an advantage was found for treatment (Nesbit and Baum 1950). This conclusion is no longer held to be valid, and is considered erroneous because of the use of an inappropriate control group. The idea that medical therapy is curative was first disputed by Scott (1959) who advocated hormonal manipulation only for pain secondary to metastatic disease. This controversy as to the place and timing of treatment is currently being investigated by the MRC in a prospective trial of delayed versus immediate orchidectomy and by the EORTC of delayed versus immediate GnRH agonist therapy. This controversy will be discussed in more detail later in this chapter.

Between 1965 and 1968 The Veterans Administration (VA) looked at 509 men with newly diagnosed, biopsy proven prostate adenocarcinoma. They showed no significant survival advantage to patients with localised disease with early hormonal intervention as compared to placebo-treated patients, although the onset of metastatic disease seemed to be delayed in the treatment arm (Byar 1973). As the median age of patients presenting with the disease was 72 years, the life expectancy of this group statistically confounds trial analysis: more than 50% of patients in the VA study died of other causes. Quality adjusted life years (QUALY) is a more meaningful parameter of treatment assessment than overall survival (Byrne 1992). The elderly median age of the patients preselects for susceptibility to the toxicities of any available therapies, as is demonstrated by the high cardiovascular mortality and morbidity of treatment with oestrogens.

Current Choice of Androgen Deprivation Therapies

The "Gold Standard" of treatment remains bilateral orchidectomy which rapidly brings down serum testosterone to one tenth of pretreatment levels. Although the surgical morbidity is relatively low many patients feel that orchidectomy is an unacceptable treatment, and this together with the lack of a survival advantage to current treatment, has fuelled the search for alternative medical therapies for prostate cancer.

Diethystilboestrol (DES) is a synthetic non-steroidal oestrogen analogue, first described in 1938 and initially promoted in the late 1940s for preventing miscarriages and preterm births. Although still commonly used, it is generally regarded as unacceptable treatment, because of its gross toxicities which range from gynaecomastia and indigestion to cardiovascular mortality. In 1967 The Veterans Administration Cooperative Urological Research Group (VACURG 1967) published their prospective analysis of a randomised study comparing orchidectomy or oestrogen therapy with placebo. Nearly 2000 patients were enrolled in these trials and although the oestrogen-treated patients appeared to have a reduced cancer mortality, this effect was more than negated by an increase in cardiovascular morbidity and mortality. The adverse changes mirror those of the oral contraceptive pill in women, in that antithrombin III levels decrease and this leads to increased platelet adhesiveness (Varenhorst et al. 1981). These effects are measurable biologically and clinically even with low dosage DES regimens, which have the added disadvantage of a lower success rate. Many clinicians argue that because oestrogen therapy is cheap, it is also a "good" medical therapy. We would argue that it may be cheap, but it is also dangerous, and that patients' lives are worth more than the 4p per day, which is the current treatment cost.

Cyproterone acetate is a progestogenic antiandrogen with complex endocrine effects. It limits the synthesis of androgens indirectly by inhibiting the production of pituitary gonadotrophins and directly within the testis. In the tumour it acts by displacing testosterone from its cytoplasmic receptor and by decreasing the formation of the nuclear androgen complex. Trials have shown it to be comparable to DES in terms of response rates and durations but to have a lower but still significant cardiovascular morbidity (De Voogt et al. 1986).

Pure antiandrogens were developed as specific testosterone receptor antagonists. Flutamide was first introduced into clinical practice in 1975 but encouraging early reports of its use as a single agent in prostate cancer have not been borne out. Flutamide has significant side effects and about 15%–20% of patients will have diarrhoea. Nevertheless these compounds are theoretically attractive as they are devoid of cardiovascular side effects and because sexual potency should be maintained. Casodex is structurally similar to flutamide and devoid of central effects. Response rates similar to orchidectomy have been described in preliminary communications (Lunglmayr 1989). Nilutamide competes for the dihydrotestosterone receptor as well as affecting the adrenal hydroxylase systems. The main role for these agents is in combination therapy, limiting the action of androgens of non-testicular origin (Neri and Kassem 1984).

Gonadotrophin Releasing Hormone Agonists

The gonadotrophin releasing hormone (GnRH) analogues were initially introduced as agents with specific effects on the pituitary–gonadal axis and potentially without the toxicities of existing therapies (Schally et al. 1983).

GnRH is a single chain hypothalamic decapeptide. Like other native neuropeptides, it is synthesised as a large-molecular-weight precursor which is cleaved enzymatically before secretion into the pituitary portal circulation. The gene encoding GnRH is on chromosome 8. A 92 amino acid protein is initially translated, which is cleaved to a 56 amino acid protein termed GAP (GnRH associated peptide). This is further cleaved to form GnRH (Yang-Feng et al. 1986). Secretion of GnRH is pulsatile and its regulation complex. The main effect of GnRH is to stimulate the synthesis of luteinising hormone (LH) and its own receptor (Marian et al. 1981). Peptides resembling GnRH appear to be synthesised or act within a number of other structures, including prostate, breast, endometrium, ovary, testis and malignant pancreatic tissue (Sharpe 1980; Hsueh and Jones 1981).

Substitution of amino acids, especially the D forms which are resistant to degradation, in positions six, nine and ten, results in a range of powerful agonists with potencies at least 1000 times greater than the native form (Schally and Coy 1977). Conversely, modifications in positions one, two and three result in a range of avid GnRH receptor competitive antagonists. These modifications lead to peptides with receptor affinities different from the native peptide. The agonists after a brief period of stimulation, lead to down-regulation of the pituitary gonadotrophs which is associated with a very marked reduction in the biosynthesis of LH and a dramatic fall in GnRH receptor numbers (Clayton et al. 1982; Smith and Conn 1984).

This down-regulation results in decreased testicular production of testosterone, which can be taken advantage of clinically to provide a medical orchidectomy. This explanation of the action of the GnRH agonists, which involves a distantly secreted "paracrine factor" may not be the entire story. There are alternative theories to explain the effects of these peptides. It has been suggested that many human hormone dependent tumours are regulated by locally produced, autocrine factors, rather than distantly produced paracrine factors. Recently, a new class of peptide receptor for gonadotrophin-releasing hormone together with its ligand has been found in normal prostate, a human hormone-sensitive prostatic cancer cell line and tumour biopsy specimens. This finding of both receptor and ligand, implies that the tumour is manufacturing a peptide that stimulates its own growth, through its own cell surface-receptor, bypassing a requirement for distantly secreted stimulus. The receptor appears not to be expressed in hormone insensitive cell lines although the ligand is (Qayum et al. 1990). In cell culture, addition of GnRH has a stimulatory effect on growth. This effect occurs without the presence of added sex steroids. These findings suggest a direct effect of GnRH analogues at the level of the tumour cells, possibly by down-regulation of their own receptors on the cell surface.

The virtual logarithmic increase of prostatic cancer incidence with age is striking in all populations (Waterhouse et al. 1982). Plasma testosterone and free testosterone decrease with age, providing a challenging paradox as regards the aetiology of prostatic cancer. As the testes involute the pituitary gonadotrophins rise. There have been a number of investigations as to whether there is a hormonal difference that predisposes to prostatic cancer. In a study of 26 patients with carcinoma of the prostate who were compared with 58 normal men and 232 patients with benign prostatic hypertrophy, significantly lower levels of LH were found in the two patient groups as compared with the controls (Hammond et al. 1977). However, Harper et al. (1976) could find no difference between patients with prostatic cancer, benign enlargement or matched controls. The British Prostate Study Group (1979) investigated circulating hormone levels in 197 patients with either metastatic or non-metastatic prostate cancer. Multivariate analysis showed no significant differences in concentrations of the gonadotrophins, sex steroids or prolactin between the two groups.

Clinical studies with GnRH Analogues

The major argument used by urologists against medical therapy is based upon the apparently greater cost. This has been based upon orchidectomy as an outpatient procedure (McClinton et al. 1989). However, the majority of orchidectomies are performed on inpatients. A recent analysis has shown the true cost for orchidectomy to be £2580 and for depot GnRH analogue therapy for the average patients illness to be £2760–£3380 (Rutqvist and Wilking 1992). This 7%–31% difference in cost negates the main argument against medical therapies, and supports the patient's right to choose GnRH analogue treatment for his condition. Early studies of the GnRH analogues investigated the activity of these peptides in prostatic cancer and established treatment regimens. These phase I/II investigations were followed by phase III studies contrasting GnRH agonist therapy with conventional treatment, which showed equivalence of peptide therapy to oestrogen treatment and orchidectomy. The Leuprolide Study Group (1984) compared the responses of 101 patients treated with 3 mg of DES daily with 98 patients treated with 1 mg of D-leu[6]-LHRH ethylamide subcutaneously daily. Responses, characterised according to National Prostatic Cancer Project Criteria were equivalent in both arms of the study. Of the leuprolide group 1% had a complete and 37% a partial response as compared to 2% and 44% in the DES group, respectively. These differences were not significant but differences in the side effects of treatment were. Peripheral oedema occurred in 23 oestrogen-treated patients as compared with eight leuprolide-treated patients. Thrombotic events occurred in seven of the DES versus one leuprolide-treated patients. Gastrointestinal toxicity was twofold greater in the oestrogen-treated group and gynaecomastia was almost 20 times more common. GnRH agonist treatment has been compared with orchidectomy in a number of studies. One of the most recent to be published, compared orchidectomy with zoladex in 358 patients. A total of 71% of the zoladex group and 72% of the orchidectomy group had either a complete or partial response. The median duration of response was 54 weeks in the zoladex group and 50 weeks in the orchidectomy patients. The median survival was 110 weeks in the analogue-treated group and 99 weeks in the orchidectomy group. There was no significant difference in response rate, remission duration or survival between the different treatments. Flare was reported in six zoladex treated patients, and was not described in the orchidectomy group. Fourteen orchidectomy patients had postoperative complications (Kaisary et al. 1991).

In the late 1980s, drug delivery systems became more sophisticated and depot formulations given every four to twelve weeks were shown to be effective (Waxman et al. 1989). Litigation between pharmaceutical companies has delayed the licensing of the longer-acting depots in the UK.

Combination Therapies

GnRH agonists given as a monotherapy, initially stimulate the pituitary–gonadal axis. This initial stimulatory action, leading to an LH and testosterone "surge" may exacerbate pain in 5%–40% of patients. In 0.1%–1% of patients obstructive uropathy or spinal cord compression is precipitated. This can be avoided by concurrent administration of an antiandrogen which is routinely recommended (Waxman et al. 1985), but as will be discussed later, whether both therapies should be continued indefinitely is a matter of contention. The phenomenon of tumour flare is an unacceptable complication of GnRH analogue therapy. It can be avoided by use of antagonists rather than agonists, because the former have no stimulatory effect. Since 1972, a large number of GnRH antagonist compounds have been synthesised (Schally et al. 1989). These peptides are more antigenic than the agonists because of their greater structural change. The first antagonists led to local oedema at the site of injection and occasional anaphylactoid reactions. More recently, newer analogues have been synthesised and tested in humans. These have structural modifications which are less immunogenic. In normal men and patients with advanced prostate cancer, rapid, full and persistent suppression of LH and testosterone levels, without obvious side effects, and without any elevation of plasma hormones followed subcutaneous administration (Gonzalez-Barcena et al. 1990). Marked inhibition of growth is also seen with these agents in Dunning R3327 rats, PC-3 and LNCaP prostate cancer cell lines. Again there is a suggestion of a direct effect at the level of the malignant cell. We await the results of clinical trials with great interest.

Total Androgen Blockade

In a disease that is androgen sensitive, it may be important to eliminate all sources of androgen. In normal men 95% of all circulating androgens are of testicular origin. In the medically castrate man the situation is different; up to 45% of androgens within the prostate itself are of adrenal origin. In this context, the concept of total androgen blockade is currently being re-investigated. This concept was espoused in the last decade by Labrie et al. (1983) but was originally proposed by Huggins and Scott (1945). Current clinical trials of total androgen blockade use a GnRH analogue to minimise testicular androgen production and antiandrogens such as flutamide to limit the effects of androgens of adrenal and dietary origins. The evidence provided by Labrie to support the hypothesis was based on the synergy of effect in a non-malignant laboratory model, early clinical results, and a non-randomised trial based on historical controls. There is little laboratory evidence to support this hypothesis. For example, flutamide in combination with D-trp^6-LHRH showed no synergistic growth inhibition in the Dunning R3327 rat prostate adenocarcinoma model as compared to flutamide alone (Redding and Schally 1985). Nevertheless, despite the lack of preclinical rationale, the National Cancer Institute (NCI) instigated a carefully conducted randomised study in which over 600 patients were eventually enrolled, comparing leuprolide and placebo with leuprolide and flutamide. A significant advantage was found to combination therapy both in terms of median time to objective progression (16 months vs 14 months $P = 0.03$) and median survival (35 months compared to 28 months $P = 0.03$) (Crawford et al. 1989). As expected this seven-month survival advantage fell far below the benefit seen in uncontrolled Phase II studies.

Other clinical trials, are currently investigating this hypothesis. The EORTC are comparing treatment with buserelin and placebo with buserelin and cyproterone acetate. The results of this trial are due for publication shortly. Discussion with the trial organiser has shown an equivalence of initial response and response duration for the two treatments (J. Klijn, personal communication). The Italian Prostatic Cancer Project randomised 373 patients with stage C and D prostate cancer to receive zoladex or zoladex and flutamide: 42% of patients treated with zoladex and 53% of patients treated with combination therapy responded ($P = 0.06$). The median time to disease progression was 18 months in the monotherapy and 24 months in the combination arm ($P = 0.09$).

The median time to death was 32 months for zoladex and 44 months in the zoladex and flutamide group ($P = 0.4$) (Boccardo et al. 1993).

It can be seen that the issue of the advantage of combination therapy over monotherapy remains contentious. Is the benefit seen worth the extra cost and associated possible side effects of the antiandrogen? No study comparing LHRH agonist monotherapy versus standard hormonal therapy has been performed with the same statistical power as the NCI one, leaving the question open as to whether combination treatment is superior to conventional therapy.

The combination of bilateral orchidectomy and nilutamide significantly prolonged life in patients as compared to bilateral orchidectomy alone (Beland et al. 1990). The results of this trial may not be significant because of the low median survival time in the control group. Bilateral orchidectomy versus zoladex and flutamide is being investigated in two trials (Iversen et al. 1990; Keuppens et al. 1990). The survival in both patient groups is similar to date.

At least six other major trials are in progress currently. The issue of the benefits of combination therapy are an eminently suitable subject for a meta-analysis. This has been undertaken and the results are awaited. Our own policy is to treat with combination therapy. This is based upon the clear advantage of antiandrogens in abrogating tumour flare, and the solidity of the results of the NCI trial.

GnRH analogues are being used in other ways to exploit their potential for targeting chemotherapy, which is based on the presence of GnRH receptors in tumours. Synthesis of GnRH analogues linked to cytotoxic radicals such as melphalan and cisplatin related metal complexes have been described (Schally et al. 1990). In experimental models these have shown high biological activity and localisation to prostate and breast. This type of targeting could be of significant practical therapeutic importance.

Prostate cancer is a relatively slowly progressive disease and its chemo-insensitivity may be partially due to a low growth fraction. In tumour models using the Dunning R33278 rat prostate adenocarcinoma, a GnRH analogue acted synergistically with both cyclophosphamide and mitozantrone causing growth inhibition (Eisenberger 1988). These results are yet to be translated into improved survival in humans (Dawson et al. 1992). In this context we are currently investigating adjuvant mitozantrone with leuprolide and flutamide in the setting of a phase III trial. Our preliminary results involving 60 patients are encouraging, and suggest a survival advantage to the mitozantrone treated group.

Relapsed Prostatic Cancer

Relapse inevitably occurs and upon relapse the expected median duration of survival is six months. Clinical escape seems to occur independently of the mode of primary or secondary androgen deprivation. Primary hormonal insensitivity is rare and "relapsed" cells remain androgen sensitive. We believe that the key to prolonging survival in this increasingly common disease is to unravel the mechanism of hormone independence. In this context, the GnRH receptors on the malignant cells, the cell/stromal interactions and the study of local paracrine and autocrine loops involving growth factors need to be investigated in more detail. Cunha et al. (1983) has shown the importance of stromal growth factors in regulation of normal prostate. Receptor independence and subsequent hormone insensitivity may be explained by continuing production of growth factors by surrounding stroma which has been shown in breast cancer in studies of MCF-7 cells (Bronzert et al. 1986). Indeed suramin, used in refractory prostate cancer, has been shown to bind to cellular receptors inhibiting platelet derived growth factor (PDGF), fibroblast growth factor (FGF), and transforming growth factor alpha (TGFα). Recent experiments with prostatic cancer cell lines have shown that growth stimulation of prostate carcinoma cells by androgens is, at least partly, mediated through polypeptide growth factors. Co-culture experiments with the androgen responsive cell line (LNCaP) show growth stimulation of the androgen receptor negative cell line (DU-145) (Knabbe et al. 1991). Furthermore, this latter effect could be blocked by polyanions such as suramin. However, prostatic cell lines may not be a good model system. The well-studied Dunning tumours have been passaged in rats for almost 30 years. LNCaP cells contain a modified androgen receptor system and have even been shown to exhibit striking growth stimulation when exposed to antiandrogens. The receptor has been shown to contain a single amino acid mutation in an essential region of its steroid binding domain (Schuurmans et al. 1991). Trials investigating LHRH analogues in combination with growth factor inhibitors such as somatostatin, or even more specific agents from the outset may increase response rates.

Summary

Androgen deprivation remains the mainstay of treatment in prostatic carcinoma but has yet to prove convincingly to have a survival benefit. Treatment can therefore only be recommended to palliate symptoms in advanced disease or within the setting of clinical trials in earlier stage cancer. There are now a large number of therapies that lead to androgen ablation and choice is dependent on toxicity profiles, ease of administration and cost. Depot LHRH agonist preparations are likely to be the most popular over the next decade but are increasingly likely to be used in combination with other therapies. The role of total androgen blockade remains undetermined and awaits the completion of clinical trials. The major challenge for treatment is to provide a survival advantage for our patients and to this end, further investigations into the fundamental biology of the prostate and its relationship to endocrine manipulation must be understood. The study of local peptide growth factors and the molecular biology of benign and malignant cells is likely to lead to an understanding of clonal escape mechanisms in transformed cells and subsequently to have a significant impact on the future choice of therapies.

References

Adolfsson J, Steineck G, Whitmore WF Jr (1993) Recent results of management of palpable clinically localised prostate cancer. Cancer 72:310–322

Beland G, Elhilali M, Fradet Y et al. (1990) A controlled trial of castration with and without nlutamide in metastatic prostatic carcinoma. Cancer 66(Suppl):1074–1079

Boccardo F, Pace M, Rubagotti A et al. (1993) Goserelin acetate with or without flutamide in the treatment of patients with locally advanced prostate cancer. The Italian Prostatic Cancer Project (PONCAP) Study Group. Eur J Cancer 29:1088–1093

British Prostate Study Group (1979) Evaluation of plasma hormone concentrations in relation to clinical staging in patients with prostate cancer. Br J Urol 51:582–589

Bronzert DA, Davidson M, Lippman M (1986) Oestrogen and antioestrogen resistance in human breast cancer cell lines. Adv Exp Med Biol 196:329–345.

Byar DP (1973) The Veterans Administration Cooperative Research Group's studies of cancer of the prostate. Cancer 32:1126–1130

Byrne M (1992) Cancer chemotherapy and quality of life. Editorial Br Med J 304:1523–1524

Clayton RN, Channabasavaiah K, Stewart JM, Catt KJ (1982) Hypothalamic regulation of pituitary gonadotrophin-releasing hormone receptors: effects of hypothalamic lesions and a gonadotrophin releasing hormone antagonist. Endocrinology 110:1108–1115

Crawford ED, Eisenberger MA, McLeod DG et al. (1989) A controlled trial of leuprolide with and without flutamide in prostatic carcinoma. N Engl J Med 321:419–424

Cunha GR, Chung CWK, Shamanz M, Tagachi O, Fuji H (1983) Hormone induced morphogenesis and growth: role of mesenchymal–epithelial interactions. Rec Prog Horm Res 39:559–598

Dawson NA, Wilding G, Weiss R et al. (1992) A pilot trial of chemohormonal therapy for metastatic prostate carcinoma. Cancer 69:213–219

De Voogt HJ, Smith PH, Pavone-Macaluso M, de Pauw M, Sucio S (1986) Cardiovascular side effects of diethylstilboestrol, cyproterone acetate, medroxyprogesterone acetate and estramustine phosphate used in the treatment of advanced prostatic cancer: results from the EORTC trials 30761 and 30762. J Urol 135:303–307

Eisenberger MA (1988) Chemotherapy for prostate carcinoma. In: NCI monographs no. 7 Government Printing Office, Washington DC, (WIH Publications 88-3005), pp. 151–163

Gonzalez-Barcena D, Vadillo-Buenfil M, Guerra-Arguero L, Carreno J, Comaru-Schally AM, Schally A V (1990) Potent antagonistic analog of LHRH (SB-7S) inhibits LH, FSH and testosterone levels in human beings. 72nd Annual Meeting. Endocrine Society Atlanta, GA, 20–23 June p 354 (Abstract 1318)

Hammond GL, Kantturi M, Maattala P, Pookka M, Vikho R (1977) Serum FSH, LH and prolactin in normal males and patients with prostatic diseases. Clin Endocrinol 7:129–135

Harper ME, Peeling WB, Crowley T et al. (1976) Plasma steroid and protein hormone concentrations in patients with prostatic carcinoma, before and during oestrogen therapy. Acta Endocrinol 85:650–664

Hsueh AJW, Jones PB (1981) Extrapituitary actions of gonadotrophin-releasing hormone. Endocrinol Rev 2:437–461

Huggins C, Hodges CV (1941) Studies in prostatic cancer. The effects of castration, of oestrogens and androgen injection on serum phosphatases in metastatic carcinoma of the prostate. Cancer Res 1:293–297

Huggins C, Scott WN (1945) Bilateral adrenalectomy in prostatic cancer; clinical features and urinary secretion of 17-ketosteroids and oestrogen. Ann Surg 122:1031–1041

Iversen P, Christensen M, Friis E et al. (1990) A phase III trial of zoladex and flutamide versus orchiectomy in the treatment of patients with advanced carcinoma of the prostate. Cancer 66 (Suppl):1058–1066

Kaisary AV, Tyrrell CJ, Peeling WB, Griffiths K (1991) Comparison of LHRH analogue (zoladex) with orchiectomy in patients with metastatic prostatic carcinoma. Br J Urol 67:502–508

Keuppens F, Dennis L, Smith P et al. (1990) Zoladex and flutamide versus bilateral orchiectomy: a randomized phase III EORTC 30853 study. Cancer 66 (Suppl):1045–1057

Knabbe C, Kellner U, Schmahl M, Voigt KD (1991) Growth factors in human prostate cancer cells: implications for an improved treatment of prostate cancer. J Steroid Biochem Mol Biol 40:185–192

Labrie F, Dupont A, Belanger A, La Coursiere Y, Raynaud JP (1983) New approaches of prostate cancer: complete instead of partial withdrawal of androgens. Prostate 4:579–594

Leuprolide Study Group (1984) Leuprolide versus diethystilboestrol for metastatic prostate cancer. N Engl J Med 311:1281–1286

Lunglmayr G (1989) Casodex (ICI 176, 334), a new non-steroidal antiandrogen: early clinical results. Horm Res 32 (Suppl):77–81

Marian J, Cooper RL, Conn PM (1981) Regulation of the rat pituitary gonadotrophin releasing hormone receptor. Mol Pharmacol 19:339–405

McClinton S, Moffat LEF, Ludbrook A (1989) The cost of bilateral orchiectomy as a treatment for prostatic carcinoma. Br J Urol 63:309–312

Neri R, Kassem N (1984) Biological and clinical properties of antiandrogens. In: Brescani F, King RJB, Lippman ME, Namer M, Raynaud JP (eds) Hormones and cancer 2. Proceedings of the second international congress on hormones and cancer. Raven Press, New York, pp 507–522

Nesbit RM, Baum WC (1950) Endocrine control of prostatic cancer: clinical survey of 1818 cases. JAMA 143:1317–1320

OPCS Monitor (1991) DU 2 91/4 Deaths by cause, 5 December

Paulson DF, Lin GH, Hinshaw W, Stephani S, Uro-Oncology Research Group (1982) Radical surgery versus radiotherapy for adenocarcinoma of the prostate. J Urol 128:502–504

Qayum A, Gullick W, Clayton RC, Sikora K, Waxman J (1990) The effects of gonadotrophin releasing hormone analogues in prostate cancer as mediated through specific tumour receptors. Br J Cancer 62:96–99

Redding TW, Schally AV (1985) Investigation of the combination of the agonist D-Trp-6-LHRH and the antiandrogen flutamide in the treatment of Dunning R3327 prostate cancer model. Prostate 6:219–232

Rutqvist LE, Wilking N (1992) Analogues of LHRH versus orchidectomy: comparison of economic costs for castration in advanced prostate cancer. Br J Cancer 65:927–929

Schally AV, Coy DH (1977) Stimulatory and inhibitory analogs of luteinizing hormone releasing hormone (LHRH). Adv Exp Med Biol 87:99–121

Schally AV, Kastin AJ, Coy DH (1983) LH-releasing hormone and its analogues: recent basic and clinical investigations. Int J Fertil 21:1–30

Schally AV, Bajusz S, Redding TW, Zalatrai A, Comaru-Schally AM (1989) Analogs of LHRH: the present and the future. In: Vickery BH, Lunenfeld V (eds) Basic aspects: GnRH analogues in cancer and in their reproduction, vol 1. Kluwer, Dordrecht, pp 5–31

Schally AV, Srkalovic G, Szende B et al. (1990) Antitumour effects of analogues of LHRH and somatostatin: experimental and clinical studies. J Steroid Biochem Mol Biol 37:1061–1067

Schuurmans ALG, Bolt J, Veldscholte J, Mulder E (1991) Regulation of growth of LNCaP human prostate tumour cells by growth factors and steroid hormones. J Steroid Biochem Mol Biol 40:193–197

Scott WW (1959) Panel discussion on some aspects of urological endocrinology. In: North Central section of the American Urological Association, Postgraduate Seminars. Cited by Thomson GJ Long term control of prostatic cancer. Surg Clin North Am 39:963–971

Sharpe RM (1980) Extra-pituitary actions of LHRH and its agonists. Nature 286:12–14

Smith WA, Conn PM (1984) Microaggregation of the gonadotrophin-releasing hormone-receptor: relations to gonadotrope desensitization. Endocrinology 114:553–559

Varenhurst E, Wallentin L, Risberg B (1981) The effects of orchidectomy, oestrogens and cyproterone acetate on the antithrombin III concentration in carcinoma of the prostate. Urol Res 9:25–28

Veterans Administration Cooperative Urological Research Group (1967) Carcinoma of the prostate treatment comparisons. J Urol 98:516–522

Waterhouse J, Ulvin C, Shamugeratram K, Powell J (1982) Cancer in five continents, Vol IV. IARC Scientific publications,

Waxman J, Man A, Hendry WF, Whitfield HN, Besser GM (1985) Importance of early tumour exacerbation in patients treated with long acting analogues of gonadotrophin releasing hormone for advanced prostate cancer. Br Med J 291:1387–1388

Waxman J, Sandow J, Thomas H, James W, Williams G (1989) A pharmacological evaluation of a new 3-month depot preparation of buserelin for prostatic cancer. Cancer Chemother Pharmacol 25:219–220

White JW (1893) The present position of the surgery of the hypertrophied prostate. Ann Surg 18:152–188

Yang-Feng TL, Seeburg PH, Francke N (1986) Human luteinizing hormone-releasing hormone gene (LHRH) is located on short arm of chromosome 8 (region 8 p11.2-p21). Somat Cell Mol Genet 12:95–100

Chapter 10

Conservative Treatment of Localised Prostate Cancer

N. J. R. George

Introduction

Prostate cancer has long been an enigma to the practising urologist. Forty years ago Franks reported, whilst attributing the original observations to Rich (1935), that the disease had apparently increased in frequency since 1900, but was a comparatively rare cause of death (1.4% of all deaths in men over 50) despite being commonly identified in autopsy specimens. He considered that at least 30% of men over 50 years had such latent or quiescent cancer (Franks 1956). Franks noted the American experience at that time to be similar to his own; later workers (Scott et al. 1969) found disease at autopsy in 57% of men over 80 years.

However, the concept of an inert or an inactive cancer is, as observed by many, not easy to accept and the inability to link apparently unequivocal histological findings with clinical progress is at the heart of the dilemma concerning treatment for prostate cancer, particularly in the elderly. A brief review of incidence and prevalence rates together with data from geographical and epidemiological studies allows an appreciation of the problems faced by clinicians wishing to avoid impaction on the twin horns of inadequate cancer therapy and surgical overtreatment for this common disease.

Variations in Incidence and Mortality

In recent years prostate cancer has developed rapidly as a cause of both medical and economic concern. In 1975, 197 700 cases were reported worldwide, the disease being the fifth most common male cancer (Parkin et al. 1984) and it may now be the most common malignancy in humans based on evidence obtained at autopsy (Dhom 1983). The disease was diagnosed in 5700 patients in 1970 and was the fourth most common male cancer in England and Wales; more recent figures indicate that it has become the second most common cause of male cancer deaths accounting for approximately 7500 deaths in 1988. New case registration has increased rapidly, and within the United Kingdom 10 820 patients were initially diagnosed in 1985 (HMSO 1975; OPCS 1989). In the north west region alone 4064 new cases of prostate carcinoma were registered between 1985 and 1989. The crude annual incidence rate was 41.9 per 100 000 (CCE 1992) and the typical rapid increase was seen after 55 years of age (Fig. 10.1). In the United States the disease is now the most commonly diagnosed cancer in elderly males, newly diagnosed cases of clinical prostate cancer having increased from 42 000 20 years ago to over 100 000 in 1990; cancer mortality increased from 14 000 to 28 500 during the same interval (Enstrom and Austin 1977; Silverberg and Lubera 1988,1989).

Worldwide, it is now well established that there are marked variations in the incidence (i.e. histologically proven disease in patients who are alive) of prostate cancer with the lowest rates being found in oriental races and the highest in US non-whites (Skeet 1976; Waterhouse et al. 1982). However, ethnic influence within particular geographical zones may show marked variation; conversly the disease is identified twice as often in men of Sweden as in those of Denmark, two races thought to share a common background.

International variations in mortality rates from prostate cancer are also well described (Dunn 1975; Waterhouse et al. 1982). Low levels are found in the Far East, Thailand, Hong Kong and Japan compared with the high rates found in the West Indes, Sweden and Norway. Marked racial differences can be observed in the United States. Mortality for blacks is twice that for whites and the disease is diagnosed at a later stage in the former population (Murphy et al. 1982; Metlin and Natarajam 1983). Although genetic variation between the races seems to offer an obvious explanation for these findings the inequality of health care provision across the population spectrum has to be

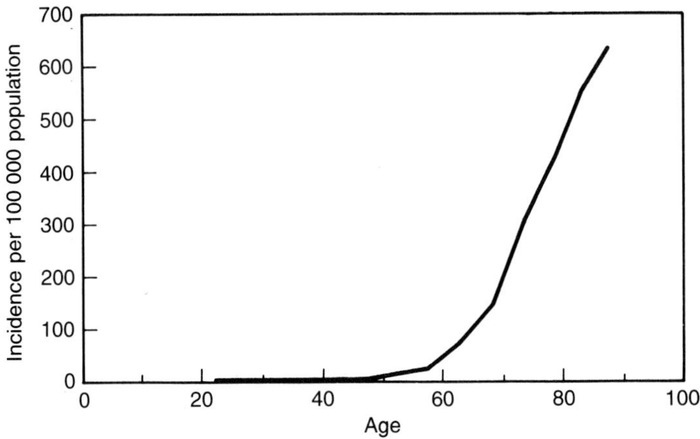

Fig. 10.1. Age-specific incidence rate of prostate cancer in the North West of England. Data from CCE (1992).

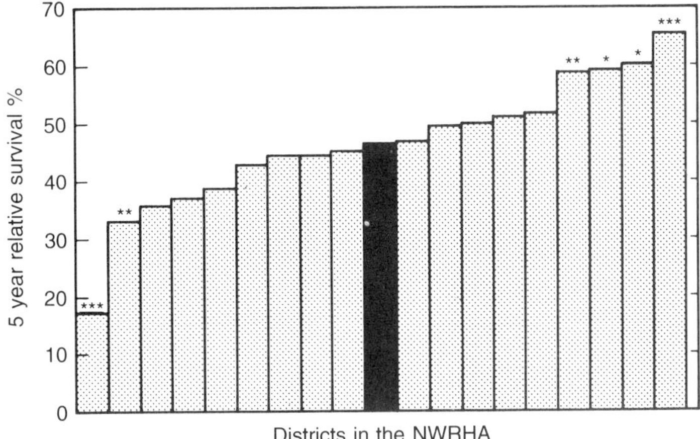

Fig. 10.2. Five-year relative survival rates across the North West Region of England in 18 districts (toned columns) as compared to the regional average (black column). Marked differences in survival within such a small area are unlikely to relate to variations in cancer biopotential alone. (Data from CCE 1992.)

considered as a possible reason for the findings. Comparative studies between US and West African blacks have to be interpreted with care bearing in mind the differing life expectation of the two populations (Jackson et al. 1977).

The incidence of clinically diagnosed disease increases more rapidly than other tumours as age progresses (Carter and Coffey 1990) being rare under 50 years, a 40-fold increase being observed by age 85 years (Fig. 10.1). The increasing health care demands of an elderly population will undoubtedly lead to further strain on already overstretched economic resources. The population of the United States over 65 years old is estimated to increase to 13.8 million males by the year 2000 from 8.4 million in 1970, an increase of 64% (US Bureau of Census 1986).

Taking such an increase in the at-risk population into account, the detection of disease and thus the resource requirement will be variably dependent on the thoroughness of clinical investigations and particularly on the sophistication of pathological processing of prostate specimens obtained at surgery. Even within a close-knit region of England with similar approaches to prostatic disease and a largely homogeneous population spectrum there is substantial incongruity in differing aspects of prostatic disease (Fig 10.2). In this case it seems likely that 5-year survival rates ranging from 17.3% to 65.4% must reflect major differences in both social and medical approaches to the condition rather than an inherent biological difference in the disease itself.

Localised Prostate Cancer

Localised prostate cancer is usually discussed in terms of clinical or latent disease. Franks described "latent" cancer as "unsuspected" cancer, the term defined as histological evidence of disease discovered at post mortem in patients dying of other certified causes (Franks 1956; Scott et al. 1969). There is little doubt as to the widespread prevalence of this form of disease, and the relationship between it and the overt clinical manifestation of the disorder is the essence of the dilemma faced by the urologist. The unknown biopotential of "unsuspected" tumours discovered following death from other causes and the undoubtedly slow growth of some neoplasms discovered during life are factors which have helped support the hypothesis of "inactive cancer". The various surveillance studies which are the subject of this chapter constitute one response to this challenge. It is also helpful to re-examine the criteria by which, in earlier years, the diagnosis of prostate cancer was established.

Latent Disease

Discovered at autopsy, evidence regarding the presence of widespread dissemination in life is often circumstantial; tests for unsuspected conditions were not usually performed in the age before the multichannel autoanalyser. Backache is common in the elderly and requests for phosphatases and skeletal surveys are unusual without clinical indications; nearly all the classical "latent" series were completed in the era prior to isotropic bone scanning. In a study representative of this era Clifton et al. (1952) reported on 49 patients with histological proof of prostate cancer. Bone marrow aspirates showed tumour cells in 9% patients despite negative skeletal surveys. Two thirds of patients were pain free. Hence in these cases the presumed "latency" of any neoplasm found incidentally at post mortem merely rests on the lack of evidence suggesting metastatic spread. Additionally most autopsy reports restrict themselves to the gland alone whereas iliac and nodes elsewhere remain unsampled or unreported (Hirst and Bergman 1954). Although the small volume and low grade of most tumours discovered at autopsy implies that spread will indeed not have occurred, historical assumptions based on retrospective material remain open to question.

Effect of Intensive Search

Despite reservations from past studies most series reporting autopsies agree that the finding of neoplastic prostatic histology in patients certified as dying from other causes is increasingly common as age progresses (Hirst and Bergman 1954). It is not surprising, bearing in mind the acknowledged multifocal nature of prostatic cancer (Hayashi et al. 1987), that a more intensive pathological search yields a higher incidence of positive findings. Early series (Halpert et al. 1963) reported on one or two sections of the gland whereas later work examining 4 mm step sections (Scott et al. 1969) observed latent disease in 41% and 57% of patients over 70 and 80 years respectively.

Geographical Variation

A number of workers have reported autopsy studies from differing geographical regions of the world in order to throw light on the distribution of latent cancer and its relationship with clinically manifest disease (Breslow et al. 1977; Guileyardo et al. 1980; Yatani et al. 1982). As will be evident from statements above, the comparability of such series will clearly depend on the age profile of patients studied as well as pathological technique employed.

Breslaw et al. (1977) reported the incidence of small carinomas (almost exclusively placed peripherally) to be approximately 12% in each of seven areas – Singapore, Hong Kong, Israel, Uganda, Jamaica, Sweden and Germany. The assessment was by means of octant count and medium and large tumours (occupying more octants) were generally found in geographic locations with a high incidence of clinical disease. It was, however, observed that many autopsies performed in Sweden were on elderly men (>75 years old) when compared with other areas (i.e., Sweden 44%, Hong Kong 19%, Uganda 8% of elderly autopsies) and thus the large cancers might merely be due to patient age rather than active tumour growth. As might be expected, autopsy technique was more thorough in Sweden than in Uganda, again a source of possible bias in the results. Yatani et al. (1982) subdivided tumours into "infiltrative" and "non-infiltrative" and found a high incidence of the former in Japanese migrants to Hawaii and in both blacks and whites in the USA; they suggested that the non-infiltrative represented the true latent or quiescent disease. Taken together, these studies show that local custom and variable socioeconomic conditions make for considerable difficulties of interpretation but nevertheless it seems reasonable to conclude that either genetic or environmental influences or both might influence conversion from latent into clinical cancer in the differing populations studied.

Clinical Disease

In contrast to latent cancer, the incidence of clinically diagnosed tumour varies widely among different international groups (Table 10.1). Age-standardised rates for Alameda black patients are almost 100 times greater than those for Chinese patients in Shanghai (Waterhouse et al. 1982). However, although it is now estimated that there may be 10 million US males with latent cancer (Carter and Coffey 1990), only a small percentage become clinically manifest each year. The increasing conversion of this "pool" of latent disease to clinically detected cancer might be explained in part by the increasing use of transurethral resection in an ageing population (Potosky et al. 1990). Furthermore, as with autopsy studies, thorough pathological search of resected material in centres with an active interest in prostate diseases might be expected to reveal increasing amounts of hitherto unsuspected (T0, stage A) cancer. Approximately a quarter of new patients presenting to one clinic were found to harbour clinically silent neoplastic change (Beynon et al. 1983).

However, it is not possible to explain the differing patterns of disease in eastern and western older males by variations in clinical or pathological practice alone. Life expectancy for Japanese males is approximately the same as that for United States males yet the age-adjusted incidence of cancer is over 15 times greater in the latter population (Silverberg 1987). Japanese men settling in Hawaii or California have a notable increase in clinical cancer

Table 10.1. Incidence of prostate cancer. Age standardised rates per 100 000 population (world standard population): based on data from Waterhouse et al. (1982)

Population	Incidence
San Fransisco Bay area	
Black	92.2
White	47.4
Chinese	18.6
Japanese	12.7
Hawaii	
White	59.7
Hawaiian	42.5
Japanese	35.9
Chinese	25.8
Scandinavia	
Sweden	44.4
Norway	38.9
Finland	27.2
Denmark	23.6
New Zealand	
Maori	39.8
Non-Maori	30.7
Singapore	
Indian	6.7
Chinese	4.8
China	
Shanghai	0.8

suggesting that environmental or other epidemiological factors are of greater significance than genetic components of the disease (Haenszel and Kurihara 1968; Dunn 1975). Conversely, reports of cancer in male relatives of patients (Steinberg et al. 1990; McWhorter et al. 1992), the worldwide predisposition of black races to the disease and the observation that ethnic groups in the same areas do not enjoy the same incidence (Table 10.1) imply that genetic influences on disease expression cannot be discounted. Diet (Carroll and Kohr 1975), body weight (Whittemore et al. 1984) and physical and sexual activity (Ross et al. 1981) are other factors which have been intensively studied in differing population groups in an attempt to identify factors responsible for conversion of histologically silent into biologically active disease.

Incidentally Diagnosed Clinical Disease

Microscopic cancer is found in approximately 10%–15% of patients undergoing resection for presumed prostatic hyperplasia, the incidence (see above) rising with the age of the patient and sectioning technique. Debate continues as to progression criteria for such stage A tumours. Epstein et al. (1986), quoting follow-up of an earlier series (Cantrell et al. 1981), originally detected progression in only one out of 49 patients with focal change as compared to

11 of 33 patients with diffuse disease; in the longer term, however, although a significant number died from other causes which thus masked the true progression rate, 16% (eight patients) had advancing disease – leading to death in six. In these cases neither the original volume nor grade of tumour predicted progression. Whether disease in socioeconomic groups able to attend centres of excellence is representative of disease in other less privileged areas of the country is an open question, bearing in mind known epidemiological data. Uncertainty regarding the outcomes of stage A or T0 disease has encouraged the widespread adoption of radical surgery to cure the disease (Epstein and Steinberg 1990), particularly in the United States and to a lesser extent in some centres of Europe. Major operative procedures naturally carry a significant risk of mortality and morbidity, particularly as the technique becomes widely adopted away from the centres of excellence.

Apart from the major cost implication, over-treatment of a proportion of patients with lesions of low biopotential will lead to an over-optimistic view of any treatment offered; introduction of the Franzen aspiration cytology technique in Sweden resulted in the incidence of prostate cancer doubling between 1958 and 1971 (Franzen et al. 1960) with resulting apparent treatment benefits (Trasti et al. 1979), probably due to inclusion of patients with lesions of questionable biopotential. Recent advice suggests that it is probably best at the present time to suppress emotional arguments about cancer surgery in favour of informed and objective endeavour to understand better the natural history of early prostate cancer (Smith and Cho 1990).

Conclusion

It seems clear that considerable doubt exists regarding the behaviour of histological identifiable prostate cancer cells. The discrepancy between the incidence of latent and clinical disease sends a clear signal that intensive research is required to describe the biological characteristics of each so as to prevent both undertreatment and overtreatment of respective patient cohorts. Although difficult to achieve, a crucial preliminary step in this investigation process is to discover whether any subgroup of patients presenting with clinical prostate cancer have "latent" survival characteristics; subsequent subdivisions might possibly be made between those with developing lower urinary tract symptoms and those asymptomatic men presenting to well-man clinics. Observational studies of the natural history of localised prostate cancer fulfil this basic research requirement.

Observational Studies in Localised Prostate Cancer

Observational studies or conservative treatment, referred to as deferred treatment or "watchful waiting" by authors anxious not to imply neglect in the follow-up of patients with neoplastic disease, has recently been the subject of heated debate. Although the variable outcome of patients with this disorder has been recognised for many years (Whitmore 1973), the marked increase in incidence described above together with the widespread application of radical surgery for the condition has prompted an energetic biological, medical and economic discussion on the merits and pitfalls of treatment. Central to the debate concerning the need for, or abuse of, radical therapy is the biological behaviour of the tumour itself and hence studies which have addressed this problem have been subjected to intense scrutiny. It should be emphasised that whereas the authors of such work might, as a result of their observations, advocate conservative or deferred treatment in certain risk groups, the true purpose of the series is to illustrate as best possible the natural history of localised disease within the context of a population based study.

It is inevitable that, in clinically based research, there will be defects in data collection to which attention must be drawn. In this context the variable incidence of prostate cancer in differing areas and other factors already mentioned will be appreciated and thus the results of studies on one population (i.e. Sweden) may not necessarily hold true for patients from another (i.e. Detroit). Macroeconomic health policy, the local medicosocial framework and surgical diagnostic techniques will determine which patients are admitted to study protocols; critical analysis will take into account both these broad factors as well as particular aspects of individual studies themselves. Hence, despite every precaution, results of such observational studies may offer only general advice and conclusions rather than specific and universal pathological guidelines.

Population Based Studies

Source of Material

It is no coincidence that three recent series (George 1988; Johansson et al. 1989, 1992; Adolfsson et al. 1992) come from countries where sociomedical policy allows information to be collected from across the population spectrum regardless of "ability to pay" or any other exclusion factor. Such data collection should hold an advantage over others in which only certain sections of the population have access to medical care; information gathered from narrow strata is unlikely to be representative of the population as a whole. Nevertheless, as previously described, even within areas of Northern Britain and Sweden significant differences occur in both the patient's and doctor's attitude to disease which need careful examination before valid conclusions can be reached and perhaps extrapolated to the study of localised prostate cancer in general.

Recruitment to Study

General Background

Within the UK until very recently (1991) the great majority of patients later found to have histological prostate cancer of any stage or grade presented with obstructive or irritative symptoms of bladder outflow tract obstruction to their primary physician, who referred on for second opinion. Recently widespread publicity in the national press about prostate disease has caused some men without symptoms to come forward but in the Manchester series (George 1988) approximately 95% of patients were symptomatic on referral and such a mode of presentation may have implications for biopotential (see below).

By contrast in Sweden a more proactive approach to public health medicine might be expected to attract patients at an early stage in their disease, perhaps influencing lead time bias. In the Karolinska study (Adolfsson et al. 1992) 172 patients were recruited in 1978–82 who were "selected from a larger group"; the authors concede no formal variables or randomisation processes were involved in selection. The study profile as compared to the overall cancer population in that area is thus not clear although it seems likely that patients were at the "mild" end of the spectrum as patients with larger tumours who refused treatment offered "were included in the series". Overall, these authors do not define the material source, i.e., symptom status, physician referral or health check clinic etc.

Recruitment to the Örebro study (Johansson et al. 1989) was from a stable population surrounding the County Hospital and although a definite statement is not made as to the reason for seeking advice it seems possible that many patients had lower urinary tract symptoms as rectal examination and Franzen fine needle aspiration was frequently performed; all other cases were discovered following transurethral resection for outflow tract symptoms but the ratio of histology to cytology is not stated.

Patient Age

The literature on prostate cancer might suggest that selection of patients from different age groups could significantly affect the outcome of observational studies. The mean ages of patients included in the Örebro study was 72 years (range <60->80 years), Stockholm Study 68 years (39–89) and Manchester 74.8 years (62–90). In this respect therefore the series appear evenly matched.

Inclusions and Exclusions from Study

Each study suffers from a number of variations from the ideal recruitment pattern which would of necessity include every case of proven prostate cancer within the population drainage area. In the Manchester study all cases were notified through the central histological laboratory and all those – regardless of stage and grade – with negative bone scans and normal acid phosphatase were put up for candidacy in the watch and wait programme. Data collection was inadequate in 19 of 152 eligible patients; severe unrelated disease precluded recruitment in 11 patients and eight refused to participate. Thirteen additional patients were withdrawn by their consultants due to anxiety concerning (usually) grade and stage. Of 120 patients entered 50% were well-, 32%

were moderately- and 18% were poorly-differentiated tumours (unpublished observations). This study therefore recruited T0–3 Nx M0 tumours which, when compared to the ideal group, were biased towards well and moderately-differentiated histological pattern.

The Karolinska group by contrast included only "small" T1–2 tumours in their study which were all diagnosed by cytological aspirate (no incidental T0 or stage A post-transurethral resection tumours). Only patients with well- and moderately-differentiated histology were recruited. Of 122 patients 109 were T2 (89%) and the tumours well-differentiated in 77 (63%); these figures have been interpreted as showing bias towards the classical well-differentiated B2 nodule recognised by many including Whitmore as heralding a good prognosis.

It is unfortunate that admission to the Örebro study was varied during 1977/79. Initially patients with T0–T2 stage were admitted but during this period only patients with well-differentiated histology were accepted; after March 1979 patients under 75 with higher grade tumours were randomised to no treatment or irradiation therapy. This fluctuating admission pattern has provided ammunition for critics, particularly in North America, to discount this otherwise thorough study, recently updated and reported in 1992.

Exclusions based on this protocol determined that 83 of 306 (27%) histologically proven cases were not admitted to the study; clearly the argument that a well-differentiated bias exists is difficult to counter. Other points of contention involve the ability to distinguish between T0 (localised) and T0 (diffuse) on Franzen biopsy and the stated limit (>25% of specimen) between these two types of incidental tumour as measured against other definitions in the literature. Nevertheless, despite these reservations this series represents a precise and thorough attempt to answer the question of local prostate cancer behaviour and with correct interpretation is undoubtedly a valuable addition to the sparse literature on the subject.

Local Progression

Local progression is perhaps the most fundamental evidence that the prostate tumour is active. No study to date has involved rectal ultrasound and hence relatively crude estimations are made by the examiner's finger. However in the UK and Swedish studies most observations were at least made by the same examiner or group of examiners; investigator variation during follow-up can clearly be a source of substantial error in such studies.

Considerable differences emerge in the progression rates of the series studied probably due both to differing definitions of progression and preselection of cases likely to progress. Johansson et al. (1989) defined progression as growth "through the capsule", i.e. attainment of T3 status. Hence lesser advance from T1–T2 would presumably not be recorded as progresson by these authors. Adolfsson's definition was>25% increase in tumour diameter as judged by previous experience of rectal examination in that patient. In the Manchester study any recorded increase of whatever type over the previous examination was recorded as evidence of local progression.

The variable bias on histological criteria for admission has been mentioned above. Bearing these factors in mind, local progression rates were seen in 84% of patients in Manchester, 55% in Stockholm and 29% in Örebro (20% if patients without bone metastases are included). In the 1992 update non-metastatic progression to T3 status was seen in 76/223 (34%) showing continuing increase with time. It is difficult not to believe that these wide variations relate to protocol criteria rather than tumour bioactivity although the differing incidence profile of disease between the two countries (Table 10.1) cannot be dismissed.

Adolfsson noticed that higher stage disease "tended to progress faster than lower stage disease" and although statistical significance was not reached the observation taken in reverse supports the contention that predominance of early stage disease in this series would result in a lower local progression rate.

Bone Metastases

Spectrum of Bone Metastases at Recruitment

It is instructive to note the composition of the patients considered for entry into the observational studies. In Örebro 654 patients were diagnosed between March 1977 and February 1984, of which 159 (24%) had positive bone scans. Figures from Stockholm are not recorded but in Manchester 54% of patients recruited in 1980–86 presented at initial diagnosis with incurable metastatic disease, a figure which has since shown little sign of reducing and which again underlines differences between the series as well as the relatively advanced form of prostate cancer found in the North West of England.

Progression to Metastases on Study

During the majority of the time that these studies were underway, detection of bony metastases was by means of clinical signs, standard X-ray films, prostatic acid phosphatase estimations and ^{99}Tc bone scanning. The imperfections of these diagnostic aids have been well described by others but it seems likely that the presence or absence of bony lesions – as opposed to the exact time of development – would be reasonably accurately recorded, particularly as all series excluded to a greater or lesser extent the high-grade histology thought responsible for most false negative acid phosphatase results. The effect of the arrival of PSA and other diagnostic techniques in the mid-1980s is discussed below.

Bone disease developed in 17/122 (14%) in the Karolinska study, 20/223 (9%) in Örebro updated to 26/223 (12%) in the 1992 report; 13/120 (11%) positive bone scans were detected in Manchester. The probability of developing disease in bone was estimated by Adolfson to be 8% and 28% at five and ten years respectively whereas in Manchester the crude mean time to scan conversion was 36 months. It is perhaps slightly surprising bearing in mind the differences noted above in admission criteria that the metastatic rate should be so similar in all three areas; additionally, in Örebro five of 20 patients (25%) developing metastases had no sign of local progression again highlighting that, whilst conventional small lesion/large lesion/metastasis bioscience wisdom may be true for a majority of cases, a significant minority exhibit eccentric biological characteristics, a view long promulgated by Whitmore and others.

Disease Specific Mortality

Whilst discussion continues about relative rates of local progression (see below) it is the age-related disease spectrum of these patients that is the fundamental cause of debate regarding the advisability or otherwise of treating prostate cancer in the elderly. Each series confirms that the great majority of deaths occur from non-prostatic causes; 40%, 31% and 37% in the Manchester, Stockholm and Örebro studies respectively (Table 10.2, Fig. 10.3). In the Örebro update 124 patients had died of non-prostatic causes (56%) and cancer specific death in these three locations was just 4%, 7% and 7% (update 8.5%). Ten-year disease specific survival in Örebro was 86.8%. Hence in essence the decision to treat in localised prostate cancer depends in great part on the age of the patient and an assessment of the likelihood of death from non-prostatic causes. These decisions have to be taken against

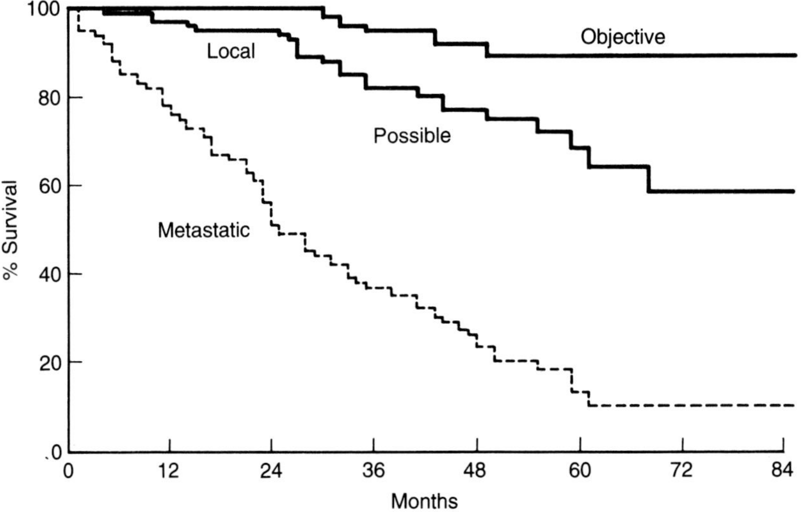

Fig. 10.3. Actuarial survival of patients excluding non-cancer deaths. Patients with localised prostate cancer (solid lines) assessed both for cases proven to have died of disease ($n=5$, objective) and for cases with severe non-prostatic illness ($n=15$, possible) or other reason for protocol violation (missed bone scan) in whom stable markers suggested prostate cancer was unlikely to be responsible for death. Both curves represented for completeness are compared with survival of 181 patients with bone scan-positive disease treated immediately after diagnosis (dotted line). Data from George (1988).

Table 10.2. Summary of essential data from observational studies in Manchester, Stockholm and Örebro. See text for details.

	George (1988)	Adolfsson (1992)	Johansson	
			1989	1992
Censored population	Total 363 M° 152	Not known	654 495	654 495
Study population	120	122	223	223
Mean age (years)	74.8	68	72	72
Excluded stage	Some T3 (physician choice)	T0 T3	T3	T3
Excluded grade	Some poor (physican choice)	Poor	Variable (see text) well diff. only 1977–79	Variable (see text) well diff. only 1977–79
Local progression defined	Any increase	>25% increase diameter	To or beyond T3	To or beyond T3
Local progression rate	84%	55%	20% (but see text)	34%
Development of bone metastases	13/120 (11%)	17/122 (14%)	20/233 (9%)	28/233 (12%)
Disease specific mortality	4%	7%	7%	8.5%
Non-cancer mortality	40%	31%	37%	47%

a background of increased longevity in the general population and for many, increased expectation of enhanced quality of life in the retirement years.

Effect of Stage and Grade

Variations in admission criteria between the two Swedish studies which reported stage and grade data account for differences in observed prognosis. In the Karolinska study grade and stage were thought not to influence progression but this is likely to be the result of recruiting only patients with small low grade T1/T2 tumours. In the Örebro study progression in incidentally discovered (T0 localised) lesions was lower than that for palpable T1/T2 tumours; although only nine patients with poor grade histology were admitted to study (4%) corrected survival was very poor, five patients dying of the disease. Well- and moderately-differentiated lesions led to survival of

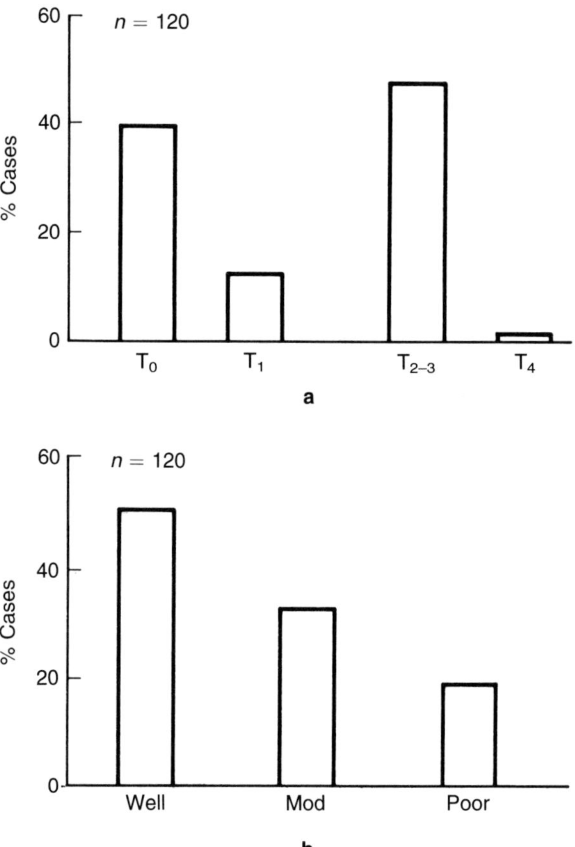

Fig. 10.4. Stage (**a**) and grade (**b**) of 120 patients entered into the Manchester study. Unpublished data from George (1988).

98% and 90% at five years respectively. Thereafter, however, the moderately-differentiated group deteriorated substantially whereas the corrected survival of patients with well-differentiated lesions remained high at 92.7% over ten years.

Unpublished data (Fig. 10.4) from Manchester initially supported the concept of a reasonable prognosis for patients with moderate grade tumours. Crude cancer specific survival at five years was 86%, 80% and 58% for well-, moderate- and poorly-differentiated lesions. Subsequent analysis, however, indicates that only well-differentiated neoplasms are maintaining their excellent survival status. There is general agreement from all studies that grade is the single most important prognostic indicator for men with localised prostate cancer.

Conclusions from Observational Studies

As inevitably will be the case when practical medicine meets theoretical ideal, each of the observational series has drawbacks. Nevertheless a realistic appraisal of shortcomings can result in the establishment of valid conclusions.

Disease Progression

Although the number of patients presenting with local symptoms in the Örebro study is not recorded, progression free survival decreases in each category of stage and grade at five and ten years. In the Manchester study, where 95% of patients presented with symptoms and all histology was obtained by means of necessary transurethral resection, 84% of patients advanced locally. These factors taken together suggest that there are few cases (probably none in Manchester) who do not advance as time progresses.

This important conclusion underscores the value of these series which have been heavily criticised as advocating "no treatment for patients with cancer". For many years the latent theory promoted by Franks (1956) has led to confusion among urologists and primary physicians. At least in the Northwest United Kingdom it is now quite clear that such a concept is no longer tenable in those patients who attend because of lower tract symptoms.

This does not of course mean that the proposition of latent or inactive tumours is dismissed. Within the UK the age and clinical state of the patients on whom the observations were made are markedly different from the asymptomatic 50-year-old North American attending his well-man clinic. Current prostatic publicity within the UK is starting to produce small numbers of similar men and there is no rational reason to suggest that tumour biopotential as seen in the elderly will apply to the younger asymptomatic man. The well-described discrepancy between autopsy prevalence and clinical incidence of the disease suggests that it remains a possibility that some men may indeed have "latent" cell types (which will not give rise to trouble in the patient's lifetime) whereas others have progressive tendencies which in time will lead to clinical manifestation and death if age and intercurrent disease do not intervene. The dilemma at present is related to the surgeon's inability to resolve this question and hence to be confident that his patient does not have a life-threatening condition.

Stage

Although not as convincing as grade, cumulative evidence from the studies suggests that T0 tumours (particularly local) have a better prognosis than those stage T2. Problems relate to the difficulty of assessment using the Franzen cytological technique (T0 local or T0 diffuse?) and the possibility that transurethral resection may in fact remove all tumour in some patients with central zone T0 lesions thus leading to a false expectation of progression. In general, however, there seems little doubt that progression increases with stage.

Grade

In the absence of adequate markers grade remains the single best indicator of likelihood to progress. Evidence from the three studies seems to suggest that only well-differentiated tumours can be expected to remain quiescent over long periods of time. Moderate- and (especially) high-grade tumours will progress at a significant rate which is likely to rule out a watchful waiting policy except in certain elderly men. Nevertheless, exceptions are widespread and whereas a classical moderately differentiated B2 nodule may be confined for years certain well differentiated tumours may rapidly metastasise; tumour heterogeneity and unrepresentative biopsy material are likely to be important in this respect.

Age

No evidence was found from the studies that age per se affected the patient's prognosis. In the Örebro series the rate of tumour advance did not differ between patients over and under 70 years of age. Many surgeons are presently taking 70 years as the "cut off" with regard to the treatment options available (i.e. suitability for radical prostatectomy) although 15-year survival with good quality of life is far from unusual at this age in the experience of many. The choice of treatment no doubt thus remains a delicate balance between the various identified risk factors in any one patient.

Treatment by Watchful Waiting

It is clear from the summary above that there is no blanket rule that can be applied to men with localised disease. In general, men over 70 years are likely to be suitable candidates for watchful waiting whereas those under 65 are not. The age of death of the patient's father as well as the patient's own age, stage, grade and coincidental medical conditions will determine the balance of the equation. At the present time it is still possible to propose that tumours detected in "well-man" clinics (presume asymptomatic) might carry a different prognosis to that in symptomatic men; however, the lack of a credible biological marker means that the surgeon must assume the worst and advise accordingly. This dilemma will clearly lead to overtreatment – possibly of large numbers of men – until the biological potential of the tumours can be identified.

Unlike the situation at the commencement of the observational studies when progression to metastases could only be assessed by regular prostatic acid phosphatase estimations and bone scanning, the clinician now has the possibility of anticipating advanced disease before it manifests as a positive scan. High definition rectal ultrasound can be very helpful in those cases

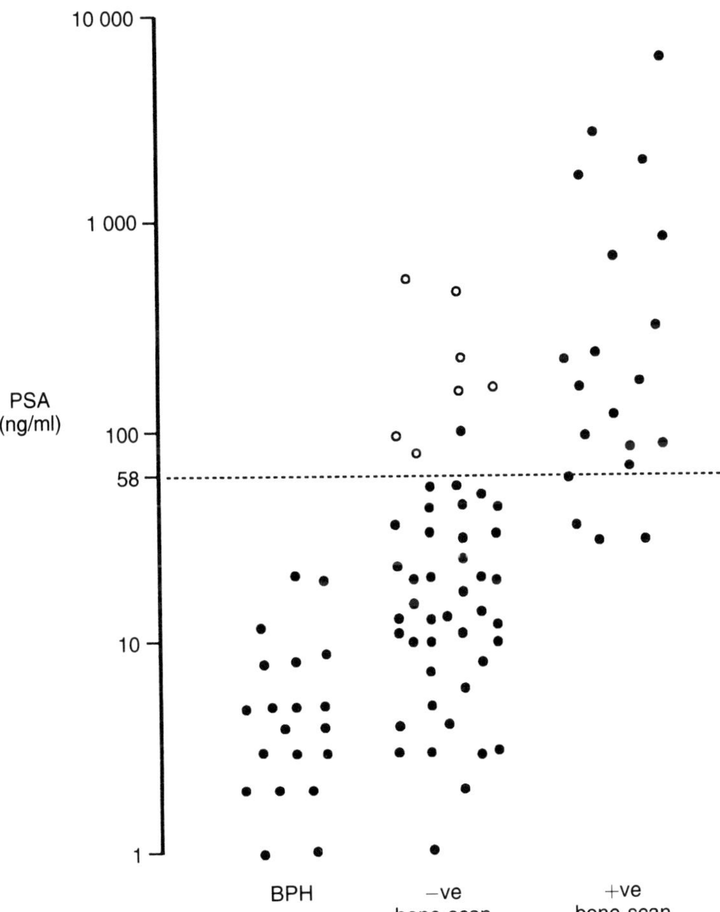

Fig. 10.5. Prostate specific antigen levels (Hybritech) in groups of patients with bone scan positive (M1) and scan negative (M0). Open circles, patients with raised acid phosphatase values; - - -, optimum cut off for disease in bone. Patients with prostate cancer compared to values from 20 patients with benign prostatic hypertrophy (BPH). Data from Pantelides et al. (1992).

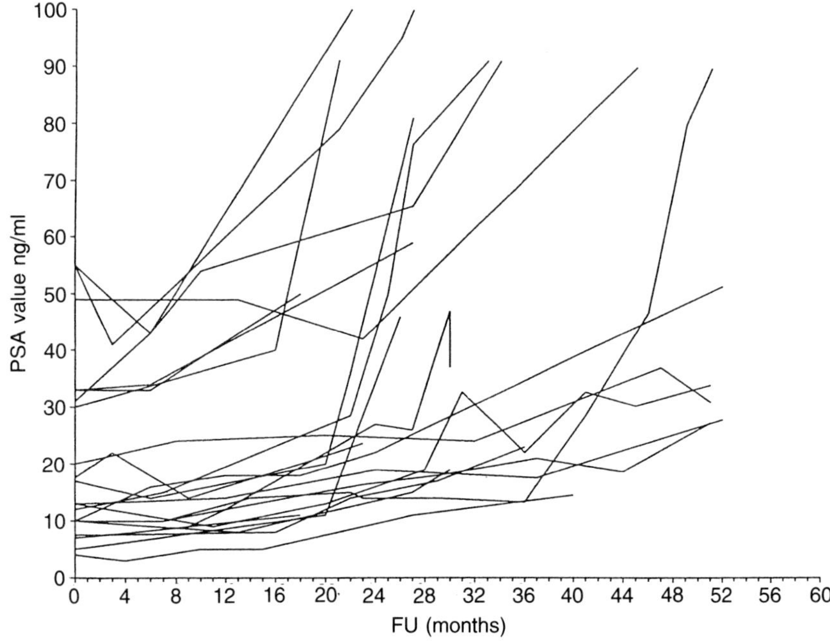

Fig. 10.6a

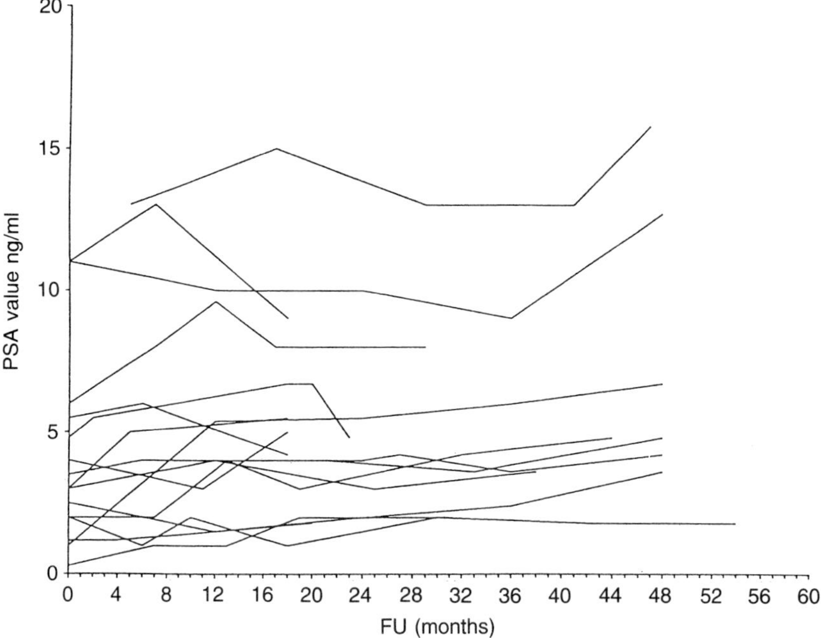

Fig. 10.6b

with paradoxical digital findings but it is probably not suited to the regular (6-monthly) monitoring of large numbers of elderly men.

Prostate specific antigen (PSA) by contrast has revolutionised the "watch and wait" clinic by obviating the need for bone scans unless marked elevation occurs. Pantelides et al. (1992) determined that a level of 58 ng/ml led to a 79% predictive accuracy for disease in bone (Fig. 10.5). Rising values measured over time usually indicate the need for intervention before bone changes occur but the concept is flawed in some cases as the PSA rise may not always be gradual (Fig. 10.6) and in these unusual cases disease advance may occur even between six-monthly visits. Despite this caveat, however, PSA has proved to be extremely helpful when monitoring patients over 65–70 years old and represents a genuine cost-effective advance in management.

It hardly needs to be stated that the medical aspects of "watchful waiting" cannot be delegated to junior members of the team. Any patient (and his wife) who knows he has a form of cancer will rightly demand that only the most experienced physician will be observing his progress. Under these conditions it has been the experience of the author that most older men, having had the full facts placed in front of them, will accept the concept of careful observation with its inherent benefits of strong psychological support and negligible morbidity. Loss of patient confidence, however, in these special circumstances can spell disaster for all and invites a litigious postscript.

Tumour Biopotential

These studies of untreated prostate cancer indicate that no advance will be made until the biopotential of any particular tumour can be assessed. To date, such a breakthrough has proved elusive and under these circumstances it is entirely to be expected that the surgeon will take a pessimistic view of any identified neoplasm, particularly in a younger man. Naturally, the identification of any particular marker in any one tumour will be of little use without the corresponding information on the patient's progress and survival. For this reason some have advocated a three-armed prospective trial comparing conservative treatment, radical prostatectomy and radiotherapy in early prostate cancer. Although prolonged survival times inevitably mean that it might be many years before a significant result emerged from such a study, the endeavour would at least allow histological material to be banked and later tested against observed progression. The pivotal role to be played by biological markers in early prostate cancer is the subject of review elsewhere in this text.

Fig. 10.6. PSA values in patients with localised prostate cancer followed without treatment divided according to whether values rose with time (a) or remain stable (b). Although the majority of slowly rising values allowed adequate warning of impending metastatic problems and thus need for treatment, a few patients suddenly advanced having previously been rising at a steady rate. Levels in stable patients were usually within the range 2–12 ng/ml at initial diagnosis. (The different scales for PSA should be noted.) (Unpublished data from Pantelides et al.)

References

Adolfsson J, Carstensen T, Lowhagen T (1992) Deferred treatment in localised prostate cancer. Br J Urol 69:183–187

Beynon L, Busuttil A, Newsham JE, Chisholm GD (1983) Incidental carcinoma of the prostate; selection for deferred treatment. Br J Urol 55:733–736

Breslow N, Chan CE, Dhom G et al. (1977) Latent carcinoma of prostate at autopsy in seven areas. Int J Cancer 20:680–688

Cantrell BB, DeKlerk DP, Eggleston JC, Boitnott JK, Walsh PC (1981) Pathological factors that influence prognosis in stage A prostate cancer, influence of extent versus grade. J Urol 125:516–520

Carroll KK, Kohr HT (1975) Dietary fat in relation to tumorigenesis. Prog Biochem Pharmacol 10:308–353

Carter HB, Coffey DS (1990) The prostate: an interesting medical problem. Prostate 16:39–48

CCE (1992) Report by the Centre for Cancer Epidemiology. North West Regional Health Authority, Manchester, UK

Clifton JA, Philipp RJ, Loduvic BS, Fowler WM (1952) Observations on occult carcinoma of the prostate gland. Am J Med Sci 224:121–130

Dhom G (1983) Epidemiologic aspects of latent and clinically manifest carcinoma of the prostate. J Cancer Res Clin Oncol 106:210–218

Dunn JE (1975) Carcinoma epidemiology in populations of the United States – with emphasis on Hawaii and California – and Japan. Cancer Res 35:3240–3245

Enstrom JE, Austin DF (1977) Interpreting cancer survival rates. Science 195:847–851

Epstein JI, Steinberg GD (1990) Significance of low grade prostate cancer on needle biopsy. Cancer 66:1927–1932

Epstein JL, Paull G, Eggleston JC, Walsh PC (1986) Prognosis of untreated state A1 prostate carcinoma: study of 94 cases with extended follow up. J Urol 136:837–839

Franks LM (1956) Natural history of prostatic cancer. Lancet ii: 1037–1039

Franzen S, Giertz G, Zajicek J (1960) Cytological diagnosis of prostate tumours by transrectal aspiration biopsy. A preliminary report. Br J Urol 32:193–196

George NJR (1988) Natural history of localised prostate cancer managed by conservative therapy alone. Lancet i:494–497

Guileyardo JM, Johnson WD, Walsh RA, Akazaki K, Correa P (1980) Prevalence of latent prostate carcinoma in the population. J Natl Cancer Inst 65:311–316

Haenszel W, Kurihara M (1968) Studies of Japanese immigrants. 1. Mortality from cancer and other diseases among Japanese in the Unites States. J Natl Cancer Inst 40:43–68

Halpert B, Sheehan EE, Schmarlhurst WR, Scott R (1963) Survey of 5000 autopsies. Cancer 16:737–742

Hayashi T, Taki Y, Ikai K, Hiura M, Kiriyama T, Shizuki K (1987) Latent and clinically manifest prostatic carcinoma. Prostate 10:275–279

Hirst AE, Bergman RT (1954) Carcinoma of the prostate in men more than 80 years old. Cancer 7:136–141

HMSO (1975) The Registrar General's Statistical Review of England and Wales 1968–1970

Jackson MA, Ahluwalia BS, Herson J (1977) Characterisation of prostatic carcinoma among blacks: a continuation report. Cancer Treat Rep 61:167–172

Johansson JE, Anderson SE, Krusemo UB, Adami H-O, Bergstrom R, Kraaz W (1989) Natural history of localised prostate cancer. Lancet i:799–803

Johansson JE, Adami HO, Andersson SO, Bergström R, Holmberg L, Krusemo UB (1992) High 10 year survival rate in patients with early untreated prostate cancer. JAMA 267:2191–2196

McWhorter WP, Hernandez AD, Meikle AW et al. (1992) A screening study of prostate cancer in high risk families. J Urol 148:826–828

Metlin C, Natarajan N (1983) Epidemiological observations from the American College of Surgeons survey on prostate cancer. Prostate 4:223–331

Murphy GP, Natarajan N, Pontes JE et al. (1982) National survey of prostate cancer in the United States by the American College of Surgeons. J Urol 127:928–934

Office of Population Censuses and Surveys (1989) Monitor DH2-89 (Cancer Research Campaign Factsheet 3.1)

Pantelides ML, Bowman SP, George NJR (1992) Levels of prostate specific antigen that predict skeletal spread in prostate cancer. Br J Urol 70:299–303

Parkin DM, Stjernswärd J, Muir CS (1984) Estimates of the worldwide frequency of twelve major cancers. Bull World Health Organ 62:163–182

Potosky AL, Kessler L, Gridley G, Brown CC, Horm JW (1990) Rise in prostatic cancer incidence associated with increased use of transurethral resection. J Natl Cancer Inst 82:1624–1628

Rich AR (1935) On frequency of occurrence of occult carcinoma of prostate. J Urol 33:215–223

Ross RK, Deapen D, Cassagrande J, Paganini-Hill A, Henderson BE (1981) A cohort study of mortality from cancer of the prostate in Catholic priests. Br J Cancer 43:233–235

Scott R, Mutchnik DL, Laskowski TZ, Schmalhorst WR (1969) Carcinoma of prostate in elderly men: growth characteristics and clinical significance. J Urol 101:602–607

Silverberg E (1987) Statistical and epidemiological data on urologic cancer. Cancer 60:692–717

Silverberg E, Lubera JA (1988) Cancer statistics. CA 38:14–15

Silverberg E, Lubera J A (1989) Cancer statistics. CA 39:3–20

Skeet R G (1976) Scientific foundations of urology. In: Williams DI, Chisholm GD, (eds) Epidemiology of urogenital tumours, vol II. Heinemann, London, pp 199–211

Smith JA, Cho Y-H (1990) Management of stage A prostate cancer. Urol Clin North Am 17:769–777

Steinberg GD, Carter BS, Beaty TH, Childs B, Walsh PC (1990) Family history and risk of prostate cancer. Prostate 17:337–347

Trasti H, Nilsson S, Peterson L-E (1979) Applied diagnostic technique: a decisive factor in the long term T-year survival rate in prostatic cancer. Br J Urol 51:135–139

US Bureau of Census (1986) Statistical Abstract of the United States 1987, 107th edn. US Government Printing Office

Waterhouse JAH, Muir CS, Shanmugaratnam K, Powell J (1982) Cancer incidence in five continents. Vol. iv, no 42. IARC Scientific Publication, Lyon

Whitmore WF (1973) Natural history of prostate cancer. Cancer 32:1104–1112

Whittemore AS, Paffenbarger RS, Anderson K, Lee JE (1984) Early precursors of urogenital cancer in former college men. J Urol 132:1256–1261

Yatani R, Chigusa K, Akazaki K, Stemmermann GN (1982) Geographical pathology of latent prostate carcinoma. Int J Cancer 29:611–616

Chapter 11

Radical Prostatectomy for Prostate Cancer

G. L. Andriole

Introduction

Prostate cancer is now estimated to be the most common cancer occurring among American men. There were more than 130 000 new cases of prostate cancer diagnosed in the United States during 1992. Prostate cancer is the third leading cause of cancer deaths among American men with more than 30 000 deaths (almost 12% of all cancer deaths) in 1992. The incidence and mortality rates of prostate cancer have been increasing over the past few years (Boring et al. 1992).

Traditionally, prostate cancer was diagnosed in men who either complained of symptoms arising from the prostate (e.g. obstruction, prostatitis, urinary infection) or a digital rectal examination suspicious for cancer. In general, only about 50% to 60% of patients whose prostate cancer is diagnosed in this manner have disease that is clinically localised to the prostate on the basis of radionuclide bone scanning and serum enzymatic prostatic acid phosphatase levels. When these patients undergo complete surgical staging by pelvic lymph node dissection and radical prostatectomy, only about one half have pathologically organ-confined disease. Therefore, when traditional means of detecting prostate cancer are employed, only about one-third of the newly diagnosed cases of prostate cancer are detected when they are truly organ-confined and potentially curable by radical prostatectomy alone. Therefore, until better forms of therapy for non-organ-confined prostate cancer are developed, the only means of decreasing the mortality from prostate cancer is to strive to detect pathologically organ-confined tumours more commonly. These considerations have provided the rationale and impetus for screening for prostate cancer.

Currently the most effective means of screening for prostate cancer appears to be the combined use of serum PSA testing and digital rectal examination (Catalona et al. 1991). If the patient has an abnormality of either of these tests, sonographically guided systematic sextant biopsies of the prostate are performed. When this approach is used to detect prostate cancer, up to 80%

tumours are pathologically organ-confined at the time of detection. Because of this enhanced ability to detect organ-confined prostate cancer as well as the heightened recognition that definitive radiation therapy often fails to control localised disease completely within the radiation fields (as evidenced by rising serum PSA levels in more than 50% of men within 5 years of treatment and by persistently positive prostatic biopsy more than one year after completion of therapy) (Stamey et al. 1989) there has been a renewed enthusiasm for radical prostatectomy as the treatment of choice for men with localised prostate cancer. Additionally, technical refinements that allow preservation of the cavernosal nerves, bloodless control of the dorsal venous complex, and improved mucosa to mucosa vesicourethral anastomotic techniques have significantly reduced the morbidity and mortality of radical retropubic prostatectomy (Walsh 1987). These refinements made nerve-sparing radical prostatectomy a much more palatable option for both surgeons and patients. Since the mid-1980s, nerve-sparing radical retropubic prostatectomy has been performed at an ever-increasing rate at a large number of centres. Because of the rising number of prostate cancer cases, nerve-sparing radical retropubic prostatectomy will likely remain an important operation for all urologic surgeons.

Selection of Patients for Radical Prostatectomy

The ideal candidates for radical prostatectomy are healthy men with a life expectancy that exceeds 10 years who have clinically organ-confined (stage T0–T2) prostate cancer. Serum enzymatic prostatic acid phosphatase is not usually necessary to stage prostate cancer. Pelvic imaging by either CT or MRI scanning should be reserved for selected patients known to be at high risk for nodal metastases (e.g. by virtue of having a large primary tumour, a poorly-differentiated tumour, or a markedly elevated serum prostate specific antigen level > 40 ng/ml). In these cases a CT or MRI scan may identify enlarged pelvic lymph nodes that may then be biopsied percutaneously or via laparoscopy. Since radical prostatectomy is infrequently indicated in patients with macroscopic nodal metastases, histological identification of lymph node metastases by any means short of open pelvic lymph node dissection spares the patient the risks and morbidity of open lymphadenectomy.

A recent report has questioned the necessity of the staging radionuclide bone scan for prostate cancer patients whose serum PSA is less than 10 or 20 ng/ml (Chybowski et al. 1991). However, during the past two years three patients have been encountered with biopsy-proven bone metastases and a serum PSA below 10 ng/ml. Therefore, a radionuclide scan is still recommended for routine staging of most men with prostate cancer.

Radical prostatectomy is not generally recommended as a curative procedure for patients with clinical stage T3 or N1 disease (Zincke et al. 1987; Steinberg et al. 1990). At some centres radical prostatectomy is performed on selected young men with clinical stage T3 disease (i.e. advanced local disease without distant spread) especially if significant endocrine "downsizing" occurs after preoperative treatment with 3–6 months of reversible hormonal therapy (such as gonadotrophic releasing hormonal analogues). Such an approach may be logical in that it tends to select patients with well differentiated, endocrine responsive tumours. It may also provide excellent long-term local control. However, firm data (especially long-term serum PSA levels) are lacking concerning its long-term therapeutic efficacy.

By a similar rationale, patients with otherwise localised disease but an isolated elevation of serum enzymatic prostatic acid phosphatase or those with N1 tumours (i.e. lymph node metastases) have occasionally been treated with radical prostatectomy alone or by combined radical prostatectomy and hormone therapy (Zincke et al. 1987; Steinberg et al. 1990). Excellent short-term, symptom-free survival has been reported at several centres with this approach. However, in this setting, the benefit of radical prostatectomy beyond local control is unclear. The prolonged survivals that have been observed in patients undergoing both radical prostatectomy and endocrine manipulation may be due to the early institution of hormonal therapy rather than to the prostatectomy.

At the other end of the spectrum of prostate cancer, controversy also exists about the need to treat aggressively patients with low volume impalpable tumours detected during simple prostatectomy. The natural history of these tumours may be indolent but the cancer progression rate at 10 years has been reported to approach 20% (Blute et al. 1986; Epstein et al. 1986). Unfortunately, there is currently no precise means of predicting which patients are at greatest risk for progression (Voges et al. 1992). In recognition of this fact and considering that there is a high probability that the tumour is pathologically organ-confined and that most patients (up to 80%) will retain potency if a nerve-sparing radical prostatectomy is performed (Epstein et al. 1988), radical prostatectomy seems appropriate for young patients with this stage of prostate cancer. In the past it has been speculated that radical prostatectomy is more difficult to perform after a transurethral prostatectomy but, with few exceptions, recent experience does not support this.

Recently, questions have also been raised regarding the necessity of definitive therapy for all men with clinical stage T1 (i.e. palpable nodule) prostate cancer. Whitmore et al. (1990) has reported a select series of 75 men with stage B disease who were followed expectantly for up to 10 years without administration of curative therapy. To be included in this study, patients were observed for one year and did not demonstrate any evidence of disease progression. Subsequent therapy, such as palliative transurethral resection, hormone manipulation and radiation, were administered only if symptoms developed and/or disease progression was demonstrated. Using this treatment strategy, the median interval to disease progression exceeded five years. Ultimately, however, 70% of patients progressed locally and about half of these patients required at least one transurethral resection of the prostate to palliate bladder outlet obstruction. One-third of the patients developed bone metastases and required hormonal therapy. Overall, 15% died of prostate cancer and 24% died of natural causes. The median 15-year actuarial survival for patients managed in this manner was 67%±12%. This was better than the predicted survival of age-matched men. Reports from Scandinavia (Johansson et al. 1989, 1992) mimic this experience: selected patients with small, well-differentiated lesions may manifest low rates of cancer progression, metastasis and death. In the 1992 report of Johansson et al., two-thirds of the men had well-differentiated lesions, 23% of whom progressed while more than half (55% and 67% respectively) of men with grade 2 or 3 lesions progressed. The profound influence of the high proportion of well-differentiated tumours on the overall outcome of the whole group of patients is further reflected in the fact that more than two-thirds of the cancer deaths occurred in the one-third of men with grade 2 or grade 3 lesions and that prostate cancer was the cause of death in only one of 12 men with grade 1 tumours but five of eight men with grade 3 tumours. Therefore, the implication of this report should not be applied to men with grade 2 or grade 3 lesions and it is evident that until an effective means of accurately determining individual tumour behaviour is available, it is difficult to predict which patients with prostate cancer will behave in a benign manner. For this reason, nerve-sparing radical retropubic prostatectomy is likely to remain the primary treatment for the majority of healthy men with clinically organ-confined prostate cancer.

Selection of Patients for Nerve-Sparing versus Traditional Radical Retropubic Prostatectomy

From the time of its original description in 1982 (Walsh and Donker 1982), questions have been raised about the wisdom of employing nerve-sparing radical prostatectomy for patients with prostate cancer. There has been concern that this procedure may compromise the surgical oncological principle of wide excision of cancer-containing organs. In particular since perineural invasion is known to be a common and often early development in men with prostate cancer, nerve-sparing techniques may result in incomplete tumour resection for some patients. This is especially true for patients with large primary tumours as the incidence of microscopic extraprostatic extension or perineural invasion in one study approached 90% (Stamey et al. 1988). In another study, some of the positive margins observed in 40% of patients may have been negative if non-nerve-sparing surgery was performed (Epstein 1990). Although the exact long-term implication of perineural invasion and microscopic capsular extension in the region of the neurovascular bundles is not exactly known, the high frequency of these occurrences is certainly cause for concern.

To examine the role of nerve-sparing radical prostatectomy in patients with clinical stage T2 prostate cancer, Bigg et al. (1990) reviewed 77 patients who underwent either bilateral (47), unilateral (26), or non-nerve-sparing (4) radical prostatectomy. The decision to sacrifice neurovascular bundle(s) was made intraoperatively on the basis of palpation. When the patient's outcome was viewed with two strict criteria of successful extirpative cancer surgery (i.e. histological demonstration of organ-confined tumour with negative urethral, bladder neck and capsular margins and an undetectable postoperative serum prostate specific antigen level), only 17 of 47 patients (36%) treated with bilateral nerve-sparing techniques and 7 of 26 (27%) patients treated with unilateral nerve-sparing techniques had the ideal outcome. Of the 24 patients who enjoyed the ideal outcome from the point of view of cancer control, 15

Table 11.1. Indications for excision of neurovascular bundle

Preoperative
Impotence
High grade tumour
High volume (bilateral) tumour
Induration of the lateral sulcus

Intraoperative
Induration of lateral sulcus detected after opening endopelvic fascia
Bundle adherent to tumour when incising lateral fascia

retained potency. Therefore, only 15 of 73 (20%) patients with stage T2 prostate cancer who underwent nerve-sparing radical retropubic prostatectomy had the optimal outcome in terms of both cancer control and preservation of potency. Nine of the 53 (17%) patients with non-organ-confined disease had their only positive margin in the region of the neurovascular bundle and may have had a negative margin if wide excision of the neurovascular bundle had been performed.

It appears on balance that a proportion of patients with clinical stage T2 prostate cancer are not well-served by nerve-sparing radical prostatectomy. Because of these considerations most urological surgeons have become less enthusiastic about performing bilateral nerve-sparing surgery in these men. However, it is important to emphasise that there is no conclusive proof that "wide excision" of neurovascular bundles will ensure negative margins (Epstein 1990), nor that the positive margins observed after nerve-sparing surgery necessarily imply a dismal prognosis. It now appears that the ideal candidates for nerve-sparing surgery are healthy, young, sexually active men with low-volume, low- or moderate-grade tumours who have prebiopsy serum PSA levels less than 10 ng/ml. Some indications for excision of neurovascular bundle(s) are shown in Table 11.1.

Technique of Nerve-Sparing Radical Retropubic Prostatectomy

Patients who are undergoing radical prostatectomy are asked to donate up to three units of autologous blood preoperatively. This approach delays surgery a few weeks but is very beneficial and reassuring to patients as it minimises the requirement for perioperative non-autologous transfusions. At our centre, we are investigating the use of erythropoietin preoperatively. It is possible that this agent, combined with intraoperative haemodilution (i.e. removal of 1 to 3 units of blood after induction of anaesthesia with reinfusion near the end of the procedure) will completely mitigate the need for autologous blood donation. With either approach, fewer than 10% of men undergoing radical prostatectomy will receive non-autologous blood products.

The patient is instructed to use a small, cleansing enema the night before surgery is due. On the morning of surgery, broad spectrum intravenous antibiotics are administered when he is sent for. As prophylaxis against thromboembolic disease, sequential compression hose stockings are placed intraoperatively and remain in use during the immediate postoperative period (3–4 days). This approach has been preferable to mini-dose heparin in reducing the rate of thromboembolic complications without predisposing patients to the wound and lymphocele complications that may occur with heparin.

Patients are placed supine with their back extended and their legs on spreader bars. The entire lower abdomen, perineum, pubis and genitalia are prepped and draped in a sterile manner. A 22 French, 30 cc balloon Foley catheter is placed. A lower midline abdominal extraperitoneal incision is made and the pelvic side walls and space of Retzius are bluntly dissected. This allows placement of a Balfour self-retaining retractor. Modified bilateral pelvic lymph node dissections are performed. All nodal tissue within the obturator fossae is removed bilaterally. It is helpful to use multiple fine haemoclips during the lymphadenectomy to minimise the chances of lymphocele formation postoperatively. If the lymph nodes show no evidence of metastatic disease, radical prostatectomy is performed.

A wide, malleable middle blade is attached to the Balfour so that it retracts the balloon of the Foley catheter cephalad. This manoeuvre places the prostate on traction and facilitates accurate division of the puboprostatic ligaments, the dorsal venous complex and the urethra. All adipose tissue is teased off the surface of the prostate and the endopelvic fascia. This is accomplished by retracting the prostate medially with a sponge stick and using a Kuttner dissector. After this is accomplished, it is usually possible to visualise the endopelvic fascia and the puboprostatic ligaments. Occasionally small veins may arise from the superficial dorsal venous complex and course superficial to the endopelvic fascia and puboprostatic ligaments. These vessels should be coagulated prior to division as bleeding may obscure the anatomy and compromise the apical dissection of the prostate. The endopelvic fascia is punctured just lateral to the prostate gland and medial to the levator muscles. A delicate right angle clamp is used to tent up the endopelvic fascia. This allows incision of the fascia alone without inadvertent injury to the veins on the capsule of the prostate. Occasionally there may be a sizeable vein traversing the space between the prostate and the levator muscle just deep to the endopelvic fascia (Fig. 11.1). These veins should be ligated with fine silk prior to dividing the puboprostatic ligaments. If adhesions have formed between the levator muscle and the lateral surface of the prostate (from inflammation, prior surgery, or biopsy) sharp dissection should be used to divide them. Once the sides of the prostate are dissected free, the puboprostatic ligaments should be sharply divided with fine scissors close to the symphysis pubis. This releases the prostate gland and allows palpation of the anterior surface of the urethra and most of the lateral surfaces of the prostate. This palpation may give the surgeon an indication that advanced disease is present and may guide his decision to perform a non-nerve-sparing prostatectomy (see above).

After the puboprostatic ligaments have been divided, the groove between the urethra and the dorsal venous complex is palpated between the thumb and forefinger of the left hand. A blunt-tipped right-angle clamp is placed from left to right between the anterior wall of the urethra and the dorsal venous complex. Care should be taken not to place this clamp too close to the anterior

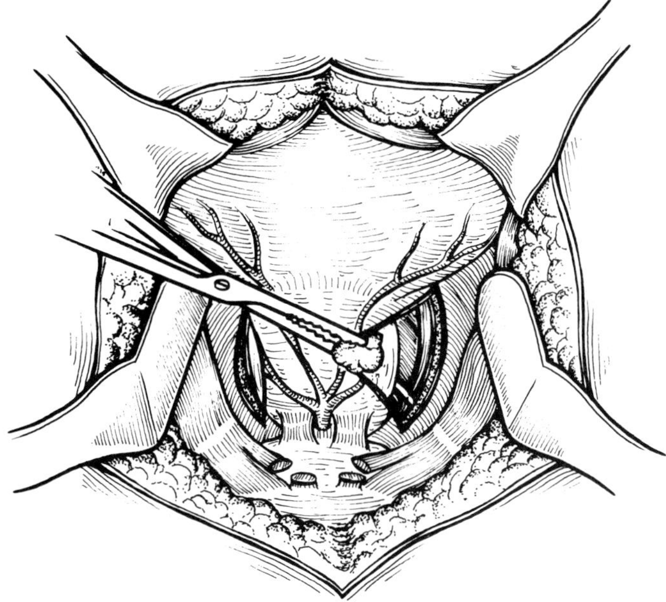

Fig. 11.1. In some individuals large veins may lie deep to the endopelvic fascia coursing between the lateral aspect of the prostate and the levator muscles. Recognition, ligation, and division of these veins is necessary if a bloodless apical dissection is to be performed.

surface of the urethra as injury to the anterior striated sphincter muscle fibres or to the urethral mucosa itself may occur. Preservation of the anterior muscle fibres is thought to be important to achieve early return of continence. After placing the right angle clamp, the space between the urethra and the dorsal venous complex is developed by gently spreading the clamp parallel to the urethra. A no. 1 polygalactan tie is placed in the jaws of the right angle, pulled through, and tied distally. Traction on the prostate with a sponge stick is often helpful in positioning the ligature distally on the dorsal venous complex. Two or three 2-0 chromic sutures may also be placed around the major branches of the dorsal venous complex as they ramify on the surface of the prostate. This prevents significant back bleeding when the dorsal venous complex is divided. To divide the dorsal venous complex, the right-angle clamp is placed above the urethra and a long-handled knife is used to divide the complex. If bleeding from the distal end of the complex occurs, downward traction on the prostate facilitates placement of a 2-0 chromic suture ligature. Care should be taken when dividing the dorsal venous complex to be certain that it is performed distal to the prostate, as occasionally portions of the anterior capsule of the prostate may inadvertently be left attached to the dorsal venous complex. This is undesirable as the additional tissue may obscure later dissection of the urethra and may be the cause of detectable serum PSA levels or of recurrent prostate cancer postoperatively.

If the dorsal venous complex has been appropriately divided, the urethra

a   **b**

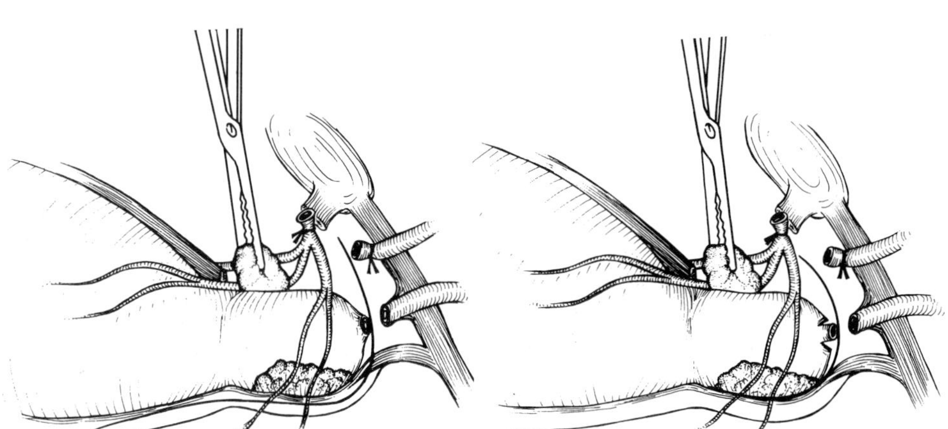

Fig. 11.2. a The correct plane of dissection between Denonvillier's fascia and the anterior rectal wall is established by completely transecting the rectourethralis muscle distal to the apex of the prostate. **b** Incorrect dissection between the prostate and Denonvillier's fascia may occur if the rectourethralis muscle is incompletely divided. A subcapsular dissection may also occur if the urethra is transected too close to the prostate.

should be clearly visible when cephalad traction on the prostate with a sponge stick is performed. The urethra should be mobilised from within the neurovascular bundles by placing fine-tipped Metzenbaum scissors just lateral to the urethra and spreading longitudinally. After this has been accomplished on both sides, a delicate right-angle clamp may be placed from right to left between the neurovascular bundles and the urethra. Gentle upward traction with this clamp, coupled with judicious spreading of the clamp tents the urethra up out of the depths of the pelvis and away from the neurovascular bundles. With a sponge stick retracting the anterior surface of the prostate cephalad, a long-handled knife is used to divide the anterior portion of the urethra 2 mm distal to the apex of the prostate. The catheter is then grasped from within the urethra with a delicate right-angle clamp and tented up as much as possible into the wound. The posterior wall of the urethra is then easily visible and may be divided with a knife. After the urethra is divided, the Foley catheter is clamped with a Kelly clamp and transected. The Kelly clamp on the catheter is secured to the drapes over the upper abdominal wall with a towel clip. This puts gentle traction on the prostate and facilitates exposure of the apex of the prostate.

The dissection of the prostatic apex is performed by dividing the rectourethralis muscle just distal to the prostate (Fig. 11.2). This is accomplished either by placing a delicate right-angle clamp underneath the muscle fibres and sharply dividing them with a knife or by cutting the fibres directly with fine-tipped scissors. If this procedure is performed properly and completely, one then enters the plane between Denonvillier's fascia and the rectum. With gentle upward traction on the prostate, sharp scissors may be used to divide the lateral pelvic fascia that invests both the prostate and the neurovascular bundle. Any remnants of the rectourethralis muscle fibres and all adhesions between Denonvillier's fascia and the anterior rectal wall should also be divided, complete division of these structures frees the prostate so that it may easily be rotated up out of the pelvis. While dividing the lateral pelvic fascia; two or three small branches of the neurovascular bundles will be encountered as they enter the middle portion of the gland. Coagulation or ligation of these is fraught with the possibility of injuring the bundle; because of this it has been our preference to divide these vessels sharply. Significant bleeding is infrequent.

With the prostate rotated up out of the pelvis, Denonvillier's fascia may be entered transversely where it overlies the seminal vesicles. To facilitate this, the fascia should initially be fulgurated with electrocautery to minimise bleeding from multiple veins that surround the ampullae of the vasa. Once the seminal vesicles are visualised, the pedicles of the prostate are easily identified immediately lateral to the seminal vesicles. The pedicles are ligated with 0 silk and transected. When performing ligature and division of pedicles, care should be taken not to place the ligature too far laterally as this may injure the neurovascular bundle or to divide the pedicle too close to the prostate (and thus leave prostatic tissue attached to the pedicle and/or expose tumour).

After both pedicles have been completely divided, a blunt right-angle clamp may be easily placed between the seminal vesicles and the bladder base and gently spread; 5 ml of indigo carmine is administered intravenously. The middle blade on the Balfour retractor is removed and the bladder is entered, transversely 3–5 mm proximal to the bladder neck. Allis clamps are placed on the bladder, a sponge stick in the bladder and a pedicle clamp between the bladder and seminal vesicles to facilitate visualisation of the posterior portion of the bladder neck and the ureteral orifices. Division of the posterior portion of the trigone is greatly simplified by spreading the pedicle clamp between the seminal vesicles and the bladder base, lifting it up slightly. After the bladder neck has been completely transected, the middle blade is replaced so that the bladder is retracted superiorly. The seminal vesicles may then be dissected out in their entirety using a delicate right-angle clamp and fine haemoclips. The ampullae of the vasa are clipped and divided.

After the specimen has been removed, the bladder neck is stomatised anteriorly with three sutures of 3- 0 chromic and repaired in a tennis racket fashion. Two layers of 2- 0 chromic (one running and one interrupted) are placed, beginning in the midline of the trigone and continuing toward the stomatised bladder neck. The last few sutures are placed so that they evert the bladder mucosa. The vesicourethral anastomosis is performed over an 18 French Foley catheter. Four to six sutures of 2- 0 chromic are placed symmetrically around the urethra. A double-armed suture is preferable as this permits atraumatic, precise placement of the sutures on both the urethral and bladder sides of the anastomosis. Eversion of the urethral stump with a sponge stick in the perineum generally exposes the complete circumference of the urethra. Care should be taken when placing the posterior sutures to avoid injuring the neurovascular bundles.

Suction drains are placed in each hemipelvis and brought out through separate stab wounds. The midline fascia and skin are closed in standard fashion.

Postoperative Care

Patients continue to wear intermittent sequential compression stockings until they are fully ambulatory, usually 18–72 h postoperatively. The closed suction drains are generally removed in 3–5 days, typically when drainage is less than 30 ml per day. Patients remain hospitalised for approximately 5 days and are discharged with a Foley catheter in place with plans to remove it in the office 14 days after surgery.

Complications of Radical Retropubic Prostatectomy

In spite of the fact that patients undergoing radical retropubic prostatectomy are often elderly, this operation can be performed with surprisingly little morbidity and almost no mortality. Although older series reported morbidity rates of over 50%, recent series suggest that fewer than one of ten patients undergoing radical retropubic prostatectomy suffer a significant complication (Boxer et al. 1977; Bahnson and Catalona 1990; Leandri et al. 1992). Similarly, the mortality of radical retropubic prostatectomy that had previously been reported to approach 3% is now estimated to be less than 1%. During the past two years more than 500 radical retropubic prostatectomies have been

Table 11.2. Early complications of radical retropubic prostatectomies performed during the last 2 years at Barnes Hospital

	No. (%)
Pulmonary embolism	9 (1.4)
Myocardial infarction	7 (1.0)
Wound infection/seroma	6 (0.9)
Lymphocele	2 (0.9)
Arrhythmia	6 (0.9)
Deep venous thrombosis	5 (0.7)
Spontaneous deflation Foley balloon	4 (0.6)
Central line sepsis/phlebitis	3 (0.4)
Retained drain	3 (0.4)
Prolonged urine leak	3 (0.4)
Clostridium difficile colitis	2 (0.3)
Prolonged ileus	2 (0.3)
GI bleeding	1 (0.1)
Ureteral injury	1 (0.1)
Rectal perforation	1 (0.1)
Cerebrovascular accident	1 (0.1)
Postoperative bleeding requiring exploration	1 (0.1)
Death (thought to be secondary to arrhythmia)	1 (0.1)

Table 11.3. Estimated late complications of radical retropubic prostatectomy

Incontinence	
Stress	3%
Total	2%
Impotence	
Partial	25%
Total	20%
Bladder neck contracture	
Requiring TUR	5%
Requiring dilation	3%

performed and the early and late complications are shown in Tables 11.2 and 11.3.

Early complications

Blood Loss

Patients undergoing radical retropubic prostatectomy typically lose approximately 1500 ml of blood with a range between 250 and 4000 ml in our series of over 500 patients. The use of regional anaesthetic techniques and temporary occlusion of the hypogastric artery have been reported to reduce blood loss, but in our experience the overall benefits have been slight. Perhaps more significant than these techniques in minimising blood loss is careful management of the dorsal venous complex with direct vision incision of the puboprostatic ligaments, and "pillars" of the prostate and careful suture ligation of the dorsal venous complex after placement of back bleeding sutures on the prostatic side.

In our experience no transfusion-related complications have been reported with the current use of autologous blood. Fewer than one out of seven patients undergoing radical retropubic prostatectomy has required non-autologous transfusion.

Rectal Injury

Rectal injury is more likely to occur in patients with high stage disease or prior rectal surgery. The reported incidence of this complication has ranged between 0 and 7%. We have experienced one such injury in the past 5 years. This low rate may be attributable to the use of direct vision incision of the rectourethralis muscle after transection of the urethra by passing the tips of a right-angle clamp underneath the fibres of the rectourethralis muscle thus tenting them away from the rectum. This manoeuvre facilitates establishment of the proper plane of dissection between the prostate and the rectum with minimal upward traction on the prostate and anterior rectal wall. If it is difficult to discern completely the fibres of the rectourethralis muscle, or if the posterior apical dissection has been begun in or near the surgical capsule of the prostate, or if there is any doubt about the proper plane of dissection between the prostate and the rectum, we prefer to remove the prostate in an antegrade (rather than a retrograde) manner. This approach allows entry into the appropriate dissection plane near the bladder neck and seminal vesicles. From this vantage, the rectum can often be directly visualised and retracted away from the prostate.

If a rectal laceration occurs, it is often possible to repair it by closing the rectum in two layers. The pelvis should be irrigated copiously, drains should be placed in the region of the laceration and the anal sphincter should be dilated to defunctionalise it temporarily. The need for a diverting colostomy in these patients depends on the size of the injury, whether the patient has received prior radiation therapy, the general condition of the patient, and the surgeon's assessment of the vascularity, viability and completeness of the rectal repair.

Ureteral Injury

There are two occasions during pelvic node dissection and radical retropubic prostatectomy when ureteral injury may occur. During the lymphadenectomy the ureter may be injured if the bladder is not completely dissected free of the pelvic side wall. During the prostatectomy per se, patients with a large median lobe may have significant J-hooking of the ureters. As such, the ureter may be injured when transecting the posterior aspect of the bladder neck. The most important aspect of managing patients with ureteral injury is intraoperative recognition. To facilitate this, it has been our practice to routinely inject 5 ml of indigo carmine intravenously at the time of transection of the bladder neck and carefully to inspect the operative field for any evidence of blue urine outside of the bladder. If a ureteral injury is recognised, it should be treated by intubated reimplantation at an appropriate site remote from the "tennis" racket repair of the bladder neck.

Thromboembolic Complications

Deep venous thrombosis and pulmonary embolism represent the most common complications of radical retropubic prostatectomy at our institution. We have noted pulmonary embolism in 3% of our patients; other series have reported higher rates. Deep venous thrombosis without pulmonary embolism is more common and may occur in up to 10% of patients. As mentioned above, we use intermittent compression hose until patients are fully ambulatory for prophylaxis against venous thrombosis. We did note a decreased incidence of thromboembolic complications in a study of patients randomly assigned to receive either mini-dose heparin or no anticoagulation preoperatively, but have not routinely used perioperative anticoagulation because of the increased complications and blood loss.

A high level of clinical suspicion should be maintained postoperatively to detect deep venous thrombosis or pulmonary embolism. Any unexplained fever, tachycardia, tachypnoea, or minimal leg tenderness or oedema should be completely evaluated with Doppler studies of the lower extremity veins, electrocardiography, arterial blood gasses, chest X-ray, and radionuclide-ventilation–perfusion scans. It has been our practice to anticoagulate patients with full-dose intravenous heparin immediately if we suspect pulmonary embolism on clinical grounds and to stop heparin if the definitive evaluation is negative. We obtain a pulmonary arteriogram if our clinical assessment and the interpretation of the ventilation–perfusion lung scan are at variance. We have not noted major haemorrhagic complications from heparin in the early postoperative period, although lymphatic drainage through the pelvic suction drains has been reported to be increased in heparinised patients.

Lymphocele

A carefully performed modified lymph node dissection including only the nodes within the obturator fossae is not associated with a high incidence of lymphatic leakage, lymphocele formation or of lymphoedema of the scrotum or lower extremities. In the past year, only two patients (less than 1%) have experienced a lymphatic complication (lymphocele formation). We attribute this low rate to careful ligation and haemoclip occlusion of lymphatic channels. Lymphoceles usually present as pelvic pain and leg swelling. The diagnosis is confirmed by pelvic CT scan or ultrasonography. Lymphoceles are treated by radiographically guided aspiration and tube drainage. Percutaneous tube placement allows the walls of the cavity to coapt. The tube may be slowly advanced out over 1–2 weeks. Alternatively, lymphocele cavities may be treated with ethanol sclerosis or marsupialisation into the peritoneal cavity.

Persistent Suction Drainage

Fluid leakage through the Jackson–Pratt drains usually ceases by day 3 or 4. Patients with persistent leakage beyond this time present a diagnostic dilemma: the fluid is may be either urine (from an injured ureter or vesicourethral anastomosis) or lymph. It is important to determine which by either testing it for creatinine concentration relative to serum creatinine or by observing it after intravenous indigo carmine administration. If the drainage is lymph, we take the drains off suction and slowly advance them out over a few days. If the fluid is urine, the leak is most likely from the vesicourethral anastomosis. We obtain a gentle, fluoroscopically guided cystogram to verify the site of leakage and its relationship to the drain and the Foley catheter. We generally take the Jackson–Pratt drain off suction and pull it away from the bladder if it appears to be too close to the site of leakage. With this approach, all such leaks have healed spontaneously within 3–4 weeks.

Retained Drain

This vexing (and embarrassing) problem occurs if the Jackson–Pratt drain has been inadvertently weakened when tying it to the skin or if it has been incorporated into a fascial closure suture. Removal of the offending suture under local anaesthesia is usually possible.

Spontaneous Deflation of Catheter Balloon

In spite of careful testing of catheter balloons prior to their use during radical retropubic prostatectomy, two patients have experienced catheter loss during the first two postoperative weeks. In both cases, loss was attributed to a small leak in the balloon, possibly caused by handling the catheter intraoperatively with forceps. We now routinely avoid any handling of the catheter by any instrument other than the gloved human hand. When this complication occurs, urgent replacement is indicated unless in the judgement of the surgeon the catheter may be left out. We do not advocate "blind" passage of a catheter through a fresh vesicoureteral anastomosis in the emergency room or the office as this may disrupt the anastomosis. Our preferred technique is to pass a floppy tipped guidewire into the bladder under flexible cystoscopic control. We then place an 18 French Councill-tip catheter over the guidewire. This is a relatively atraumatic means of replacing the Foley catheter. We have not observed incontinence among patients whose catheter has been misplaced.

Other Complications

Other complications such as myocardial infarction, cardiac arrhythmia, and gastrointestinal bleeding occasionally occur following radical retropubic prostatectomy. Additionally, there are reports in the literature of anastomotic suture granulomas and of Ogilvie's syndrome in patients who have undergone radical retropubic prostatectomy.

Late Complications

The major late complications of radical retropubic prostatectomy are loss of sexual function, incontinence or bladder neck contracture.

Bladder Neck Contracture

Bladder neck contracture has been reported to occur in up to a quarter of the patients undergoing radical prostatectomy. The incidence has not been stratified to the type of vesicourethral anastomotic technique. It has become our preference to carefully stomatise the bladder neck with fine chromic sutures and to perform a meticulous mucosa-to-mucosa anastomosis over an 18 French silastic Foley catheter. With use of this technique, our anastomotic stricture rate is 4%. Most of the patients who develop these strictures are managed in the office with one or more dilations employing direct vision placement of a guidewire or filiform with subsequent coaxial or "follower" dilation. A minority of patients with bladder neck contracture have required outpatient transurethral resection or incision of the stricture. Great care should be taken when performing a transurethral incision or resection of the stricture as incontinence may occur.

Incontinence

Total urinary incontinence is an infrequent complication of nerve-sparing radical retropubic prostatectomy. This is probably because of improved recognition of the anatomy of the pelvic floor musculature and performance of an accurate mucosa-to-mucosa vesicourethral anastomosis. Those patients who do experience incontinence after radical prostatectomy should be evaluated urodynamically, as an unstable bladder rather than sphincter dysfunction may cause or contribute significantly to the incontinence. Patients with total incontinence after radical prostatectomy who do not have bladder instability are given the option of management with either a Cunningham clamp, condom catheter or placement of an artificial urinary sphincter. The latter procedure usually is more satisfactory for the patient. We have not observed sufficient success with Teflon injection to increase urethral resistance. Patients with bladder instability after radical prostatectomy may respond to appropriate pharmacological agents.

Approximately 2% of patients have required precautionary pads because of occasional stress incontinence after radical retropubic prostatectomy. Pharmacological agents may be beneficial to these patients, and we usually do not resort to artificial sphincter placement in such patients. The use of adjuvant radiation therapy for patients with detectable serum PSA levels and/or positive margins after radical prostatectomy does not seem permanently to worsen the continence, although during and shortly after therapy temporary incontinence may occur. It has been our practice to delay postoperative radiation therapy until the patient has achieved continence.

Potency

Preservation of sexual potency by nerve-sparing techniques is dependent both on the age of the patient and the stage of the disease. Young men with stage A tumours should enjoy return of sexual function within 6 months up to 90% of the time whereas older patients near the age of 70 years with clinical or pathological stage B2-lesions are less frequently potent postoperatively. Most patients who regain potency begin to do so within 3 months of surgery with full erections requiring up to 18 months to return. Some patients are potent almost immediately after removing the catheter. The wide range of time for the return of potency makes it difficult to predict early which patients who have a technically satisfactory nerve-sparing procedure will retain potency postoperatively.

Patients who are not potent 12 months postoperatively are counselled to undergo further testing and treatment either with intracorporal injection of vasodilators or use of vacuum erection devices. Alternatively, placement of a penile implant may be advised.

Alternatives to Radical Retropubic Prostatectomy

Radical retropubic prostatectomy has the advantages of allowing lymph node staging and excision of the prostate with preservation of sexual function in many patients. Radical perineal prostatectomy may also be appropriate for selected patients, but has the disadvantages of necessitating a separate approach (either laparoscopy or open lymphadenectomy) (Frazier et al. 1992) to sample the pelvic lymph nodes. If sexual function is not a consideration, the combined use of laparoscopic node dissection and radical perineal prostatectomy may be appropriate. Additionally, refinement of technique and innovation of instrumentation may one day make laparoscopic prostatectomy a reality (Schuessler et al. 1992). Until then, however, young men who are sexually active and who have localised prostate cancer are most appropriately treated with nerve-sparing radical retropubic prostatectomy.

Long-Term Results of Radical Prostatectomy in Controlling Cancer

Radical prostatectomy has long been regarded as an effective treatment for patients with organ-confined prostate cancer (Elder et al. 1982; Gibbons et al. 1989; Lepor et al. 1989; Stein et al. 1992; Paulson et al. 1990). Whether this will remain true today when serum PSA levels are routinely monitored after radical prostatectomy is not yet known. It is clear that postradical prostatectomy patients with a detectable serum PSA will almost invariably manifest clinical evidence of recurrence (up to 2 years after initial PSA detection). Many such patients will have detectable local tumour persistence especially if ultrasound-guided biopsy of the vesicourethral anastomosis is performed (Abi-Aad et al. 1992). Fortunately, it appears that only a minority of men after radical prostatectomy will have detectable PSA, especially if careful preoperative selection has been performed. More than 85% of patients who have pathologically organ-confined prostate cancer (that is, no evidence of microscopic capsular penetration, urethral or bladder or seminal vesical involvement, and pathologically confirmed negative lymph nodes) have undetectable postoperative PSA values. Long-term follow-up of those patients suggests that only 5%–10% are destined to develop detectable PSA levels. Almost three-quarters of the patients destined to demonstrate detectable serum PSA levels appear to do so within the first year after surgery and almost 90% do so within 3 years.

Patients with microscopically advanced disease may also manifest high rates of complete tumour control. In our series, approximately 70% of patients with either capsular penetration alone or positive margins alone, have undetectable postoperative PSA values 2 years after surgery. Seminal vesical invasion, however implies a worse prognosis; only about half the patients have undetectable postoperative serum PSA values at 2 years.

These findings suggest that the disease-control capabilities of radical prostatectomy are excellent if pathologically organ-confined tumours are treated. The presence of any histological finding of advanced disease correlates with a progressively higher probability of disease recurrence (Table 11.4). Whether any form of early adjuvant treatment after radical prostatectomy for pathological stage T3 patients is effective is uncertain. Radiation therapy in this setting will result in undetectable PSA levels for up to 50% of men with pathological stage T3 disease and detectable postoperative PSA, but long-term disease control and survival after radiation therapy in this setting has not been proven.

Table 11.4. Estimated frequency of detectable PSA levels 5 years after radical prostatectomy

Pathologic stage	%
Organ-confined	10–15
Microscopic capsular penetration or positive margins only	30–35
Seminal vesicle invasion	50–60
Lymph node metastasis	90

Conclusion

Radical prostatectomy has emerged as an acceptable treatment for patients with clinically organ-confined prostate cancer. As early detection programmes become more widely implemented, a higher proportion of patients diagnosed with prostate cancer will have pathologically organ-confined disease. Radical prostatectomy is the ideal therapy for these patients as it is associated with low morbidity, complication and failure rates.

References

Abi-Aad AS, MacFarlane MT, Stein A et al. (1992) Detection of local recurrence after radical prostatectomy of a prostate specific antigen and transrectal ultrasound. J Urol 147:952–955

Bahnson RR, Catalona WJ (1990) Complications of radical retropubic prostatectomy. In: Smith, Erlich (eds) The complications of urologic surgery. W. B. Saunders, Philadelphia, pp 386–394

Bigg SW, Kavoussi LR, Catalona WJ (1990) Role of nerve-sparing radical prostatectomy for clinical stage B2 prostate cancer. J Urol 144:1420–1424

Blute ML, Zincke H, Farrow G (1986) Long-term follow-up of young patients with Stage A adenocarcinoma of the prostate. J Urol 136:840–843

Boring C, Squires TS, Tang T (1992) Cancer statistics, 1992. CA 42:29

Boxer RJ, Kaughman JJ, Goodwin WE (1977) Radical prostatectomy of carcinoma of the prostate: 1951 through 1976. A review of 329 patients. J Urol 117:208–214

Catalona WJ, Smith DS, Ratliff TL et al. (1991) Measurement of prostate specific antigen in serum as a screening test for prostate cancer. N Eng J Med 324:1156–1161

Chybowski FM, Larson J, Bergstrah EJ, Oesterling JE (1991) Predicting radionuclide bone scan findings in patients with newly diagnosed untreated prostate cancer: prostate specific antigen is superior to all other clinical parameters. J Urol 145:313–318

Elder JS, Jewett HJ, Walsh PC (1982) Radical-perineal prostatectomy for clinical Stage B2 carcinoma of the prostate. J Urol 127:704

Epstein JI (1990) Evaluation of radical prostatectomy capsular margins of resection: the significance of margins designated as negative, closely approaching and positive. Am J Surg Pathol 14:626–632

Epstein JI, Paull G, Eggelston JC et al. (1986) Prognosis of untreated Stage A1 prostatic carcinoma: a study of 94 cases with extended follow-up. J Urol 136:837–839

Epstein JI, Oesterling JE, Walsh PC (1988) The volume and anatomic location of residual tumor in radical prostatectomy specimens removed for Stage A1 prostate cancer. J Urol 139:975–979

Frazier HA, Robertson JE, Paulson DF (1992) Radical prostatectomy: the pros and cons of the perineal versus retropublic approach. J Urol 147:888–890

Gibbons RP, Correa RJ, Brannen GE et al. (1989) Total prostatectomy for clinically localized prostate cancer: long term results. J Urol 141:564

Johansson JE, Adami HO, Andersson SO et al. (1989) Natural history of localized prostatic cancer: population based study in 223 untreated patients. Lancet i:799–803

Johansson JE, Adami HO, Andersson SO et al. (1992) High 10 year survival rate in patients with early untreated prostate cancer. JAMA 267:2191–2196

Leandri P, Rossignol G, Gautier J et al. (1992) Radical retropublic prostatectomy: morbidity and quality of life experience with 620 cases. J Urol 147:883

Lepor H, Kimball AW, Walsh PC (1989) Cause specific actuarial survival analysis: a useful method for reporting survival data in men with clinically localized carcinoma of the prostate. J Urol 141:82

Paulson DF, Moul JW, Walther PJ (1990) Radical prostatectomy for clinical Stage T_1–$T_2N_0M_0$ prostatic adenocarcinoma: long term results. J Urol 144:1180

Schuessler WW, Kavoussi LR, Clayman RV et al. (1992) Laparoscopic radical prostatectomy: initial case report. J Urol 147:246A

Stamey TA, McNeal JE, Freiha FS et al. (1988) Morphometric and clinical studies of 68 radical prostatectomies. J Urol 139:1235–1241

Stamey TA, Kabalin JN, Ferrari M (1989) Prostate specific antigen in the diagnosis and treatment of adenocarcinoma of the prostate. III Radiation treated patients. J Urol 141:1084

Stein A, deKernion JB, Smith RB et al. (1992) Prostate specific antigen level after radical prostatectomy in patients with organ confined and locally extensive prostate cancer. J Urol 147:942

Steinberg GD, Epstein JI, Piantodos IS, Walsh PC (1990) Management of Stage D1 adenocarcinoma of the prostate: the Johns Hopkins experience 1974 to 1987. J Urol 144:1425–1433

Voges GE, McNeal JE, Redwine EA et al. (1992) The predictive significance of substaging Stage A prostate cancer (A1 versus A2) for volume and grade of total cancer in the prostate. J Urol 147:858

Walsh PC (1987) Radical prostatectomy: preservation of sexual function. Cancer control: the controversy. Urol Clin North Am 14:663

Walsh PC, Donker PJ (1982) Impotence following radical prostatectomy: insight into etiology and prevention. J Urol 128:492–497

Whitmore WF, Warner JA, Thompson IM (1990) Expectant management of localized prostatic cancer. Cancer 67:1091–1096

Zincke H, Utz DC, Thule PM et al. (1987) Treatment options for patients with Stage D1 adenocarcinoma of the prostate. Urology 30:307–315

Chapter 12

Overview of Renal Parenchymal Cancer

A. W. S. Ritchie

Introduction

Whilst we await the elusive magic bullet, research, trials and debate continue across a broad spectrum of issues in renal cancer and this overview aims to update the reader with recent trends and studies as an introduction to three specific chapters related to renal malignancy – molecular genetic aspects of Wilms' tumour and renal carcinoma, the role of conservative surgery and immunotherapy of metastatic disease.

The role of genetic and cytogenetic changes in the genesis of renal tumours has not yet been unravelled for renal carcinoma (Meloni et al. 1992). The most frequent abnormalities are a loss or rearrangement of material in 3p or an extra chromosome 7 (Maloney et al. 1991). A review of the available evidence for cytogenetic abnormalities in Wilms' tumour and renal carcinoma is presented in Chapter 13.

The presentation of renal carcinoma has been modified by the widespread use of high quality ultrasound imaging in the abdomen and retroperitoneum. A much higher proportion of diagnoses are being made as a chance finding. In a survey of incidental renal carcinoma in Japan, a dramatic increase in the number of incidentally found tumours was noted. Out of an analysis of 1428 cases, 20 were found by chance in 1980 and this figure had increased to 338 in 1988. The tumours were detected at routine health examination or during investigation for other diseases. The method of detection was ultrasound in 68%, CT in 22% and IVU in 6%. The tumours were localised to the kidney in 76% and the mean tumour diameter was 5.4 cm. The 5-year survival was 86.3% when deaths from other malignancies were excluded. Patients whose tumours were found by health check and by ultrasound had better survival (Aso and Homma 1992).

It is likely that these figures are representative of other parts of the globe and these findings have some important implications in relation to our lack of detailed knowledge of the natural history of these early tumours and how they should be managed (see below). The findings are, however, not unexpected when viewed in the light of post-mortem evidence of a large number of renal tumours which are never diagnosed during the patient's life (Hellsten et al. 1981, 1983).

The place of parenchymal preserving surgery and the need for a lymph node dissection are areas of continuing debate and are now being subjected to clinical trial.

In metastatic disease, chemotherapy has been put in its place. Yagoda (1989) has reviewed 41 new single agent chemotherapeutic agents given to 2309 patients with advanced disease between 1983 and 1989. Only 5% responded (95% confidence intervals of 4%–5%). The "culprit" for this obvious treatment failure is the multidrug resistant gene *mdr*1 (Fojo et al. 1987).

The lack of progress with conventional cytotoxic chemotherapy has been a stimulus to renewed exploration of the place for treatment with biological response modifiers. This area has seen the major investment of effort in recent years and yields a small but predictable pattern of response. The treatment is, however, very expensive and unpleasant for the patient and needs refinement to improve the therapeutic ratio and identify those most likely to benefit. At present it appears that the patient with low volume lung metastases and good performance status is the most likely candidate for response. Neidhart et al. (1991) have reported a response rate of 44% after treatment with interferon in patients with lung only metastases. Unfortunately, the majority of patients with metastatic renal carcinoma do not fall into this category and continue to die of their disease.

These controversial areas in management will be covered in more detail in response to questions posed by clinicians.

Do All Renal Tumours Need to be Treated?

This question can be posed at both ends of the spectrum of renal carcinoma. Are incidentally diagnosed small tumours simply conventional renal cancers which have been found early or do they represent a distinct disease entity with different biological characteristics? The work of Hellsten et al. (1981, 1983) indicates that some renal tumours remain silent throughout the host's life. Conversely, lesions of less than 3 cm in diameter, which used to be labelled as adenomas, can manifest aggressive behaviour with the production of metastases. Without reliable prognostic indicators, the pressure will be on the clinician to treat all such lesions in patients who are fit for surgery, but close follow-up in those not being removed, may yield valuable information on their natural history. At the other end of the spectrum, is the patient with metastatic disease and an asymptomatic primary. Here the treatment recommended may depend more on which surgeon the patient goes to, than any more logical selection process.

If the patient is to have biological therapy, the conventional wisdom is that the tumour should be removed before starting such therapy. The reasons put forward to support this policy are that debulking the total disease burden will allow biological therapy to be more effective. The primary tumour may act as an immunological sump and prevent access of immunologically active cells to metastases. The primary may also act as a continued source of metastatic deposits. This conventional wisdom has recently been challenged in a small study (12 patients) in which patients were treated with one course of a combination of interleukin-2 and α-interferon before removal of the primary. Further treatment was given after the nephrectomy if and when the patient was fit enough. There were three partial responders and no patient responded after nephrectomy who had not responded before nephrectomy (Spencer et al. 1992). This interesting finding certainly merits further investigation as the approach has some advantages. The systemic treatment need not be delayed by the time taken to recover from nephrectomy. Even marginal increases in creatinine levels may limit the maximum dose of treatment after nephrectomy and unresolved infection can delay biological treatment for several weeks. The other pragmatic advantage is that response to treatment could be used as a selection factor for nephrectomy, thus sparing some patients the need for this procedure until local symptoms develop.

Is Radical Nephrectomy Necessary for Every Tumour?

Without the increasing number of small tumours being found by chance, this question may have been seen as a bit of an academic nicety. The results of renal parenchymal preservation are reviewed and discussed in Chapter 15.

The debate surrounding the use of conservative surgery in the presence of a normal contralateral kidney does, however, need to be answered and has now been put to trial in an EORTCMRC group study, which randomises patients with tumours of less than 5 cm in diameter and a normal opposite kidney to radical nephrectomy with lymph node sampling or partial nephrectomy and lymph node sampling. Frozen sections of suspicious margins or abnormal-sized lymph nodes are strongly recommended and close follow-up has been incorporated into the study. Critical to the widespread adoption of partial nephrectomy will be the number of local recurrences and the morbidity of the procedure. The ability to get negative margins may be helped by use of intraoperative ultrasound (Assimos et al. 1991) but *ex vivo* dissection studies suggest that preoperative investigations usually underestimate the extent of disease. Radical nephrectomy has a low incidence of local complications whereas partial nephrectomy is attended by the risks of urinary fistulae and secondary haemorrhage. If the trial can provide clear answers to these questions, then our management strategy will have advanced.

Does Regional Lymph Node Dissection Make any Difference to Survival?

The presence of lymph node metastases has a significant adverse effect (10%–25% 5-year survival) on patient survival (Marshall 1986). It remains possible, however, that some patients with low volume regional and juxta-regional nodes may be rendered tumour free by formal lymph node dissection. This certainly was the implication of the results of Robson et al. (1969) who were strongly in favour of an extended node dissection and whose results, of approximately 35% 5-year survival for N+ patients, have not been reproduced. It is noteworthy that Robson used mediastinoscopy to identify the presence of lymphatic metastases in the superior mediastinum (see below).

The debate requires information on the incidence of positive nodes in order to determine what proportion of patients may benefit from node excision. The incidence of positive nodes is dependent on the source of the material and the enthusiasm of the pathologist for step section analyses. A review of surgical reports has shown that regional node metastases are found in association with 5%–10% of tumours confined by the renal capsule, approximately 30% of tumours extending through the renal capsule and 50% of those with distant metastases (Pizzocaro 1986). Post-mortem studies show a higher incidence of node metastases and indicate that positive regional nodes correlate with node metastases above the diaphragm (Hellsten et al. 1983). Furthermore, distant nodes such as in the axilla or inguinal groups may contain tumour when the regional nodes are negative (Hulten et al. 1969). This erratic pattern of lymphatic dissemination of tumour means that the benefit of formal lymphadenectomy is unlikely to be considerable, although some authors claim a 3%–10% improvement in survival in retrospective analyses (Marshall 1986). Recently, Herrlinger et al. (1991) have reported better survival in 320 patients having a "systematically extended lymph node dissection" than in 191 patients having a "facultative dissection". Facultative was used to indicate that either no nodes were taken, or only a few were taken for staging purposes. No additional operative risk was noted as a result of the extended node dissection. Unfortunately the patients were not randomised to one or other type of node dissection and no data were presented to indicate that the two groups of patients were similar.

The controversy surrounding node dissection may be answered by a further EORTC randomised study, which compares nephrectomy with and without lymph node dissection and which has recruited well. It is possible that this study will identify subgroups of patients, such as those with higher T category, as being likely to benefit from the node dissection.

Is There a Place for Embolisation?

Following a report by Almgard et al. (1973), renal arterial embolisation has been used and adapted in the management of renal tumours. Interventional radiological techniques have been used to reduce the blood supply prior to nephrectomy, to deliver drugs and microcapsules of drugs and to palliate symptoms in patients with inoperable tumours. The possibility that tumour infarction may enhance host defence mechanisms was reported by Swanson et al. (1980) and stimulated great interest in the use of embolisation. In 1982

60% of UK urologists were using this technique (Ritchie and Chisholm 1983). The kidney being an end organ with a clearly defined blood supply seems, at first glance, an ideal candidate for embolisation. Experience has shown, however, that whereas complete infarction of the normal renal parenchyma can be achieved reliably, tumour infarction is less predictable. The reason is that tumours parasitise extra blood supply from initially small renal capsular vessels and are therefore not dependent on the main arterial supply. This phenomenon is well demonstrated in the aortogram phase of renal arteriography, where substantial extrarenal blood supply of large tumours can be demonstrated. This fact has limited use of embolisation as an aid to the surgeon in large vascular tumours. In addition, the early promise of the embolisation and delayed nephrectomy protocol was not sustained (Swanson et al. 1983) and increasing awareness of the morbidity of embolisation has meant that interest in and use of the technique has waned. The technique still has an occasional place, however, and can be of value in the management of troublesome symptoms in patients who are deemed inoperable. Highly selective embolisation of branch arteries can also be used in patients where preservation of blood supply to normal renal parenchyma is necessary.

Simple deprivation of blood supply is only one part of angiographic approaches in the management of renal carcinoma. The use of radioactive seeds and microencapsulated chemotherapeutic agents has also been described. Kato et al. (1989) reported the use of chemoembolisation with mitomycin C in 173 patients. The median total dose given was 20 mg with a range of 5–120 mg. Gelfoam embolisation was combined in 129 patients to limit the loss of the micro capsules via arteriovenous fistulae in the tumour.

A non-randomised comparison of survival in 76 evaluable patients with stage 1–3 disease was made with 62 patients having nephrectomy without chemoembolisation. There was no difference in survival in those with stage 1 disease but the survival of those with stage 2 and 3 disease was significantly better in those having preoperative chemoembolisation. In spite of the latter results, this approach has not been adopted widely – most likely as a result of the perceived complexity of the approach and lack of clear benefit for the majority of patients.

The use of biological agents in microcapsule form, may be worthy of exploration as a method of delivering high doses to large primary tumours.

Do the Benefits of Biological Response Modifiers Justify Their Use?

Traditional approaches to solid tumour immunotherapy were based on attempts to stimulate host immune activity by use of tumour "vaccines" with or without adjuvants. Agents such as BCG, transfer factor, polymerised tumour cells (with or without *C. parvum*) immune RNA, thymosin fraction 5 and tumour necrosis factor have all been reported with little activity over and above the spontaneous disease fluctuation seen with renal carcinoma (Ritchie and deKernion 1989). Recombinant DNA technology has permitted the production of large quantities of "purified" biological response mediators and modifiers, which have formed the basis for a new era of biological therapy.

Interferons are included under the heading of immunotherapy although their mechanism of action is not clearly understood. Interferon alpha has emerged as more effective, in renal carcinoma, than interferon beta or gamma and results in a modest but predictable response rate.

The reports by Rosenberg (1988) of the use of high dose interleukin-2 (IL-2 with and without primed lymphocytes) and the responses engendered in patients with renal carcinoma and melanoma produced an explosion of interest in "biological" therapy. Of particular interest for the use of IL-2, and to a lesser extent interferon, were the complete responders – a new phenomenon in the field of metastatic renal carcinoma. With wider use and an appreciation of the morbidity and mortality related to this treatment approach, the enthusiasm has subsided. The production and administration of lymphokine activated killer (LAK) cells or tumour infiltrating lymphocytes (TIL) has proved too complex, expensive and time consuming to be practical on a large scale. Alternative approaches have included subcutaneous administration of IL-2, combination of IL-2 with interferons and cytotoxic agents such as vinblastine, 5-FU and mitomycin C. The results of such treatments are reviewed in Chapter 14.

A novel approach to getting the drug to the metastases has been reported by Huland et al. (1992). These authors report on six patients treated by inhalation of natural IL-2 using a nebuliser five times per day. The inhalational therapy was supported by low dose IL-2 and subcutaneous interferon. There were no complete responses but lung metastases responded in five of five patients. Vascular leakage and pulmonary oedema, the "bugbear" of high dose IV treatment, was not seen.

This and other combinations and routes of administration of biological therapy will doubtless evolve empirically but the direction for biological therapy does require some consideration.

Even the use of single agent immunotherapy in laboratory animals is complex and our understanding of the precise mechanisms of action is limited. If these complexities are projected to the clinical situation and added to the variable behaviour of metastatic renal carcinoma then the assessment of treatment results becomes difficult. This assessment process is made nearly impossible when combination therapy with three or more agents and different schedules are reported. Dissection of the important components from the less important needs a huge investment in time and basic immunological research. Who will pay?

Putting the issue of mechanisms of action aside, it also seems logical to try and rationalise use of such expensive and toxic agents. Both interferon alpha and interleukin-2 have been licensed for use in metastatic renal carcinoma in the UK and other European countries. Both agents have been licensed without evidence from definitive phase 3 trials. The evidence of response used to support their licence has come mostly from phase 2 studies which deliberately restricted recruitment to patients with good performance status – a well-known favourable prognostic factor in this disease. In such selected patients, interferon will produce complete responses of variable duration in 2% and partial response in 14% (Horoszewicz and Murphy 1989). Side effects will be seen in all patients including responders and non-responders and there are no reliable controlled data to suggest any improvement in survival.

If biological therapies are to have a role for general use, it is important that response rates in selected patients are put into the context of the total population of patients with metastatic disease and are assessed along with quality of life (during and after treatment) and survival. Only randomised studies comparing the "active" treatment with standard therapy, will yield the necessary information.

References

Almgard LE, Fernstrom I, Haverling M, Ljungqvist A (1973) Treatment of renal adenocarcinoma by embolic occlusion of the renal circulation. Br J Urol 45:474–479

Aso Y, Homma Y (1992) A survey of incidental renal cell carcinoma in Japan. J Urol 147:340–343

Assimos DG, Boyce WH, Woodruff RP, Harrison LH, McCullough DL, Kroovand RL (1991) Intraoperative renal ultrasonography: a useful adjunct to partial nephrectomy. J Urol 146:1218–1220

Fojo AT, Shen DW, Mickley LA et al. (1987) Intrinsic drug resistance in human kidney cancer is associated with expression of a human multidrug resistance gene. J Clin Oncol 5:1922–1927

Hellsten S, Berge T, Wehlin I (1981) Unrecognised renal cell carcinoma. Clinical and diagnostic aspects. Scand J Urol Nephrol 8:269–272

Hellsten B, Berge T, Linell F (1983) Clinically unrecognised renal carcinoma: aspects of tumour morphology, lymphatic and haematogenous metastatic spread. Br J Urol 55:166–170

Herrlinger A, Schrott KM, Sigel A (1991) What are the benefits of extended dissection of the regional renal lymph nodes in the therapy of renal cell carcinoma? J Urol 146:1224–1227

Horoszewicz JS, Murphy GP (1989) An assessment of the current use of human interferons in therapy of urological cancers. J Urol 142:1173–1180

Huland E, Huland H, Heinzer H (1992) Interleukin-2 by inhalation: local therapy for metastatic renal cell carcinoma. J Urol 147:344–348

Hulten L, Rosencrantz T, Wahlquist L et al. (1969) Occurrence and localization of lymph node metastases in renal carcinoma. Scand J Urol Nephrol 3:129–133

Kato K, Sato K, Abe R, Moriyama M (1989) The role of embolization/chemoembolization in the treatment of renal cell carcinoma. In: Murphy GP, Khoury S (eds) Therapeutic progress in urological cancers. Alan R. Liss, New York, pp 697–705

Maloney KE, Norman RW, Lee CLY, Millard OH, Welch JP (1991) Cytogenetic abnormalities associated with renal cell carcinoma. J Urol 146:692–696

Marshall FF (1986) Lymphadenectomy for renal cell carcinoma. In: deKernion JB, Pavone-Macaluso M (eds) Tumors of the kidney. Vol 13 International perspectives in urology. Williams and Wilkins, Baltimore, pp 87–97

Meloni AM, Bridge J, Sandberg AA (1992) Reviews on chromosome studies in urological tumors. 1. Renal tumors. J Urol 148:253–265

Neidhart JA, Anderson SA, Harris JE et al. (1991) Vinblastine fails to improve response of renal cancer to interferon alpha-n1: high response rate in patients with pulmonary metasases. J Clin Oncol 9:832–837

Pizzocaro G (1986) Lymphadenectomy in renal adenocarcinoma. In: deKernion JB, Pavone-Macaluso M (eds) Tumors of the kidney. Vol 13 International perspectives in urology. Williams and Wilkins, Baltimore, pp 75–86

Ritchie AWS, Chisholm GD (1983) Management of renal carcinoma – a questionnaire survey. Br J Urol 55:591–594

Ritchie AWS, deKernion JB (1989) The immunobiology of renal carcinoma. In: Chisholm GD, Fair WR (eds) Scientific foundations in urology, 3rd edn. Heinemann Medical, London, pp 540–548

Robson CJ, Churchill BM, Anderson W (1969) The results of radical nephrectomy for renal cell carcinoma. J Urol 101:297–301
Rosenberg SA (1988) Immunotherapy of cancer using interleukin-2: current status and future prospects. Immunol Today 9:58–62
Spencer WF, Linehan M, Walther MM et al. (1992) Immunotherapy with interleukin-2 and alpha interferon in patients with metastatic renal cell cancer with in situ primary cancers: a pilot study. J Urol 147:24–30
Swanson DA, Wallace S, Johnson DE (1980) The role of embolization and nephrectomy in the treatment of renal cell carcinoma. Urol Clin North Am 7:719–
Swanson DA, Johnson DE, von Eschenbach AC, Chuang VP, Wallace S (1983) Angioinfarction plus nephrectomy for metastatic renal cell carcinoma – an update. J Urol 130:449–452
Yagoda A (1989) Chemotherapy of renal cell carcinoma: 1983–1989. Semin Urol 7:199–206

Chapter 13

Molecular Genetics of Wilms' Tumour and Renal Cell Carcinoma

E. R. Maher

It is now generally accepted that cancer is caused by an accumulation of genetic mutations. However, only a small proportion of cancer-associated gene mutations are inherited (i.e. are germline mutations); the majority of gene mutations in cancer cells are acquired (somatic mutations) and are secondary to environmental carcinogens such as radiation, cigarette smoking or chemicals. Almost all human cancers occur in both sporadic and inherited forms (Hodgson and Maher 1992), and it appears that mutations in a restricted number of genes are involved in the genesis of both sporadic and inherited cancers. Consequently, the identification of the genetic mutations responsible for familial cancers has become an important step in understanding the molecular pathology of human carcinogenesis. In familial cancer syndromes, although an inherited germline mutation accounts for the cancer predisposition, this alone is not sufficient to produce a tumour and additional acquired mutations are also necessary. In this chapter the molecular pathology of Wilms' tumour and renal cell carcinoma is discussed with particular emphasis on how the investigation of rare inherited cancer syndromes is contributing towards understanding the molecular genetics of these tumours.

Molecular Genetics of Cancer: General Aspects

Cancer is caused by abnormalities in the genetic mechanisms which control cellular growth and proliferation. Normal cellular growth and differentiation is coordinated by controlling the activity of genes which have (a) a positive effect on growth and proliferation (these are known as *proto-oncogenes*), or (b) a negative effect on cell growth and proliferation (the so-called *tumour suppressor genes or antioncogenes*). It is estimated that, on average, between four and six genetic mutations are necessary to transform a normal cell into a malignant cell. These mutations occur in both proto-oncogenes (producing an oncogene) and in tumour suppressor genes.

Oncogenes are derived from normal cellular genes called proto-oncogenes and act dominantly to induce or maintain cell transformation. More than 40 proto-oncogenes or oncogenes have been reported, and oncogenes may promote cell transformation by a variety of mechanisms such as encoding growth or transcription factors (e.g. *myc*), or by interfering with the g-protein signal transduction pathway (e.g. *ras* family) (Bishop 1991).

Mutations which inactivate a tumour suppressor gene will remove a negative control on cellular growth and proliferation. There is now abundant evidence that the mutations of tumour suppressor genes are of critical importance in human carcinogenesis. The evidence for this comes from three broad lines of enquiry: (a) cell fusion studies; (b) identification of inherited cancer syndrome genes; and (c) the detection of allele loss in human cancers.

Harris et al. (1969) demonstrated that the fusion of malignant cells with normal cells resulted in a non-malignant hybrid cell. This suggested that the malignant cells had lost a normal cellular control mechanism which could be replaced by a normal cell, and that tumorigenicity behaved as a recessive genetic trait. Further evidence for the existence of specific tumour suppressor genes is provided by experiments in which single chromosomes or part of a chromosome have been introduced into a tumour cell line and shown to suppress tumorigenicity (see below).

The concept of a class of tumour suppressor genes was further advanced by

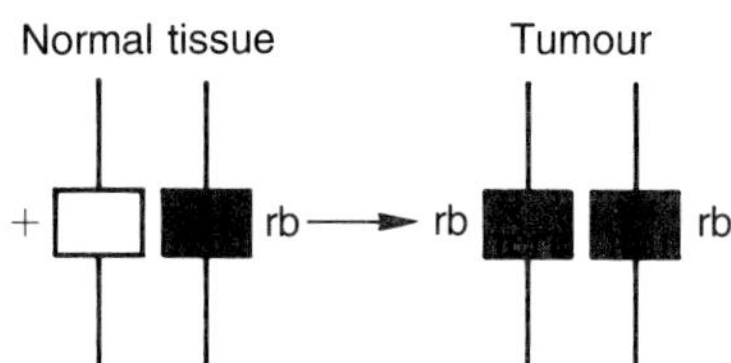

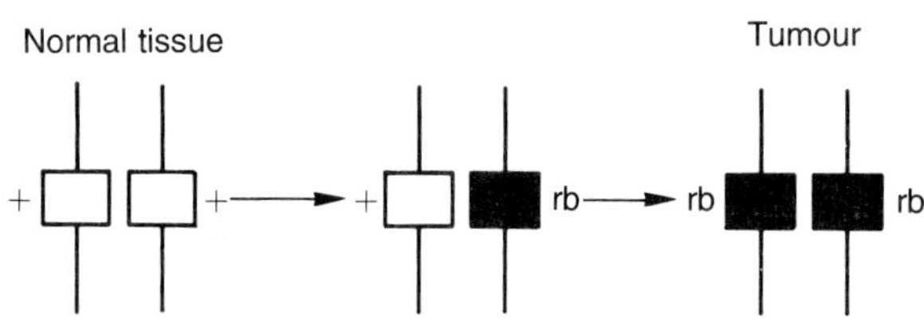

Fig. 13.1. "One hit" and "two hit" mutation models of retinoblastoma. The normal allele of the retinoblastoma tumour suppressor gene is indicated by "+", and the mutated allele by "rb". Children with bilateral tumours have inherited one rb allele. If the normal allele is mutated the cell is homozygous for the rb mutation and a tumour develops. Sporadic cases (which are always unilateral) have two normal alleles and two mutational events (hits) are necessary for a tumour to develop.

studies of retinoblastoma. This rare childhood tumour occurs sporadically in most cases, but about 30% of affected children have multiple tumours or have inherited the susceptibility to retinoblastoma as a dominant trait. Knudson (1971) analysed the age of onset of unilateral retinoblastoma and predicted that retinoblastoma could arise from two rate-limiting steps (mutations). A different pattern was found for children with multiple tumours; there was an earlier age at diagnosis and the data fitted a one step mutation model. It was later suggested that retinoblastoma was initiated by mutations at both alleles of a single locus. Children with multiple tumours were predicted to have inherited a germline mutation of one allele so that only one somatic mutation of the other allele was necessary for retinoblastoma to develop (Fig. 13.1). In unilateral sporadic tumours both alleles were inactivated by acquired mutations. Mutations of the retinoblastoma gene are therefore recessive at a cellular level, since one normal allele can prevent tumorigenesis and tumours only develop from retinoblasts with homozygous mutations. This model explains the earlier age of onset and occurrence of multiple tumours in patients with germline mutations. The retinoblastoma gene was later mapped to chromosome 13 and further evidence for this model was provided by reports of chromosome 13 deletions and allele loss in retinoblastoma tumour tissue (Fig. 13.2). The isolation and characterisation of the retinoblastoma gene

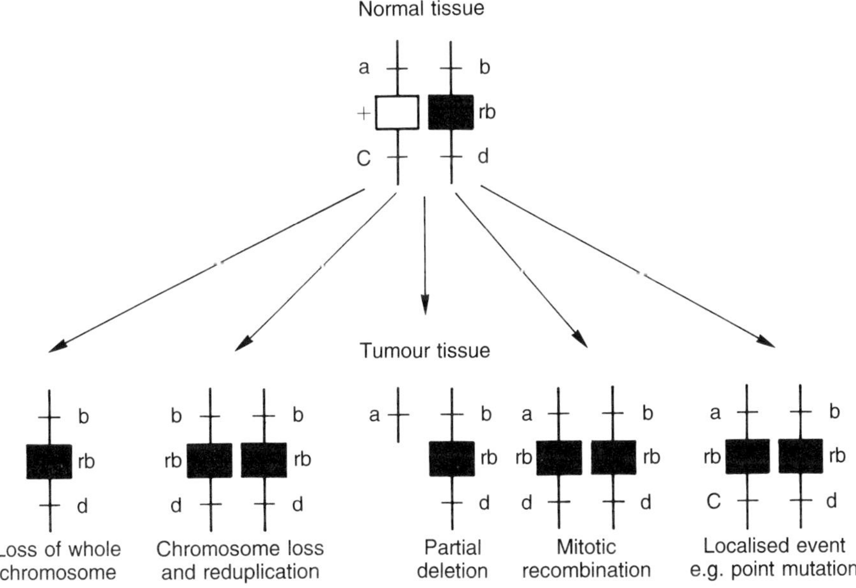

Fig. 13.2. Tumour allele loss in the retinoblastoma model of tumorigenesis. Mechanism of tumour suppressor gene inactivation in retinoblastoma. The normal allele of the retinoblastoma tumour suppressor gene is indicated by "+", and the mutated allele by "rb". Note that the individual is heterozygous (a/b and c/d) at two arbitrary marker loci either side of the retinoblastoma locus. The normal tumour suppressor gene allele (+) has been lost in the tumour cells. Note that allele loss may also occur at the marker loci depending on the precise mutational event. For further details see Cavanee et al. (1983).

(Friend et al. 1986), allowed the confirmation of the retinoblastoma-tumour suppressor gene hypothesis shown in Fig. 13.1. This model of tumorigenesis with loss of both alleles at a single locus has become a paradigm for a class of recessive tumour suppressor genes. However, not all tumour suppressor genes comply with this model and alternative, more complex, models have been proposed as in Wilms' tumour (see below). The detection of cytogenetic deletions or chromosome specific allele loss has become a widely used approach to mapping tumour suppressor genes in a wide variety of inherited and sporadic cancers including Wilms' tumour and renal cell carcinoma (Fig. 13.2).

Wilms' Tumour

Wilms' tumour accounts for 8% of all childhood cancers and affects approximately 1 in 10 000 children. The median age at diagnosis is 3–4 years and 80% of patients present before 5 years of age. Approximately 5% of cases have bilateral tumours and this subgroup has an earlier age of onset (mean 30 months).

Pathology

Wilms' tumour is thought to be derived from a mesenchymal renal stem cell (metanephric blastema). Islands of cells resembling metanephric blastema (nephrogenic rests) may persist into infancy and are found in 1% of normal infant kidneys, but in up to 40% of kidneys with unilateral Wilms' tumour and almost 100% of bilateral cases (Beckwith et al. 1990). Nephrogenic rests have been categorised into perilobar (PLNR) and intralobar rests (ILNR). It appears that tumours associated with ILNR have an earlier age at onset and higher frequency of associated congenital abnormalities than those associated with PLNR. The resemblance of Wilms' tumour cells to renal stem cells suggested that the Wilms' tumour gene might have a role in kidney development.

Genetic Predisposition to Wilms' tumour

Most cases of Wilms' tumour are sporadic, but a small proportion of affected children are genetically predisposed. A genetic predisposition to Wilms' tumour is seen in association with (a) WAGR syndrome, (b) Drash syndrome, (c) Beckwith–Wiedemann syndrome, (d) hemihypertrophy, (e) familial Wilms' tumour, (f) Perlman nephroblastomatosis. An increased incidence of congenital genitourinary abnormalities has been noted among children with Wilms' tumour.

The WAGR syndrome consists of Wilms' tumour (W), aniridia (A), genitourinary abnormalities (G), and mental retardation (R). Up to a third of children with sporadic aniridia develop Wilms' tumour. Most children with the WAGR syndrome have cytogenetically visible chromosome 11 deletions involving band 11p13 (Fig. 13.3). This observation formed the basis for the assignment and subsequent isolation of a Wilms' tumour suppressor gene from chromosome 11p13. WAGR syndrome is uncommon (<2% of all children with Wilms' tumour), and shows incomplete penetrance with only 50% of AGR patients developing Wilms' tumour (Narahara et al. 1984).

Drash syndrome is a rare disorder characterised by male pseudohermaphroditism, Wilms' tumour and characteristic glomerulonephropathy causing progressive renal failure. Not all patients have the complete triad and nephropathy plus Wilms' tumour or urogenital abnormalities is sufficient to make the diagnosis. Wilms' tumour in Drash syndrome presents early (mean 18 months) and is usually bilateral (Jadresic et al. 1991). Gonadoblastoma may also occur.

Beckwith–Wiedemann syndrome has an estimated incidence of 1 in 14 000, and is characterised by exomphalos or umbilical hernia, macroglossia, gigantism, earlobe grooves or helical rim pits, visceromegaly (liver, kidney, spleen), cryptorchidism, occasional cardiac defects and neonatal hypoglycaemia. Most published cases are reported to be sporadic, but familial Beckwith–Wiedemann syndrome is well recognised. In these cases inheritance appears to be autosomal dominant with incomplete penetrance, but there is wide variation in expression. There are at least seven sets of monozygotic twins discordant for Beckwith–Wiedemann syndrome (Olney et al. 1988). Penetrance

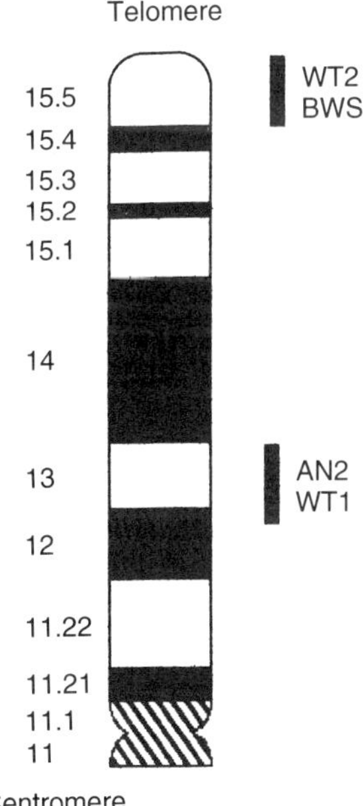

Fig. 13.3. Idiogram of the short arm of chromosome 11 (11p) showing the localisations of the WT1 and aniridia (AN2) genes (chromosome 11p13), and the WT2 and Beckwith–Wiedemann syndrome (BWS) genes.

is more complete when the mother is the transmitting parent. A possible explanation for these findings is genomic imprinting and further evidence for this effect is the detection of uniparental disomy (two paternally derived chromosomes 11) in sporadic Beckwith–Wiedemann syndrome (Henry et al. 1991). Patients with Beckwith–Wiedemann syndrome are at increased risk of several embryonal neoplasms, the most frequent of which is Wilms' tumour (Wiedemann 1983). There appears to be an association between hemihypertrophy and neoplasia in Beckwith–Wiedemann syndrome: 12.5% of all children with Beckwith–Wiedemann syndrome have hemihypertrophy, but 40% of those with tumours.

Less than 1% of Wilms' tumour patients have an affected relative. Familial predisposition to Wilms' tumour is inherited as an autosomal dominant trait with incomplete penetrance (Matsunaga 1981).

Molecular Genetics

Molecular genetic analysis of Wilms' tumour from sporadic and genetically predisposed individuals has provided evidence for three Wilms' tumour genes (named WT1, WT2 and WT3). The first two genes (WT1 and WT2) have been mapped to the short arm of chromosome 11, but a gene for familial Wilms' tumour (WT3) has been excluded from this region. The WT1 gene has been isolated, but many aspects of Wilms' tumorigenesis have not yet been fully delineated.

WT1: Isolation and Function

The detailed analysis of constitutional chromosome 11 deletions in children with the WAGR syndrome localised the Wilms' tumour (WT1) and aniridia (AN2) genes to a small region of distal chromosome 11p13. Molecular genetic analysis of sporadic Wilms' tumour identified a group of tumours with chromosome 11 allele loss restricted to 11p13, providing further evidence of a Wilms' tumour suppressor gene in this region. Extensive physical mapping of the target region culminated in the isolation of the same candidate gene by two independent groups (Call et al. 1990; Gessler et al. 1990). This gene (now called WT1) encodes a DNA binding protein with four zinc finger domains. The WT1 gene product DNA binding recognition site is similar to that recognised by the early growth response-1 (EGR-1) gene product (Rauscher et al. 1990). It has been suggested that the WT1 gene product may function as a tissue specific antagonist of EGR-1 or other similar transcriptional activators (Morris et al. 1991).

Reports of Wilms' tumours with homozygous mutations of WT1 have established WT1 as the Wilms' tumour suppressor gene in 11p13 (Cowell et al. 1991; Huff et al. 1991). The finding of somatic WT1 mutations in nephrogenic rests (Park et al. 1993), suggests that inactivation of WT1 is an early event in the pathogenesis of Wilms' tumour. However, unlike retinoblastoma only a small proportion of Wilms' tumours have been demonstrated to have homozygous WT1 gene mutations and there is clear evidence that other genes can be involved in the pathogenesis of Wilms' tumour (see below).

In addition to functioning as a Wilms' tumour suppressor gene and its presumed role in fetal glomerular differentiation, the increased frequency of genital anomalies in children with bilateral Wilms' tumour led to suggestions that the WT1 gene might have a role in normal genital development (van Heyningen et al. 1990). Confirmation of this hypothesis has come from studies of children with the rare Drash syndrome. All 10 patients investigated by Pelletier et al. (1991a) were found to have WT1 gene mutations which reduced the DNA binding activity of the WT1 protein (nine mutations affected zinc finger 3 and one zinc finger 2). In addition, Wilms' tumours from three patients, and a juvenile granulosa cell tumour from one patient were found to have homozygous WT1 mutations. It is of interest that the genital abnormalities in Drash syndrome are more severe than those in the WAGR syndrome. Therefore the presence of an abnormal protein would appear to be more harmful than a simple reduction in dosage. This suggests that the WT1 gene mutations in Drash syndrome have a dominant-negative effect and the abnormal protein interferes with the function of the normal protein encoded by the remaining normal allele. As would be expected for a gene with a role in the development of the urogenital system, Pritchard-Jones et al. (1990) found specific WT1 mRNA expression during nephrogenesis and in the developing gonad.

WT2: A Wilms' Tumour Gene in Chromosome 11p15.5

The existence of a second Wilms' tumour gene in chromosome 11p15.5 was suggested by (a) molecular genetic analysis of Wilms' tumours, and (b) the association of Wilms' tumour with Beckwith–Wiedemann syndrome. The chromosome 11p15.5 Wilms' tumour gene has been named WT2, but it is not clear whether WT2 and the Beckwith–Wiedemann syndrome gene are identical or separate genes.

Henry et al. (1989) analysed two tumours from patients with WAGR syndrome and found chromosome 11 allele loss restricted to 11p15, and Koufos et al. (1989) reported three Wilms' tumours in which there was loss of heterozygosity (allclc loss) (because of mitotic recombination) at chromosome 11p15, but not at more proximal loci. These findings implicated acquired mutations of a gene (WT2) in chromosome 11p15.5 in a subset of Wilms' tumours. In addition, suppression of tumorigenicity by the introduction of a normal chromosome 11 into a Wilms' tumour cell line appears to be mediated by the 11p15.5 region and not 11p13 (Dowdy et al.1991).

The increased frequency of Wilms' tumour in patients with Beckwith–Wiedemann syndrome has been described. Familial Beckwith–Wiedemann syndrome has been mapped to chromosome 11p15.5 by genetic linkage studies (Koufos et al. 1989; Ping et al. 1989), and some sporadic cases are associated with chromosomal duplications of this region. In such cases the duplicated material is of paternal origin (Henry et al 1991). This finding led to suggestions that genomic imprinting effects may be important in the pathogenesis of Beckwith–Wiedemann syndrome. Further evidence for this hypothesis is the finding of uniparental disomy for chromosome 11p15.5 markers in some sporadic Beckwith–Wiedemann syndrome cases (Henry et al. 1991). Chromosome 11p15.5 shows homology to distal chromosome 7 in the mouse, and Ferguson-Smith et al. (1991) have demonstrated that mice with uniparental disomy for chromosome 7 are abnormally large (as are children with Beckwith–Wiedemann syndrome). The insulin-like growth factor gene (IGF-II) maps to chromosome 11p15.5 in humans and distal chromosome 7 in the mouse. In the mouse only the IGF-II gene on the paternally inherited chromosome is expressed (De Chiara et al. 1991; Ferguson-Smith et al. 1991), and so uniparental paternal disomy for distal chromosome 7 results in overexpression of IGF-II and fetal overgrowth. Could Beckwith–Wiedemann syndrome be caused by overexpression of IGF-II? Although there is some evidence for this suggestion, the Beckwith–Wiedemann gene has not yet been identified (Little et al. 1991).

A Wilms' tumour gene and the Beckwith–Wiedemann syndrome locus both map to chromosome 11p15.5. Are they identical and could IGF-II be WT2? Loss of IGF-II imprinting, so that both alleles of the IGF-II gene are expressed, is frequent in sporadic Wilms' tumour (Ogawa et al. 1993; Rainier et al. 1993). Although overexpression of IGF-II might be oncogenic, reports of chromosome 11p15.5 allele deletions in some Wilms' tumours, and the suppression of tumorigenicity produced by introducing a chromosome 11p15.5 fragment into a Wilms' tumour cell line are all in favour of WT2 being a tumour suppressor gene rather than a proto-oncogene.

WT3: Another Wilms' Tumour Gene

The rarity of familial Wilms' tumour has prevented large-scale family linkage studies; however, genetic linkage studies in four large Wilms' tumour families excluded the predisposing gene from the p13 and p15.5 regions of chromosome 11 (Grundy et al. 1988; Huff et al. 1988; Schwartz et al. 1991). This established the existence of a third Wilms' tumour gene (named WT3) which has not yet been localised. Pelletier et al. (1991b) have reported a father–son pair with Wilms' tumour (and hypospadias and cryptorchidism in the son) associated with a germline WT1 mutation. Therefore familial Wilms' tumour may be caused by mutations in either WT1 or WT3. The rarity of familial Wilms' tumour may be related to the association of genital malformations (causing reduced reproductive fitness) with WT1 mutations.

Mechanism of Wilms' Tumorigenesis

Knudson and Strong (1972) analysed the age at diagnosis of unilateral and bilateral Wilms' tumour. As for retinoblastoma, the statistical analysis was consistent with a two-hit and one-hit model of tumorigenesis respectively. However, the molecular genetic studies described above have demonstrated that Wilms' tumorigenesis is more complex than that of retinoblastoma. In retinoblastoma inherited and acquired mutations involve both alleles of a single locus. In Wilms' tumour mutations at one or more of three loci (WT1, WT2, WT3) can be involved. A minority of Wilms' tumours are homozygous for WT1 mutations (as in retinoblastoma), but many are not. The finding of chromosome 11 allele loss restricted to 11p15.5 in Wilms' tumours from patients with a constitutional 11p13 deletion (Henry et al. 1989; Jeanpierre et al. 1990), illustrates that a two-hit model for Wilms' tumorigenesis does not require the two hits to occur at a single locus. Further complexity is suggested by the observation that chromosome 11 allele loss in sporadic Wilms' tumour occurs more frequently on maternal chromosome 11 than the paternally derived homologue. Thus any model of the molecular pathogenesis of Wilms' tumour must allow for genomic imprinting effects and the possibility that a "first hit" might be inactivation by imprinting of a paternally inherited allele of a Wilms' tumour suppressor gene (Ferguson-Smith et al. 1990; Feinberg 1993). In addition the WT1 protein may repress expression of the IGF-II gene (Knudson 1993).

Wilms' tumour is heterogeneous with respect to genetic predisposition, histopathology and molecular genetics. Beckwith et al. (1990) have attempted to make some correlations between the clinical and histopathological findings. They reported that ILNRs are more common in patients with WAGR and Drash syndromes, whereas PLNRs are more common in Wilms' tumours from children with Beckwith–Wiedemann syndrome. However Park et al. (1993) detected somatic WT1 mutations an ILNR and in a PLNR. Further research is needed to determine if the molecular pathology of Wilms' tumour can be correlated with the histopathological and clinical findings.

Summary

The molecular pathology of Wilms' tumour is complex and does not conform to the retinoblastoma paradigm. Although the WT1 Wilms' tumour suppressor gene has been characterised and demonstrated to have a central role in normal renal and genital development, the detailed function of the WT1 gene product has not yet been elucidated. Two other genes (WT2 and WT3) have been implicated in Wilms' tumorigenesis, and further loci may also be involved (Kaneko et al. 1991).

Renal Cell Carcinoma

Renal cell carcinoma accounts for almost 90% of malignant kidney tumours. Approximately 10% of renal cell carcinomas are classified as papillary and these differ from non-papillary tumours not only in their morphology but also in molecular pathology (see below).

Genetic Predisposition to Renal Cell Carcinoma

Familial cases of renal cell carcinoma are infrequent, and account for about 1% of all cases (Maher and Yates 1991). Two main groups of inherited renal cell carcinoma can be distinguished: (a) those which occur as part of von Hippel–Lindau disease and (b) those with "pure" inherited renal cell carcinoma and no additional features (a minority of which will have constitutional chromosome 3 rearrangements). Recently it has been suggested that patients with tuberose sclerosis have an increased incidence of early onset renal cell carcinoma (Washecka and Hanna 1991).

Von Hippel–Lindau disease is the most frequent cause of inherited renal cell carcinoma. This is an autosomal dominant disorder with a minimal birth incidence of 1/36 000 (Maher et al. 1991a). A wide variety of tumours have been reported in von Hippel–Lindau disease, but the most frequent manifestations are retinal angioma (60% of patients), cerebellar (60%), spinal (13%–44%) and brainstem haemangioblastoma (18%), renal cell carcinoma (28%) and phaeochromocytoma (7%) (Maher et al. 1990a). Renal cell carcinoma is the presenting feature in only 10% of patients with von Hippel–Lindau disease, but the risk of an affected patient developing renal cell carcinoma increases to 70% by age 60 years (Maher et al. 1990a). As with other familial cancer syndromes, patients with von Hippel–Lindau disease not only have a greatly increased risk of renal cell carcinoma, but also develop tumours at an early age (mean 44 years compared to 62 years in sporadic cases), and frequently develop multiple tumours (Fill et al. 1979; Maher et al. 1990b). In addition, multiple renal cysts are frequent in von Hippel–Lindau disease and have been found in up to 76% of patients (Horton et al. 1976). These cysts may be precancerous and in patients with multiple renal cysts a continuum from simple benign cysts to frank renal cell carcinoma may be seen (Solomon and Schwartz 1988).

Familial renal cell carcinoma without additional features also occurs: the literature contains 23 reports of 105 patients with familial renal cell carcinoma (Maher and Yates 1991). The mean age at diagnosis of patients with inherited renal cell carcinoma is 48 years (Erlandsson et al. 1988) similar to the mean age at diagnosis of renal cell carcinoma in von Hippel–Lindau disease. The most likely mode of inheritance is autosomal dominant with age-dependent penetrance, vertical transmission being observed in 17 of 29 families available for analysis. A kindred reported by Cohen et al. (1979) contained ten affected patients in three generations, but here there was an association between renal cell carcinoma and a balanced 3:8 translocation with breakpoints at 3p14.2 and 8q24.1 (Fig. 13.4). Renal cell carcinoma was only seen in translocation carriers, each of whom had an 87% risk of developing renal cell carcinoma by 60 years of age. There are no other reports of familial renal cell carcinoma being associated with constitutional chromosome translocations but sporadic cases associated with balanced translocations between chromosomes 3 and 6, and 3 and 12 have been reported (Kovacs and Hoene 1988; Kovacs et al. 1989a). In both cases the affected patients developed multiple tumours at an early age. The multiple atypical renal cysts seen in von Hippel–Lindau disease do not appear to be a prominent feature of other forms of inherited renal cell carcinoma. Apart from multicentricity the histopathological appearances of all forms of inherited renal cell carcinoma are similar to those of non-familial tumours.

Molecular Genetics

It is now clear that mutations of genes on the short arm of chromosome 3 have a primary role in the pathogenesis of familial and non-familial cases of

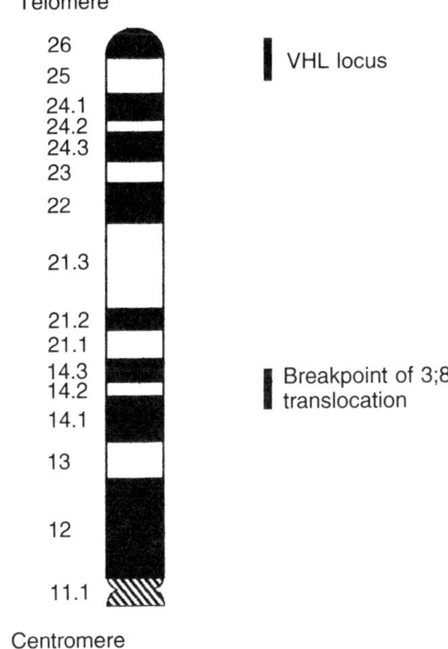

Fig. 13.4. Idiogram of the short arm of chromosome 3 (3p) showing the positions of the von Hippel–Lindau disease gene (VHL), and the breakpoints in the chromosome 3p translocations described by Cohen et al. (1979) and Kovacs et al. (1989a) (for details see text).

non-papillary renal cell carcinoma. Nevertheless full details of the molecular mechanisms of renal cell tumorigenesis have not yet been elucidated.

Molecular Pathology of Inherited Renal Cell Carcinoma

Statistical analysis of the age-at-diagnosis of renal cell carcinoma in von Hippel–Lindau disease and other forms of familial renal cell carcinoma (Erlandsson et al. 1988; Maher et al. 1990a) is compatible with a one-hit and two-hit model of tumorigenesis as described for retinoblastoma and Wilms' tumour (Knudson 1971; Knudson and Strong 1972). The von Hippel–Lindau disease gene has maps to the p25–p26 region of chromosome 3 (Fig. 13.4) (Hosoe et al. 1990; Maher et al. 1991b; Seizinger et al. 1991), and was isolated by a positional cloning strategy (Latif et al. 1993). The finding of germ-line deletions and inactivating mutations in VHL patients (Latif et al. 1993, unpublished observations) is consistent with the VHL disease gene functioning as a tumour suppressor gene. The precise biochemical function of the VHL protein has not yet been elucidated, but there is evidence that it may be a membrane-bound glycoprotein (Latif et al. 1993).

Cytogenetic and molecular genetic studies of renal cell carcinomas from von Hippel–Lindau disease patients have consistently demonstrated chromosome 3p deletions or allele loss (King et al. 1987; Tory et al. 1989; Kovacs

and Kung 1991; Crossey et al. 1994). However, many von Hippel–Lindau
disease associated renal tumours show large regions of chromosome 3 allele
loss which include not only the region of the von Hippel–Lindau disease
locus but also regions of chromosome 3p which may contain other tumour
suppressor genes. Kovacs and Kung (1991) analysed 28 renal cell carcinomas
from two patients with von Hippel–Lindau disease. The most common
cytogenetic abnormalities detected were unbalanced translocations between
chromosomes 3p and 5q, resulting in partial monosomy for the short arm of
chromosome 3 from 3p13 or 3p11. Kovacs and Kung (1991) suggested that the
von Hippel–Lindau disease gene is responsible only for the development of
renal cysts and not for the initiation of renal cell carcinoma (which results from
the loss of another renal cell carcinoma suppressor gene on chromosome 3p).
However, several findings suggest that this is incorrect and that the model of
tumorigenesis in VHL-associated tumours is similar to that in retinoblastoma.
First, some VHL disease tumours have small regions of allele loss restricted to
chromosome 3p25-p26 (Crossey et al. 1994). Second, in familial cases the allele
loss involves the chromosome 3p inherited from the nornal parent (Tory et al.
1989; Crossey et al. 1994), and in patients with germ-line VHL gene deletions
there is loss of the non-deleted allele (Richards et al. 1994)

Familial renal cell carcinoma not caused by von Hippel–Lindau disease
is rare, but usually shows autosomal dominant inheritance (Maher and
Yates 1991). Cohen et al. (1979) described a remarkable family in which
ten members developed renal cell carcinoma at a median age of 45 years.
Affected family members had inherited a balanced translocation between
chromoosme 3 (breakpoint at 3p14.2 (Wang and Perkins 1984), Fig. 13.4)
and chromosome 8. If the association of renal cell carcinoma with the familial
3;8 translocation reported by Cohen et al. (1979) is caused by inactivation of
one allele of a tumour suppressor gene at the chromosome 3 breakpoint,
then chromosome 3p must contain at least two loci for familial renal cell
carcinoma. One locus is the von Hippel–Lindau disease gene at 3p25-p26,
and the other is more proximal at 3p14.2 (Wang and Perkins 1984) (Fig. 13.4).
Molecular genetic analysis of renal cancers from the t(3;8) family reveal that
the derivative chromosome 3 and not the normal chromosome 3 is lost in the
tumour cells. If the translocation breakpoint at 3p14.2 does represent the first
hit in a two-hit mutation model, there is no information regarding the target
gene for the second hit. Additional support for a renal cell carcinoma gene
at 3p13-p14 is provided by Kovacs et al. (1989a) who described a patient with
multiple bilateral renal cell carcinoma and a constitutional 3;6 translocation
(breakpoint between 3p13 and 3p14), and Pathak et al. (1982) who reported a
patient with familial renal cell carcinoma and normal constitutional karyotype
but a chromosome 3;11 translocation (breakpoint at 3p13 or 3p14) in tumour
cells. However, detailed analysis of chromosome 3 breakpoints in the 3;8 and
3;6 translocations reported by Cohen et al. (1979) and Kovacs et al. (1989a)
respectively, has revealed that the breakpoints differ and appear unlikely to
affect a single locus (Kovacs, personal communication). Therefore although
it is widely assumed that the 3;8 translocation disrupts a renal cell carcinoma
tumour suppressor gene at 3p14.2, the evidence for this is not conclusive.
Recently Boldog et al. (1993) have reported the isolation of a novel gene from
the chromoosme 3;8 translocation breakpoint, but mutations of this gene have
not yet been reported in familial or sporadic renal cell carcinomas.

Molecular Pathology of Sporadic Renal Cell Carcinoma

Renal Cell Carcinoma Tumour Suppressor Genes on Chromosome 3

The mapping of von Hippel–Lindau disease gene to the short arm of chromosome 3 and the consistent finding of chromosome 3 specific aberrations in cytogenetic and molecular studies of sporadic renal cell carcinoma (Zbar et al. 1987; Kovacs et al. 1988), clearly suggests that chromosome 3p contains one or more genes with a key role in the pathogenesis of renal cell carcinoma. Confirmation of this hypothesis was provided by Shimizu et al. (1990) who reported that the introduction of a normal chromosome 3p modulated the tumorigenicity of a human renal cell carcinoma cell line.

What are the sites of the renal cell carcinoma tumour suppressor gene(s) on chromosome 3p, and do they correspond to the regions of the von Hippel–Lindau disease gene (3p25-p26) or the 3;8 translocation breakpoint (3p14.2)? The most frequent cytogenetic abnormalities detected in sporadic renal cell carcinoma are terminal deletions and unbalanced translocations (resulting in partial monosomy of chromosome 3p) with breakpoints in the region 3p11-p21 (Kovacs et al. 1988). In molecular genetic studies of sporadic renal cell carcinoma the most frequent change is allele loss from chromosome 3p21->pter (Zbar et al. 1987; Kovacs et al. 1988; Bergerheim et al. 1989). This includes the region to which the von Hippel–Lindau disease gene has been localised (3p25-26) but the region of the 3;8 translocation breakpoint (3p14.2) is not always included in the region of allele loss. However, Teyssier et al. (1986) reported a sporadic renal cell carcinoma in which there was a interstitial deletion of chromosome 3p which apparently did not include the region containing the von Hippel–Lindau disease gene. Van der Hout et al. (1991) suggested that the critical region for chromosome 3p allele loss in sporadic renal cell carcinoma is 3p21-3p24.3. The von Hippel–Lindau disease gene and the 3;8 translocation breakpoint both map outside this region and this finding would suggest the existence of a third renal cell carcinoma suppressor gene on the short arm of chromosome 3. However, it should be noted that individual tumours showed patterns of chromosome 3p allele loss which would include either the von Hippel–Lindau disease gene or the 3;8 translocation breakpoint and their results could be explained by the presence of only two renal cell carcinoma genes. Yamakawa et al. (1991) have reported two commonly deleted regions in sporadic renal cell carcinoma, at 3p13-p14 and at 3p21. Therefore, investigations of chromosome 3p allele loss in sporadic renal cell carcinomas would appear to suggest that at least three loci on chromosome 3p (at 3p14, 3p21 and 3p25-p26 (von Hippel–Lindau disease gene)) can be involved in the genesis of renal cell carcinoma. The cloning of the VHL disease gene and the finding of somatic mutations in renal cell carcinoma cell lines and primary tumours (Latif et al. 1993, unpublished observations) has demonstrated the VHL disease tumour suppresssor gene is probably the major renal cell carcinoma gene on chromosome 3p, but the status of the other two putative tumour suppressor genes remains to be defined.

Several other human cancers are associated with chromosome 3p allele loss including small and non-small lung cell carcinoma, and uterine and breast cancer and it is not yet known if there is any relationship between mutations in the VHL disease gene and other possible renal cell carcinoma genes on chromosome 3p and those associated with other forms of human cancer. In this context it is interesting to note that Hibi et al. (1992) have recently suggested that there might be three chromosome 3p tumour suppressor genes (at 3p25-p26, 3p21 and 3p14-centromere) involved in the pathogenesis of lung cancer.

Other Genetic Alterations in Renal Cell Carcinoma

Chromosome 3p aberrations appear to be an early and specific event in the molecular pathogenesis of non-papillary renal cell carcinoma. Nevertheless, human carcinogenesis usually involves multiple genetic alterations and muta-tions of other tumour suppressor genes and proto-oncogenes might also be expected. Morita et al. (1991a) demonstrated chromosome 3p allele loss in 64% of renal cell carcinomas, but about 30% of tumours showed loss of heterozygosity on chromosomes 5q, 6q, 10q, 11q, 17p and 19p suggesting that these regions may also contain tumour suppressor genes involved in renal carcinogenesis. Anglard et al. (1991) reported frequent (88%) chromosome 3p allele loss in early and late renal cancers, but chromosome 11p, 13 and 17 allele loss was only found in advanced tumours. Morita et al. (1991b) found that chromosome 5q allele loss (commonly in the region of the MCC (mutated in colon cancer) and APC (familial adenomatous polyposis gene) tumour suppressor genes) was correlated with the incidence of distant metastasis. The retinoblastoma and p53 tumour suppressor genes map to chromosomes 13 and 17 respectively, and might be the target for the allele losses detected by Anglard et al. (1991). Ishikawa et al. (1991) found two of 32 primary renal cell carcinomas did not express retinoblastoma protein and Oka et al. (1991) reported that 60% (6 of 10 cases) of renal cancers had p53 gene loss.

The possible role of oncogenes in renal carcinogenesis has also been inves-tigated. Increased expression of the epidermal growth factor receptor gene (Sargent et al. 1989; Gomella et al. 1990; Ishikawa et al. 1990), and the H-*ras* oncogene (Fujita et al. 1988) have been reported in renal cell carcinomas. In addition, c-*myc* oncogene expression may occur and is inversely related to the degree of tumour differentiation (Weidner et al. 1990).

In summary, non-familial renal cell carcinogenesis is associated with multi-ple genetic alterations. Mutations of the VHL disease tumour suppressor gene (and possibly other tumour suppressor genes on chromosome 3p) are an early event, but mutations of other tumour suppressor genes and proto-oncogenes may occur as later events in most cases.

Molecular Pathology and Histopathology of Renal Tumours

Attempts to correlate renal tumour histology with the results of molecular genetic analysis have clearly demonstrated that chromosome 3p allele loss is a feature of non-papillary renal cell carcinoma but not of papillary tumours, oncocytoma or cortical adenoma (Dal Cin et al 1989; Kovacs et al 1989b, c; Brauch et al. 1990; Presti et al. 1991). Presti et al. (1991) and Ogawa et al. (1991) have suggested that chromosome 3 allelle loss is a specific feaure of clear cell non-papillary cancer but not other forms of non-papillary tumours.

Interestingly, VHL gene mutations are most common in clear cell renal cell carcinomas. Further research on the correlations between molecular genetic and histopathological analyses of renal cancers may produce a more coherent classification of renal cell carcinoma than current histopathological methods.

Glossary

Allele: an alternative form of a gene or DNA marker at a single locus.

Allele loss: tumour suppressor gene mutations result in loss of the normal allele at the given locus. In addition, if the mutational event is not localised there may also be allele loss at adjacent DNA marker loci (Fig. 13.2). The detection of chromosome specific allele loss in tumour tissue enables the localisation of tumour suppressor genes to be identified.

Chromosomal localisation: the regional localisation of a locus is described by (a) chromosome, (b) short or long arm (p or q), (c) band. For example, a gene mapping to chromosome 11p13 is on the short arm of chromosome 11 in band 13 (Fig. 13.3).

Genomic imprinting: altered gene function of an allele depending upon the parent of origin.

Heterozygous: two different alleles at a given locus.

Homozygous: identical alleles at a given locus.

Locus: the position of a gene or DNA marker on a chromosome.

Uniparental disomy: inheritance of both homologues of a chromosome from a single parent with loss of the chromosome inherited from the other parent, e.g. an individual with uniparental paternal disomy for chromosome 11 will have inherited both chromosome 11s from their father.

References

Anglard P, Tory K, Brauch H et al. (1991) Molecular analysis of genetic changes in the origin and development of renal cell carcinoma. Cancer Res 51:1071–1077

Beckwith JB, Kiviat NB, Bonadio JF (1990) Nephrogenic rests, nephroblastomatosis and the pathogenesis of Wilms' tumor. Pediatr Pathol 10:1–36

Bergerheim U, Nordenskjöld M, Collins VP (1989) Deletion mapping in human renal cell carcinoma. Cancer Res 49:1390–1396

Bishop JM (1991) Molecular themes in oncogenesis. Cell 64:235–248

Boldog FL, Gemmill RM, Wilke CM et al. (1993). Positional cloning of the hereditary 3;8 chromosome translocation breakpoint. Proc Natl Acad Sci USA 90:8509–8513

Brauch H, Tory K, Linehan WM et al. (1990) Molecular analysis of the short arm of chromosome 3 in five renal oncocytomas. J Urol 143:622–624

Call KM, Glaser T, Ito CY et al. (1990) Isolation and characterization of a zinc finger polypeptide gene at the human chromosome 11 Wilms' tumor locus. Cell 60:509–520

Cavanee WK, Dryja TP, Phillips RA et al. (1983) Expression of recessive alleles by chromosomal mechanisms in retinoblastoma. Nature 305:779–881

Cohen AJ, Li FP, Berg S et al. (1979) Hereditary renal cell carcinoma associated with a chromosomal translocation. N Engl J Med 301:592–595

Cowell JK, Wadey RB, Haber DA et al. (1991) Structural rearrangements of the WT1 gene in Wilms' tumour cells. Oncogene 6:595–599.

Crossey PA, Foster K, Richards FM et al. (1994) Molecular genetic investigation of the mechanism of tumourigenesis in von Hippel–Lindau disease: Analysis of allele loss in VHL tumours. Human Genet (in press)

Dal Cin P, Gaeta J, Huben R et al. (1989) Renal cortical tumors. Cytogenetic characterization. Am J Clin Pathol 92:408–414

De Chiara TM, Robertson EJ, Efstratiadis A (1991) Parental imprinting of the mouse insulin-like growth factor II. Cell 64:849–859

Dowdy SF, Fasching CL, Araujo D et al. (1991) Suppression of tumorigenicity in Wilms' tumor by the p15.5-p14 region of chromosome 11. Science 254:293–295

Erlandsson R, Boldog F, Sümegi J, Klein G (1988) Do human renal cell carcinomas arise by a double-loss mechanism? Cancer Genet Cytogenet 36:197–202

Feinberg AP (1993) Genomic imprinting and gene activation in cancer. Nature Genet 4:110–113

Ferguson-Smith AC, Reik W, Surani MA (1990) Genomic imprinting and cancer. Cancer Surv 9:487–503

Ferguson-Smith AC, Cattanach BM, Barton SC, Breehey CV, Surani MA (1991) Embryological and molecular investigations of parental imprinting on mouse chromosome 7. Nature 351:667–670

Fill WL, Lamiell JM, Polk NO (1979) Radiographic manifestations of von Hippel–Lindau disease. Radiology 133:289–291

Friend SH, Bernards R, Rogelj S et al. (1986) A human DNA segment with properties of the gene that predisposes to retinoblastoma and osteosarcoma. Nature 323:643–644

Fujita J, Kraus MH, Onoue H et al. (1988) Activated H-ras oncogenes in human kidney tumors. Cancer Res 48:5251–5255

Gessler M, Poustka A, Cavenee W, Neve RL, Orkin SH, Bruns GA (1990) Homozygous deletion in Wilms' tumours of a zinc-finger gene identified by chromosome jumping. Nature 343:774–778

Gomella LG, Anglard P, Sargent ER, Robertson CN, Kasid A, Linehan WM (1990) Epidermal growth factor receptor gene analysis in renal cell carcinoma. J Urol 143:191–193

Grundy P, Koufos A, Morgan K, Li FP, Meadows AT, Cavenee WK (1988) Familial predisposition to Wilms' tumour does not map to the short arm of chromosome 11. Nature 336:374–376

Harris H, Miller OJ, Klein G, Worst P, Tachibam T (1969) Suppression of malignancy by cell fusion. Nature 223:363–368

Henry I, Grandjouan S, Couillan P et al. (1989) Tumor-specific loss of 11p15.5 alleles in del11p13 Wilms' tumor and in familial adrenocortical carcinoma. Proc Natl Acad Sci USA 86:3247–3251

Henry I, Bonaiti-Pellie C, Chehensse, Beldjord C, Schwartz C, Utermann G, Junien C (1991). Uniparental disomy in a genetic cancer-predisposing syndrome. Nature 351:665–667

Hibi K, Takahashi T, Yamakawa K et al. (1992) Three distinct regions involved in 3p deletion in human lung cancer. Oncogene 7:445–449

Hodgson SV, Maher ER (1993) A practical guide to human cancer genetics. Cambridge University Press, Cambridge.

Horton WA, Wong V, Eldridge R (1976) Von Hippel–Lindau disease. Arch Intern Med 136:769–777

Hosoe S, Brauch H, Latif F et al. (1990) Localization of the von Hippel–Lindau disease gene to a small region of chromosome 3. Genomics 8:634–640

Huff V, Compton DA, Chao LY, Strong LC, Geiser CF, Saunders GF (1988) Lack of linkage of familial Wilms' tumour to chromosomal band 11p13. Nature 336:377–378

Huff V, Miwa H, Haber DA et al. (1991) Evidence for WT1 as a Wilms' tumor (WT) gene: intragenic germinal deletion in bilateral WT. Am J Hum Genet 48:997–1003

Ishikawa J, Maeda S, Umezu K, Sugiyama T, Kamidono S (1990) Amplification and overexpression of the epidermal growth factor receptor gene in human renal-cell carcinoma. Int J Cancer 45:1018–1021

Ishikawa J, Xu HJ, Hu SX et al. (1991) Inactivation of the retinoblastoma gene in human bladder and renal cell carcinomas. Cancer Res 51:5736–5743

Jadresic L, Wadey RB, Buckle B, Barratt TM, Mitchell CD, Cowell JK (1991) Molecular analysis of chromosome region 11p13 in patients with Drash syndrome. Hum Genet 86:497–501

Jeanpierre C, Antignac C, Beroud C et al. (1990) Constitutional and somatic deletions of two different regions of maternal chromosome 11 in Wilms' tumor. Genomics 7:434–438

Kaneko Y, Homma C, Maseki N, Sakurai M, Hata (1991) Correlation of chromosome abnormalities with histological and clinical features in Wilms' and other childhood renal tumors. Cancer Res 51:5937–5942

King CR, Schimke RN, Arthur T, Davoren B, Collins D (1987) Proximal 3p deletion in renal cell carcinoma cells from a patient with von Hippel–Lindau disease. Cancer Genet Cytogenetic 27:345–348

Knudson AG (1971) Mutation and cancer: statistical study of retinoblastoma. Proc Natl Acad Sci USA 68:820–823

Knudson AG (1993) Antioncogenes and human cancer. Proc Natl Acad Sci USA 90:10914–10921

Knudson AG, Strong LC (1972) Mutation and cancer: neuroblastoma and phaeochromocytoma. Am J Hum Genet 24:514–532

Koufos A, Grundy P, Morgan K et al. (1989) Familial Wiedemann–Beckwith syndrome and a second Wilms' tumor locus both map to 11p15.5. Am J Hum Genet 44:711–719

Kovacs G, Hoene E (1988) Loss of der(3) in renal carcinoma cells of a patient with constitutional t(3;12). Hum Genet 78:148–150

Kovacs G, Kung HF (1991) Nonhomologous chromatid exchange in hereditary and sporadic renal cell carcinomas. Proc Natl Acad Sci USA 88:194–198

Kovacs G, Erlandsson R, Boldog F et al. (1988) Consistent chromosome 3p deletion and loss of heterozygosity in renal cell carcinoma. Proc Natl Acad Sci USA 85:1571–1575

Kovacs G, Brusa P, De Riese W (1989a) Tissue-specific expression of a constitutional 3;6 translocation: development of multiple bilateral renal-cell carcinomas. Int J Cancer 43:422–427

Kovacs G, Wilkens L, Papp T, de Riese W (1989b) Differentiation between papillary and nonpapillary renal cell carcinomas by DNA analysis. J Natl Cancer Inst 81:527–530

Kovacs G, Welter C, Wilkens L, Blin N, Deriese W (1989c) Renal oncocytoma. A phenotypic and genotypic entity of renal parenchymal tumors. Am J Pathol 134:967–971

Latif F, Tory K, Gnarra J et al. (1993) Identification of the von Hippel–Lindau disease tumour suppressor gene. Science 260:1317–1320

Little M, van Heyningen V, Hastie N (1991) Dads and disomy and disease. Nature 351:609–610

Maher ER, Yates JR (1991) Familial renal cell carcinoma: clinical and molecular genetic aspects [editorial]. Br J Cancer 63:176–179

Maher ER, Yates JRW, Harries R et al. (1990a) Clinical features and natural history of von Hippel–Lindau disease. Q J Med 77:1151–1163

Maher ER, Yates JRW, Ferguson-Smith MA (1990b) Statistical analysis of the two stage mutaion model in von Hippel–Lindau disease and in sporadic cerebellar haemangioblastoma and renal cell carcinoma. J Med Genet 27:311–314

Maher ER, Iselius L, Yates JRW et al. (1991a) Von Hippel–Lindau disease: a genetic study. J Med Genet 28:443–447

Maher ER, Bentley E, Yates JRW et al. (1991b) Mapping of the von Hippel–Lindau disease locus to a small region of chromosome 3p by genetic linkage analysis. Genomics 10:957–960

Matsunaga E (1981) Genetics of Wilms' tumor. Hum Genet 57:231–246

Morita R, Ishikawa J, Tsutsumi M et al. (1991a) Allelotype of renal cell carcinoma. Cancer Res 51:820–823

Morita R, Saito S, Ishikawa J et al. (1991b) Common regions of deletion on chromosomes 5q, 6q, and 10q in renal cell carcinoma. Cancer Res 51:5817–5820

Morris JF, Madden SL, Tournay OE, Cook DM, Sukhatme VP, Rauscher FJ (1991) Characterization of the zinc finger protein encoded by the WT1 Wilms' tumor locus. Oncogene 6:2339–2348

Narahara K, Kikkawa K, Kimira S et al. (1984) Regional mapping of catalase and Wilms' tumor-aniridia, genitourinary abnormalities and mental retardation triad loci to the chromosome segment 11p13. Hum Genet 66:181–185

Ogawa O, Kakehi Y, Ogawa K, Koshiba M, Sugiyama T, Yoshida O (1991) Allelic loss at chromosome 3p characterizes clear cell phenotype of renal cell carcinoma. Cancer Res 51:949–953

Ogawa O, Eccles MR, Szeto J et al. (1993) Nature 362:749–751

Oka K, Ishikawa J, Bruner JM, Takahashi R, Saya H (1991) Detection of loss of heterozygosity in the p53 gene in renal cell carcinoma and bladder cancer using the polymerase chain reaction. Mol Carcinog 4:10–13

Olney AH, Buehler BA, Waziri M (1988) Wiedemann–Beckwith syndrome in apparently discordant monozygotic twins. Am J Med Genet 29:491–499

Park S, Bernard A, Bove KE et al. (1993) Inactivation of WT1 in nephrogenic rests, genetic precursors to Wilms' tumour. Nature Genet 5:363–367

Pathak S, Strong LC, Ferrell RE, Trindade A (1982) Familial renal cell carcinoma with a 3:11 chromosome translocation limited to tumor cells. Science 217:939–941

Pelletier J, Breuning W, Kashtan CE et al. (1991a) Germline mutations in the Wilms' tumor suppressor gene are associated with abnormal urogenital development in Denys-Drash syndrome. Cell 67:437–447

Pelletier J, Bruening W, Li FP, Haber DA, Glaser T, Housman DE (1991b) WT1 mutations contribute to abnormal genital system development and hereditary Wilms' tumour. Nature 353, 431–434

Ping AJ, Reeve AE, Law DJ, Young MR, Boehnke M, Feinberg AP (1989) Genetic linkage of Beckwith–Wiedemann syndrome 11p15. Am J Hum Genet 44:720–723

Presti Jr JC, Rao PH, Chen Q et al. (1991) Histopathological, cytogenetic, and molecular characterization of renal cortical tumors. Cancer Res 51:1544–1552

Pritchard-Jones K, Fleming S, Davidson D et al. (1990) The candidate Wilms' tumour gene is involved in genitourinary development. Nature 346:194–197

Rainier S, Johnson LA, Dobry CJ, Ping AJ, Grundy PE, Feinberg AP (1993) Relaxation of imprinted genes in human cancer. Nature 362:747–749

Rauscher FJ, Morris JF, Tournay SE, Cook DM, Curran T (1990) Binding of the Wilms' tumor locus zinc finger protein to the EGR-1 consensus sequence. Science 250:1259–1262

Richards F M, Crossey P A, Phipps M E et al. (1994) Detailed mapping of germline deletions of the von Hippel–Landau disease tumour suppressor gene. Hum Mol Genet 3:595–598

Sargent ER, Gomella LG, Belldegrun A, Linehan WM, Kasid A (1989) Epidermal growth factor receptor gene expression in normal human kidney and renal cell carcinoma. J Urol 142:1364–1368

Schwartz CE, Haber DA, Stanton VP, Strong LC, Skolnick MH, Housman DE (1991) Familial predisposition to Wilms' tumor does not segregate with the WT1 gene. Genomics 10:927–930

Seizinger BR, Smith DI, Filling-Katz MR et al. (1991) Genetic flanking markers refine diagnostic criteria and provide insights into the genetics of von Hippel–Lindau disease. Proc Natl Acad Sci USA 88:2864–2868

Shimizu M, Yokota J, Mori N et al. (1990) Introduction of normal chromosome 3p modulates the tumorigenicity of a human renal cell carcinoma cell line YCR. Oncogene 5:185–194

Solomon D, Schwartz A (1988) Renal pathology in von Hippel–Lindau disease. Hum Pathol 19:1072–1079

Teyssier JR, Henry I, Dozier C, Ferre D, Adnet JJ, Pluot M (1986) Recurrent deletion of the short arm of chromoosome 3 in human renal cell carcinoma: shift of the c-raf locus. J Natl Cancer Inst 77:1187–1195

Tory K, Brauch H, Linehan M et al. (1989) Specific genetic change in tumours associated with von Hippel–Lindau disease. J Natl Cancer Inst 81:1097–1101

Van der Hout AH, van der Vlies P, Wijmenga C, Li FP, Oosterhuis JW, Buys CHCM (1991) The region of common allelic losses in sporadic renal cell carcinoma is bordered by the loci D3S2 and THRB. Genomics 11:537–542

van Heyningen V, Bickmore WA, Seawright A et al. (1990) Role for Wilms' tumor gene in genital development? Proc Natl Acad Sci USA 87:5383–5386

Wang N, Perkins KL (1984) Involvement of band 3p14 in t(3;8) hereditary renal carcinoma. Cancer Genet Cytogenet 11:479–480

Washecka R, Hanna M (1991) Malignant renal tumours in tuberous sclerosis. Urology 37:340–343

Weidner U, Peter S, Strohmeyer T, Hussnätter R, Ackermann R, Sies H (1990) Inverse relationship of epidermal growth factor receptor and HER2/neu gene expression in human renal cell carcinoma. Cancer Res 50:4504–4509

Wiedemann HR (1983) Tumours and hemihypertrophy associated with Wiedemann–Beckwith syndrome. Eur J Pediatr 141:129–130

Yamakawa K, Morita R, Takahashi E, Hori T, Ishikawa J, Nakamura Y (1991) A detailed deletion mapping of the short arm of chromosome 3 in sporadic renal cell carcinoma. Cancer Res 51:4707–4711

Zbar B, Brauch H, Talmadge C, Lineham M (1987) Loss of alleles of loci on the short arm of chromosome 3 in renal cell carcinoma. Nature 327:721–724

Chapter 14

Immunotherapy in the Management of Metastatic Renal Cell Carcinoma

K. B. Pittman and P. J. Selby

Introduction

Adenocarcinoma or renal cell carcinoma (RCC) is the most common cancer arising in the adult kidney and accounts for approximately 1.5% of cancer deaths in Western society. Approximately 50% of patients with renal cancer will have advanced or metastatic disease at the time of diagnosis. These patients have less than a 5% chance of 3-year survival. Of the patients who have early stage, "resectable" lesions at diagnosis, the recurrence rate remains 10% even after 10 years (McNichols et al. 1981; Myers and Gloeckler 1989). A number of factors have been found to determine the prognosis of patients with either recurrent or metastatic RCC. Most studies indicate that the important predictors of survival are performance status, duration of disease-free survival following nephrectomy, and the number of different metastatic sites with some finding the size of metastases, weight loss, sedimentation rate and fever to be important (Elson et al. 1988; de Forges et al. 1988; Palmer et al. 1992). Until the recent advent of biological therapies the options for treating advanced RCC were limited to palliative nephrectomy or resection of metastases, iatrogenic embolisation of the kidney to alleviate pain and bleeding, palliative radiotherapy, hormonal therapy (which has an objective response rate of less than 5%) and cytotoxic chemotherapy. Vinblastine, the most active cytotoxic agent in RCC produces objective responses in approximately 15%–20%; these responses are usually short lived (Linehan et al. 1989).

The clinical behaviour of RCC is very variable. The disease frequently progresses steadily but there are numerous documented reports of spontaneous regression of the tumour, as well as reports of metastatic tumour regression following excision of the primary tumour, and regression of metastatic disease following angioinfarction of the primary tumour. The occurrence of spontaneous regressions of renal cancer may be used as an argument in favour of exploring immunotherapy in this tumour. However, a critical analysis of the literature is not very encouraging. Possinger et al. (1988) reviewed the literature and we are aware of five other papers (Patel et al. 1978; Waters et al. 1979; McNichols et al. 1981; Yamashita et al. 1989; Oliver et al. 1989), so that collectively 11 spontaneous remissions are reported in 2411 patients (0.46%).

Initial studies of immunological modulation in RCC followed the observation that tumour regression occasionally occurred following periods of acute immune activation, as occurs following acute bacterial infection. Preliminary attempts at augmenting immune response included such immune stimulation as the administration of bacillus Calmette–Guérin (BCG) to patients with RCC (Morales and Eidinger 1976). Other treatments included the use of autologous antitumour vaccines (Neidhart et al. 1980), transfer factor (Montie et al. 1982), xenogenic immune RNA (Richie et al. 1984), and certain immunomodulatory drugs such as cimetidine and coumarin (Marshall et al. 1987).

The recent developments in immunotherapy are largely due to the expanding knowledge of the structure and functions of the cytokines. Moreover, the further development of lymphocyte ex vivo culture models has advanced the knowledge of the local immune response and has increased the potential scope for combining different biological response modifiers.

There is now a steadily increasing body of data that assesses the role of numerous types of immunological approaches to the problem of advanced RCC. This chapter summarises the more relevant clinical data and discusses the prospects for further application of biological response modifiers in the management of RCC.

Interferons

Interferons (IFNs) are a group of naturally occurring glycoproteins which were discovered in the supernatants of virally infected cells (Isaacs and Lindemann 1957). It was found that the IFNs protected the cells from superinfection by other viruses. Therefore, by definition, all IFNs have the capacity to induce an antiviral state in the host. Three major classes of IFNs have been delineated. Interferon-alpha (IFN-alpha) is produced by leucocytes and macrophages. Interferon-beta (IFN-beta) is produced by fibroblasts and epithelial cells. Interferon-gamma (IFN-gamma) is produced by activated T lymphocytes. All the interferons have antiviral and antiproliferative activity as well as acting synergistically with other cytokines (Kurzrock et al. 1991). These actions have prompted much interest in the potential use of IFNs for the treatment of viral disease, immunological disorders and malignancy.

The exact mechanism for these immune (and antitumour) activities is not yet clear. However, it is likely to be related to the effects of interaction with specific interferon receptors, with modulation of gene expression, which in turn alters the structure and function of different populations of cells resulting in: (a) a decrease in the proliferating activity of cells; (b) a decrease in oncogene product formation; (c) alteration of the expression of cell surface antigen, particularly HLA; (d) modulation of the immune system (both up- and down-regulation, depending on the dose); (e) inhibition of the replicating capacity of DNA and RNA viruses and (f) modulation of cell differentiation (Shearer and Taylor-Papadimitriou 1987; Kurzrock et al. 1991). The heterogeneity of the activity of interferons is even more complex when taking into account the concomitant effects of the other cytokines which also influence immune function. It seems likely that the various individual antitumour activities of the interferons are of varying significance depending on dose regimens and tumour type.

Interferon was the first available cytokine and was initially produced by cellular extraction. Now, most of the IFN used in clinical practice and research is manufactured using recombinant DNA technology. These IFNs are virtually identical to the endogenous counterparts. The $t_{1/2}$ for rIFN administered intravenously (IV) as a bolus is approximately 5 h for rIFN-alpha 2a (Roferon) and 2.5 h for rIFN-alpha 2b (Intron A). IFN may be given by any parenteral route but the majority of patients treated with IFNs receive subcutaneous (SC) or intramuscular (IM) injections. The bioavailability of rIFN-alpha given this way is 80% with protracted absorption and elimination, so that the biological effects are considerably longer compared to the IV route. Host neutralising antibodies against rIFN-alpha develop in 10%–20% of patients and may affect biological activity.

IFN has been shown to be active in a large number of human malignancies. The very best results in the clinical setting have occurred with certain haematological malignancies, especially hairy cell leukaemia (Quesada et al. 1984). Other encouraging response rates are seen in chronic myeloid leukaemia (Kurzrock et al. 1989), and certain non-Hodgkin's lymphomas (Foon et al. 1984; Bunn et al. 1986). IFN has also been evaluated in a wide range of non-haematological malignancies either alone or in combination with other biological agents or conventional cytotoxic agents.

A large number of patients with advanced RCC have been treated with purified and recombinant interferons in a large number of relatively small studies. The type of interferon used, the dose and frequency of administration is varied. These variables, along with differing combinations with cytotoxic agents or other biological agents make data analysis difficult. The initial studies using IFN in RCC suggested response rates of 20% or more (Table 14.1). In retrospect it is likely that the IFN preparations used

Table 14.1. Natural leucocyte interferon therapy in advanced RCC

Author	Year	Dose (MU)	Route	Schedule	Number evaluable	CR/PR	%RR
Quesada et al.	1983	3	IM	daily	50	3/10	26%
DeKernion et al.	1983	3	IM	5×/week	43	1/6	16%
Magnusson et al.	1983	4–16	IM	daily	7	0/0	0%
Kirkwood et al.	1985	1	IM	daily	14	0/0	0%
		10	IM	daily	16	1/2	19%
Edsmyr et al.	1985	3	IM	daily	11	1/2	27%
					141	6/20	18%

in these studies (leucocyte IFN) contained significant impurities, possibly other cytokines capable of augmenting the tumour response. This may be important when considering the role of combinations of biological agents. When the purified lymphoblastoid and recombinant IFNs (with measurable increased biological activity) became available and were used, the initial high response rates were never subsequently achieved (Tables 14.1 and 14.2).

rIFN-alpha has been most widely studied. The overall response rate to rIFN-alpha is approximately 15% with a complete response rate of approximately 2% (Table 14.3). When examining those studies which reported the higher response rates, it seems that the daily dose rates of between 5 and 10 megaU produce higher response rates than doses less than 5 megaU per day. It also seems likely that continuous interferon schedules (either daily or 3 days per week) are of more value than those schedules that contain lengthy breaks in treatment (Selby 1989). Favourable clinical characteristics are closely associated with improved response rates. Patients of good performance status, who have had the primary tumour resected, and who have predominantly pulmonary metastases generally have the best clinical outcome. This is in contrast to patients of poor performance status, with either unresected primary tumours or locally recurrent disease, and patients with metastases in the liver and other non-pulmonary sites, who tend to have low rates of tumour response. The majority of patients who respond to rIFN-alpha will show some evidence of response within 2 months of commencing therapy. The median duration of response is 8 months, with a range between the various studies of 3–12 months.

Most patients who receive IFN experience fever, myalgia and general "flu-like" symptoms after IFN administration. Often these symptoms can be partially or completely alleviated by the use of simple agents such as paracetamol. Occasionally these "acute" reactions are severe enough to warrant withdrawal of therapy. With increasing doses and prolonged treatment with IFN, severe lethargy, anorexia and weight loss, diarrhoea,

Tables 14.2. Natural lymphoblastoid interferon therapy in advanced RCC

Author	Year	Dose (MU)	Route	Schedule	Number evaluable	CR/PR	%RR
Neidhart et al.	1984a	5/m²	IM	3×/week	33	0/5	15%
Neidhart et al.	1984b	3→20	IM	d1–10q 3/52	23	1/4	22%
		5→50	IM	d1–5q 3/52	9	0/2	22%
Marumo et al.	1984	3	IM	daily	18	0/1	6%
Vugrin et al.	1985	3/m²	IM	3×/week	21	0/1	5%
Vugrin et al.	1986	30/m²	IV	3×/week	16	0/0	0%
Umeda and Niijima	1986	5	IM	daily	73	1/16	23%
Trump et al.	1987	3→20/m²	IM	d1–10q 3/52	39	0/5	13%
Eisenhauer et al.	1987	30→100	IV	weekly	37	0/4	11%
Fujita et al.	1988	3	IM	daily	24	2/4	25%
					293	4/42	16%

Table 14.3. Interferon-alpha therapy in advanced RCC

Author	Year	Dose (MU)	Route	Schedule	Number evaluable	CR/PR	%RR
Krown et al.	1983	50	IM	3×/week	37	0/5	14%
Einzig et al.	1984	3→36	IM	daily	62	0/7	11%
Quesada et al.	1985	2/m²	IM	daily	15	0/0	0%
		20/m²	IM	daily	41	1/11	29%
Kuzmits et al.	1985	10	IM	daily	8	1/0	13%
Schnall et al.	1986	3→36	IM	daily	22	0/1	5%
Fossa et al.	1986	18→36	IM	daily	2	0/1	50%
Kempf et al.	1986	2/m²	SC	3×/week	10	0/0	0%
		30/m²	IV	5×/week	10	0/1	10%
Umeda and Niijima	1986	6–10	IM	3–5 days/week	45	1/7	18%
		3→36	IM	daily	108	2/13	14%
Scheithaurer et al.	1987	10	IM	daily	18	1/1	11%
Buzaid et al.	1987	3→36	IM	daily	22	0/5	23%
Muss et al.	1987	2/m²	SC	3×/week	51	1/4	10%
Figlin et al.	1988	3→36	IM	d1–5q 1/52	19	1/4	26%
Foon et al.	1988	2/m²	SC	3×/week	21	0/1	5%
Otto et al.	1988	IM	1m	3×/week	42	0/7	17%
Porzolt et al.	1988	2	SC	d1–5q 1/52	18	1/1	11%
Marshall et al.	1989	1	SC	daily	16	0/4	25%
Fossa et al.	1992	18	IM	3×/week	53	1/5	11%
					666	11/81	14%

cytopenias and elevation of liver function tests may become significant. Certainly with prolonged treatment, marked lassitude can be very distressing as can the occasional neuropsychiatric effects (Quesada et al. 1986). Several studies have been undertaken to evaluate the effect of corticosteroids given concurrently with the IFN. There is some evidence to suggest that this approach may alleviate many of the unpleasant side effects without any significant diminution in response rate (Abdi 1988).

Several phase I studies of rIFN-beta suggest that the maximally tolerated dose of rIFN-beta is between five- to tenfold higher than rIFN-alpha (Rinehart et al. 1986). The initial hopes of being able significantly to increase the IFN dose and therefore produce higher rates of response were not fulfilled. Although higher doses of rIFN-beta may be administered with considerably less toxicity, and antitumour effects are seen, the response rates of metastatic RCC at the higher doses is not significantly different from response rates using the more conventional doses of rIFN-alpha (Rinehart et al. 1986; Kinney et al. 1990). Similarly the response rates of rIFN-gamma are no better than rIFN-alpha (Tables 14.4 and 14.5). In vitro studies suggested that the combination of IFN-alpha and IFN-gamma resulted in synergistic antiviral and antiproliferative activity and several centres have performed trials of combinations of interferons in the treatment of RCC (Foon et al. 1988; Geboers et al. 1988; Quesada et al. 1988; deMulder et al. 1990). Response rates varied from 0 to 25% with toxicity similar to the known

Table 14.4. Interferon-beta therapy in advanced RCC

Author	Year	Dose (MU)	Route	Schedule	Number evaluable	CR/PR	%RR
Rinehart et al.	1986	0.1–150	IV	3×/week	15	0/2	13%
Kish et al.	1986	3→30	IV	daily	16	0/1	6%
Kinney et al.	1990	45–1000	IV	3×/week	25	1/4	20%
					56	1/7	14%

single agent interferon toxicity data. A summary of interferon trials in RCC is depicted in Tables 14.1–14.5. At present, there is no convincing evidence that IFN-beta or IFN-gamma given alone or in combination with other IFNs is any more efficacious than IFN-alpha given as a single agent.

Interferons have also been used in combination with a number of cytotoxic agents. The most frequently evaluated of the cytotoxic agents is vinblastine (VLB), as this agent produces the highest single agent response rate in RCC (approx. 15%) (Table 14.6). The doses, dose scheduling and routes of administration vary widely in the various trials with the response rates varying from 0–40% (mean response rate of approx. 18%). The toxicity of the combinations of interferons and cytotoxics is significantly greater than interferons alone. Fossa et al. (1992) have reported an important randomised prospective trial of 178 patients in which IFN-alpha 2a at a dose of 18 MU IM three times each week was compared to the same dose of IFN plus vinblastine 0.1 mg/kg IV every three weeks. The response rate was 11% for IFN alone and 24% for IFN plus VLB. Unfortunately, there was no advantage in survival for the combination therapy and it showed enhanced toxicity.

The use of interferons in combination with other biological response modifiers in advanced RCC will be considered later in the chapter.

Table 14.5. Interferon-gamma

Author	Year	Dose (MU)	Route	Schedule	Number evaluable	CR/PR	%RR
Takaku et al.	1987	8–12	IV/IM	daily	32	0/2	6%
		40	IV	d1–5q 2/52	30	1/5	20%
Quesada et al.	1987	5–20	IV	daily	14	0/1	7%
		0.2–1	CIV	daily	16	0/1	6%
Rinehart et al.	1987	0.01–75	IV	2×/week	13	0/0	0%
Garnick et al.	1988	0.2–60	IV	d1–7q 3/52	41	1/3	10%
Foon et al.	1988	1	SC	3×/week	21	0/1	5%
Kuebler et al.	1989	0.25	CIV	daily (4 wks)	27	0/0	0%
Grups and Frohmuller	1989	5	IV	d1–8q 3/52	9	0/3	33%
Brunstch et al.	1990	1	IV	daily	40	0/1	3%
					243	2/17	8%

Table 14.6. Combination of interferon/vinblastine in advanced RCC

Author	Year	Number evaluable	CR/PR	%RR
Figlin et al.	1985	23	0/3	13%
Fossa et al.	1986			
Fossa and DeGaris	1987	40	0/10	25%
Neidhart et al.	1987	82	5/4	11%
Cetto et al.	1988	26	1/7	31%
Bergerat et al.	1988	40	1/16	43%
Sertoli et al.	1989	20	0/2	10%
Schornagel et al.	1989	54	0/10	19%
Kellokumpu-Lehtinen and Nordman	1990	20	3/3	30%
Fossa et al.	1992	66	1/15	24%
		371	11/70	22%

Variable dose/schedule for both interferon and vinblastine.

Interleukin-2

Interleukin-2 (IL-2) is a cytokine produced by activated T cells that plays a central role in immune regulation. It was originally described as a T cell growth factor present in the conditioned media of mitogen-stimulated lymphocytes (Morgan et al. 1976). It is known to have a wide variety of actions including inducing the growth of activated T cells, inducing further lymphokine production by T cells and inducing cytotoxic T cell activity. Essentially it finely regulates the maturation and subsequent development of T cells. It also has a stimulatory effect on B cells and macrophages. Moreover, lymphoid cells incubated with IL-2 develop a capacity to lyse fresh tumour cells (lymphokine-activated killer or "LAK" cells). In vivo it appears that IL-2 production is closely controlled and mechanisms for its rapid elimination exist so that IL-2 activity is normally under fine control. It is believed that these biological activities occur following IL-2 interaction with cell surface receptors of differential affinity. The IL-2 is internalised into the cell and induces a variety of changes in gene expression (Lotze 1991).

These biological activities of IL-2 are potentially very important in the organism's control of neoplasia and experiments in vivo using IL-2 in rodent tumours confirmed the antitumour activity (Lafreniere and Rosenberg 1985; Papa et al. 1986; Mule et al. 1987). The murine tumour experimental data reveal that liver and lung metastases from a variety of tumours can be inhibited by IL-2 administration; the degree of inhibition of tumours appears to be proportional to the immunogenicity of the tumour and to the dose of IL-2 administered. The antitumour effect of concomitantly administered LAK cells appears to be augmented by IL-2 proportionate to the IL-2 dose.

The biological actions of IL-2 which are important from a toxicity point of view include the development of the vascular/capillary leak syndrome. The exact mechanism of this important effect is not known but it may be due to the development of inflammatory mediators such as oxygen free radicals, vasoactive amines or metabolites of the arachidonic acid cascade. Alternatively it may be due to IL-2 inducing other cytokines, which are able to act directly on the vascular endothelium or participate in associated interactions within a cytokine cascade. This so-called cytokine cascade can activate many arms of the cellular immune system which may produce a variety of apparently pathological rather than physiological responses (Rosenstein et al. 1986; Winklehake and Gauny 1990; Siegel and Puri 1991). Whatever the exact cause of this syndrome, it appears to be a response of the host immune cells as experimental evidence suggests that it can be blocked by agents such as cyclophosphamide. Clinically toxic effects are manifest by fevers and chills, pruritus and rash, nausea and vomiting, diarrhoea, hyperbilirubinaemia, oliguria with elevated creatinine and weight gain, significant hypotension and occasionally dyspnoea and cytopenias. These side effects appear to be proportional to dose. The overall $t_{1/2}$ following IV bolus administration of recombinant IL-2 (rIL-2) is 30–60 min. More prolonged serum levels can be achieved using the intraperitoneal (IP), IM or SC route. Antibodies to rIL-2 can occasionally be detected in the serum; however the impact of these antibodies on IL-2 activity has not been fully defined (Lotze et al. 1985).

The early clinical reports of IL-2 use by Rosenberg et al. (1987) were very exciting. A group of 72 patients with advanced/metastatic RCC were treated with maximally tolerated IL-2 IV infusions with IL-2 stimulated autologous lymphocytes (or LAK cells). In this group, eight complete responses were documented with 17 partial responses, for a total response rate of 35%. This response rate was more than double the average response rates for the best alternative therapy for RCC at the time. It should be added here that the toxicity associated with this original study was significant with approximately 70% of patients requiring vasopressor therapy and 5% needing assisted ventilation. Further studies using the same regimen were performed to confirm the effectiveness of the approach. Certainly tumour responses were seen in these follow-up studies (approx. 16%), but the initial response rate of 35% has never been matched (West et al. 1987; Fisher et al. 1988). Since these initial studies, there have been many subsequent studies involving IL-2 alone in RCC, with variations in dose, route of administration, and frequency/duration of administration. Concurrently there have been many trials in which IL-2 has been combined with LAK cells, or used in combination with other biological response modifiers (Philip et al. 1989; Abrams et al. 1990; Bukowski et al. 1990; Gaynor et al. 1990; Koretz et al. 1991).

There are no completed prospective randomised trials to examine the clinical efficacy of IL-2 in RCC. However, there is now a substantial body of data which have emerged from five major non-randomised clinical trials performed during the period 1986–1990 that studied IL-2 both alone and in combination with LAK cells in RCC (Jones et al. 1992). Patient eligibility for each of the trials was similar. Patients were all required to have histologically confirmed advanced or metastatic RCC, measurable and/or evaluable disease, an ambulatory performance status of ECOG 0–1 and normal (as defined by each institution) leucocyte and platelet counts, and bilirubin and creatinine. Patients with a history or evidence of cardiovascular disease were excluded from the studies as were patients with serious infections, contraindications to pressor agents, major organ allografts, and corticosteroid dependence. Pregnant or lactating women were also excluded.

The IL-2 administration regimen for all five studies was similar and followed the regimen devised by West et al. (1987) consisting of two five-day continuous intravenous infusions at a dose of 18×10^6 IU/m²/day separated by a rest period. In the LAK studies, leucophereses were carried out during the rest period in order to obtain sufficient peripheral blood mononuclear cells for ex vivo generation of LAK cells. The induction schedule was repeated after three weeks, if there was no rapid disease progression. Maintenance treatment consisted of up to four cycles of IL-2 18×10^6 IU/m²/day for five days, repeated at four weekly intervals in patients with stable disease or better commencing three weeks after the second induction cycle. One study allowed a 50% dose escalation of IL-2 above 18×10^6 IU/m²/day. Dose reduction and cessation schedules were similar in all studies.

In the group of patients who received concurrent LAK cells, after the aphereses were completed the lymphocytes collected were cultured in medium containing IL-2 to generate the LAK cells. These cells were reinfused with the second 5-day infusion of IL-2.

In the three studies in which IL-2 was used in conjunction with LAK cells 95 patients were evaluable for response. Five complete responses were documented (5%), and seven partial responses were seen, for a total response rate of 18%. In the two studies in which IL-2 was used alone, 193 patients were evaluable for response. Of these, there were eight complete responses (4%) and 20 partial responses for an overall response rate of 15%. In both groups the median duration of complete remission (for the small number of patients who achieved CR) has not yet been reached. The median duration of partial remission is approximately 1 year. For the majority of patients receiving IL-2, there was no decline in performance status following treatment. Only 5%–6% stated improved performance status, whereas 60% had stable performance status. When analysing the patients' performance status compared with the tumour response to the IL-2 therapy, there was a significant association between response data and performance status. It is important to note that in the group being analysed, the large number of patients with stable performance status is very relevant as the majority of patients entered into the trials were of good performance status to start with.

In these single-arm studies, the lack of a concurrent prospective randomised control group makes survival analysis very difficult. An available option was to use a database accumulated by the Eastern Collaborative Oncology Group from serial chemotherapy studies. While acknowledging the limitations of this approach, the analysis of the group of patients treated with IL-2 compared with the retrospective control group suggested that use of IL-2 was associated with a significant improvement in survival. For all prognostic groups combined, the median survival for those patients treated with IL-2 was 350 days compared with 250 days in the historical control group. The 3-year survival for those patients treated with IL-2 was 19% compared with 4% in the control group. When the patients were stratified into prognostic groups according to performance status, time from diagnosis to treatment and number of sites of metastases it became apparent that the survival advantage was seen predominantly in the best prognostic groups. An example of a good partial response to

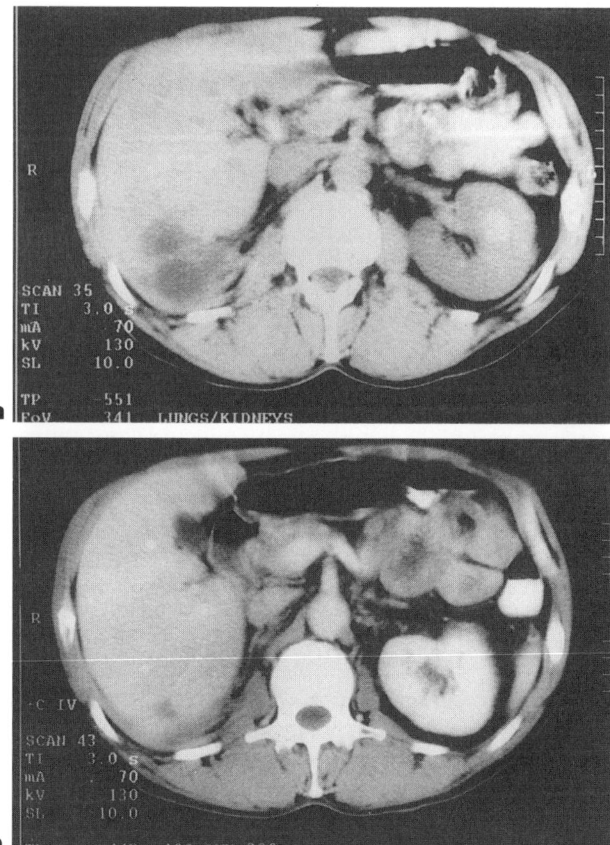

Fig.14.1. Scan of a patient with metastatic renal cell carcinoma involving left kidney (**a**). Following a total of 20 days infused IL-2 (**b**), the renal lesion has disappeared and the liver lesion has also significantly regressed. Remission is continuous at 6 months.

IL-2 alone is shown in Fig. 14.1. There was no significant difference in the impact on survival of the use or non-use of LAK cells (Palmer et al. 1992).

The efficacy of the treatment in terms of absolute numbers of patients achieving a complete response is modest. However, it seems that in that good/low risk group of patients the probability of response is quite significant, and the probability of surviving 2 years appears to be improved by approximately 25%. Conversely those patients of poorer performance status, with bulky or multisite disease, and with a short time interval between initial diagnosis and diagnosis of recurrent disease had no survival advantage in this analysis of this regimen of treatment.

These data support the hypothesis that IL-2 prolongs survival but may be the subject of unidentified variations in patient prognostic features between the IL-2 and chemotherapy studies. They must be interpreted cautiously and should not curtail further research.

Interleukin-2 Plus Interferon

In vitro studies have shown IFNs to be synergistic with IL-2 in stimulating NK activity and in increasing the expression of IL-2 receptors (Brooks et al. 1985; van de Griend et al. 1986). Preclinical animal model data had also demonstrated synergy between IL-2 and IFN-beta (Iigo et al. 1988). Therefore apart from the attraction of combining two agents that are known to be individually effective in RCC, there is reasonable scientific basis for using this particular combination. A review of results of 13 different studies involving the combination of IL-2 and IFN suggests that this combination does produce responses at least comparable to IL-2 alone (Table 14.7). The dose of both IL-2 and IFN varied as did the method of administration, as many of the studies were phase I studies. The time between treatments was also highly variable. Of the 371 patients evaluable for response in these studies, there were 16 complete responders and 54 partial responders, for an overall response rate of 19%. There are no clear trends as to whether there is any significant dose–response relationship. Although three studies which produced the highest rate of complete responses both gave the treatment 4–5 days per week for 4–6 weeks at a time. At present there are not enough data to determine whether or not the treatment confers survival advantage. However, it seems that the combination is tolerated as well as the IL-2 administered alone.

As with many of the studies using biological therapies, there has been little consensus as to exactly how and in what combination the IL-2 and the IFN should be administered. Analysis of such uncontrolled data becomes difficult, and therefore firm conclusions regarding the combination cannot be safely reached. Phase III studies are now under way attempting to answer the

Table 14.7. Combination of interleukin-2 and interferon in advanced RCC

Author	Year	Number evaluable	CR/PR	%RR
Tamura et al.	1989	26	0/0	0%
Paolozzi et al.	1989	50	0/2	4%
Rosenberg et al.	1989	35	4/7	31%
Markowitz et al.	1989	14	0/3	21%
Krigel et al.	1990	22	1/5	27%
Hirsh et al.	1990	12	3/3	50%
Morant et al.	1990	6	0/2	33%
Figlin et al.	1990	22	0/7	32%
Bartsch et al.	1990	19	0/3	16%
Lindemann et al.	1990	24	1/0	4%
Atzpodien et al.	1991	34	4/6	36%
Demchak et al.	1991	29	0/5	17%
Pichert et al.	1991	6	0/0	0%
		371	11/70	22%

Variable dose/schedule for both interferon and interleukin

question of whether the combination of IL-2 and IFN is more effective in the treatment of advanced RCC than IL-2 alone.

Ex vivo Cultured Lymphocytes (Adoptive Cellular Therapy)

Lymphokine-activated killer cells (LAK cells) are essentially any lymphocytes which are ex vivo incubated with IL-2 and subsequently develop the capacity to lyse fresh and cultured tumour cells (Lotze et al. 1981). LAK cells may arise from a heterogeneous population of cells; however most LAK precursors are null cells, and the most potent LAK activity is by cells that prior to activation were natural killer (NK) cells. The cellular lytic activity observed in LAK cells is non-specific although normal autologous cells are not lysed (Topelian and Rosenberg 1991).

In clinical trials, systemic treatment with LAK cells has invariably been given concurrently with IL-2, and the encouraging results of this combination in RCC have been discussed earlier in this chapter. It is difficult to determine exactly what role the ex vivo cultured and reinfused LAK cells play in these responses as it is now known that IL-2 alone produces significant response rates which are comparable to LAK/IL-2 therapy in RCC.

Tumour-infiltrating lymphocytes (TIL) are T cells which infiltrate tumours in vivo and can be isolated and cultured with IL-2. TILs may exhibit MHC specific tumour cells lysis and studies in vitro suggest that they are far more potent in producing tumour regression in comparison with LAK cells (Rosenberg et al. 1986). Early studies using TILs and IL-2 in metastatic melanoma produced some encouraging results (Lotze et al. 1981; Kradlin et al. 1989). There has been considerable difficulty in developing the in vitro TIL culture to the stage when it may be used in human trials. Larger-scale cultures (required for human clinical studies) may have the problem of poor homogeneity of the T-cell population so that the specific cytotoxicity is diminished.

Even so, some small clinical trials have already examined the feasibility of this approach in RCC. As with many such pilot studies, the treatment regimens were variable and the numbers of patients actually treated were very small (Topelian et al. 1988; Kradlin et al. 1989; Bukowski et al. 1991). However, objective tumour responses were seen in these trials. There is difficulty in interpreting the early results as it is certainly unclear as to which of the agents is actually effective, i.e. TILs, LAKs, or IL-2. What can be concluded is that it seems likely that this approach is feasible in the clinical setting.

Tumour Necrosis Factor

Tumour necrosis factor (TNF) is a protein secreted by macrophages in response to infection. As TNF was found to produce haemorrhagic necrosis in experimental tumours, while leaving normal tissues intact, it was soon being tested in clinical trials. The exact mechanism of TNFs antitumour activity is not known; certainly it has apparent direct cytotoxic and antiproliferative effects on many tumour cell lines. These effects are quite variable in different tumour cell lines and the reasons for this variability are unclear. In addition, TNF has been shown to act synergistically with many cytotoxic chemotherapy agents, as well as interferons. The indirect effects of TNF which are important in vivo include: inducing secondary mediators such as IL-1 and IL-6; endothelial activation leading to capillary leak syndrome; induction of a procoagulant state; increased chemotaxis of neutrophils; lymphocyte activation and monocyte–macrophage activation (Spriggs 1991).

Recombinant TNF has a $t_{1/2}$ of approximately 16 min after IV bolus injection (Blick et al. 1987). However, slower clearance seems to occur with higher IV bolus doses (Selby et al. 1987). Significant toxicity of TNF in phase I studies included hypotension, constitutional symptoms (fever, rigors, fatigue, anorexia), alteration of liver function tests, and occasional leucocytosis (Kumura et al. 1987). Attempts to achieve sustained levels of recombinant TNF with continuous IV infusion have been unsuccessful (Sherman et al. 1988). TNF has also been administered via the intramuscular and intraperitoneal routes. Similar toxicity profiles for each of these routes of administration have been observed.

The overall response rate of various tumours to single agent TNF given intravenously is less than 5%. A phase II study of TNF in RCC (Skillings et al. 1992) produced two responses from 22 evaluable patients but was associated with considerable toxicity. As synergy between TNF and a number of cytokines has been observed in vitro, there have been a number of small trials using the combination of TNF and other cytokines. Low response rates were again observed and the combination of cytokines produced significant toxicities (Smith et al. 1991; Negrier et al. 1992). Larger studies using TNF and its combinations are required to assess properly what role TNF may play in the management of RCC.

Cimetidine/Coumarin

In 1987 a great deal of interest was created by the first report of the combination of cimetidine and coumarin in metastatic RCC (Marshall et al. 1987). This combination was based on earlier work with the two agents both in murine models and in clinical trials with metastatic melanoma (Osband et al. 1981; Thornes and Lynch 1983). The theoretical basis for activity of cimetidine is the supposed antagonism of the H_2 receptor on T suppressor cells (Gifford et al. 1980; Thornes and Lynch 1983). The theory for the immunological modulating capacity of coumarin is even less well substantiated. There is a mixed body of animal model and in vitro data which show some immunomodulatory or immunoaugmentary effect of coumarin and coumarin derivatives (Thornes et al. 1968; Friedman 1981). The initial report by Marshall et al. (1987) in which 45 patients were treated with cimetidine and coumarin suggested an objective response rate of 33%. As this combination was very easily administered, with virtually no side effects, it became an attractive combination to consider using in patients with advanced RCC.

Follow-up studies using this combination have failed to confirm the efficacy shown in the original trial. Three studies with a total of 103 patients demonstrated a response rate of only 4% (Dexeus et al. 1990; Glynne-Jones et al. 1990; Herrman et al. 1990). In one of the studies in which immunological assessment was concurrently undertaken, there was no significant enhancement of any immunological parameters. With the lack of demonstrable efficacy and with the exact immunological mechanism of the two agents being questioned, enthusiasm for this combination has waned.

Conclusions/Prospects

Biological therapy for renal cancer remains in its infancy. Interferon and IL-2 and to a lesser extent tumour necrosis factor will produce regressions of renal cancers and some of these may be long lasting. However, the majority of patients appear not to have remissions of their tumours and the impact from survival for any agent remains unproven despite the encouraging results described for our comparison to matched non-concurrent controls. Other agents which have significant immune modulation effects in this class include interleukin-6 which appears to have an antitumour effect in solid tumour transplantable model systems perhaps particularly in synergy with other agents in some experimental systems. Further research to evaluate interleukin-6 in the laboratory and possibly in the clinic is indicated.

The ability to produce regressions of renal cancers should not be dismissed lightly. This tumour is resistant to most chemotherapy and for most patients is inexorably progressive resulting in early death once recurrence or metastasis has occurred. Further progress will probably depend on a better biological understanding of the effects of these agents on cancers and some ability to predict which patients will benefit. This may come from biological studies of the tumours or the patient's ability to mount effective immune responses.

Research into biological therapy should continue with cautious clinical research where possible making use of randomised prospective trials and laboratory research to unravel the proper basis for the use of these powerful, potentially effective and potentially highly toxic new anticancer therapies.

References

Abdi EA (1988) Combination of interferon and prednisone in human cancer. Eur J Cancer Clin Oncol 24:723–724

Abrams JJ, Rayner AA, Wierik PH et al. (1990) High dose recombinant interleukin-2 alone: a regimen with limited activity in the treatment of advanced renal cell carcinoma. J Natl Cancer Inst 82:1202–1206

Atzpodien J, Korfer A, Menzel T et al. (1991) Home therapy using recombinant human IL-2 and IFN-alpha2b in patients with metastatic renal cell carcinoma. Proc Am Soc Clin Oncol 10:177

Bartsch HH, Adler M, Ringert RH et al. (1990) Sequential therapy of recombinant interferon-alpha (IFN-A) and recombinant interleukin-2 (IL-2) in patients with advanced renal cell carcinoma (RCC). Proc Am Soc Clin Oncol 9:143

Bergerat JP, Herbrecht R, Defour P et al. (1988) Combination of recombinant interferon alpha 2A and vinblastine in advanced renal cell carcinoma. Cancer 62:2320–2324

Blick M, Sherwin SA, Rosenbaum M et al. (1987) Phase 1 study of recombinant tumour necrosis factor in cancer patients. Cancer Res 47:2986–2989

Brooks CG, Holscher M, Urdel D (1985) Natural killer activity in cloned cytolytic T-lymphocytes: regulation by interleukin-2, interferon and specific antigen. J Immunol 135:1145–1152

Bruntsch U, de Mulder PH, ten Bokkel Huinink WW et al. (1990) Phase 2 study of recombinant human interferon-gamma in metastatic renal cell carcinoma. J Biol Response Mod 9:335–338

Bukowski RM, Goodman P, Crawford ED et al. (1990) Phase 2 trial of high dose intermittent interleukin-2 in metastatic renal cell carcinoma: a Southwest Oncology Group study. J Natl Cancer Inst 82:143–146

Bukowski RM, Sharfman W, Murthy S et al. (1991) Clinical results and characterization of tumour infiltrating lymphocytes with or without recombinant interleukin-2 in human metastatic renal cell carcinoma. Cancer Res 51:4199–4205

Bunn PA, Ihde DC, Foon K (1986) The role of recombinant interferon-alpha-2a in the therapy of cutaneous T-cell lymphoma. Cancer 57:83–91

Buzaid AC, Robertone A, Kisola C et al. (1987) Phase 2 study of interferon alpha-2a recombinant (Roferon A) in metastatic renal cell carcinoma. J Clin Oncol 5:1083–1089

Cetto GL, Franceschi T, Turrina G et al. (1988) Recombinant alpha-interferon and vinblastine in metastatic renal cell carcinoma: efficacy of low doses. Semin Surg Oncol 4:184–190

de Forges A, Rey A, Klink M et al. (1988) Prognostic factors of adult metastatic renal carcinoma: a multivariate analysis. Semin Surg Oncol 4:149–154

DeKernion B, Sarna G, Trinidada A et al. (1983) The treatment of renal cell carcinoma with human leukocyte alpha interferon. J Urol 130:1063–1066

Demchak P, Atkins M, Sell K et al. (1991) Phase-2 study of interleukin-2 (IL-2) and interferon alpha-2a (IFN-a) outpatient therapy for metastatic renal cancer. Proc Am Soc Clin Oncol 10:175

deMulder PH, Debruyne FM, Franssen MP et al. (1990) Phase 1/2 study of recombinant interferon alpha and gamma in advanced progressive renal cell carcinoma. Cancer Immunol Immunother 31:321–324

Dexeus FH, Logothetis CJ, Sella A et al. (1990) Phase 2 study of coumarin and cimetidine in patients with metastatic renal cell carcinoma. J Clin Oncol 8:325–329

Edsmyr F, Eposti PL, Andersson L et al. (1985) Interferon therapy in disseminated renal cell carcinoma. Radiother Oncol 4:21–26

Einzig AI, Krown SE, Oettgen HF (1984) Recombinant leukocyte A interferon (rIFN-A) in renal cell cancer (RCC). Proc Am Soc Clin Oncol 3:227

Eisenhauer EA, Silver HK, Venner PM et al. (1987) Phase 2 study of high dose weekly intravenous human lymphoblastoid interferon in renal cell carcinoma. A study of the National Cancer Institute of Canada Clinical Trials group. Br J Cancer 55:541–543

Elson PJ, Witte RS, Trump DL (1988) Prognostic factors for survival in patients with recurrent or metastatic renal cell cancer. Cancer Res 48:7310–7313

Figlin R, Citron M, Whitehead R et al. (1990) Low dose continuous infusion recombinant human interleukin-2 (rhIL-2) and Roferon-A; an active outpatient regimen for metastatic renal cell carcinoma (RCCa). Proc Am Soc Clin Oncol 9:142

Figlin RA, DeKernion JB, Maldazys J et al. (1985) Treatment of renal cell carcinoma with alpha (human leukocyte) interferon and vinblastine in combination: A Phase 1/2 trial. Cancer Treat Rep 69:263–267

Figlin RA, DeKernion JB, Mukamel E et al. (1988) Recombinant interferon alpha-2a in metastatic renal cell carcinoma: assessment of antitumour activity and anti-interferon antibody formation. J Clin Oncol 6:1604–1610

Fisher RI, Coltman CA, Doroshaw JH et al. (1988) Metastatic renal cell cancer treated with interleukin-2 and lymphokine activated killer cells. Ann Intern Med 108:518–523

Foon KA, Sherwin SA, Abrams GR et al. (1984) Treatment of advanced non-Hodgkin's lymphoma with recombinant leukocyte A interferon. N Engl J Med 311:1148–1152

Foon K, Doroshaw J, Bonnem E et al. (1988) A prospective randomised trial of α-2B-interferon, δ-interferon or the combination in advanced metastatic renal cell carcinoma. J Biol Response Mod 7:540–545

Fossa SD, DeGaris ST (1987) Further experience with recombinant interferon alpha-2a with vinblastine in metastatic renal cell carcinoma. Int J Cancer 1 (suppl 1):36–40

Fossa SD, DeGaris ST, Heier MS et al. (1986) Recombinant interferon alpha-2a with or without vinblastine in metastatic renal carcinoma. Cancer 57:1700–1704

Fossa S, Martinelli G, Otto U et al. (1992) Recombinant interferon alpha-2a with or without vinblastine in metastatic renal cell carcinoma: results of a European multi-centre phase III study. Ann Oncol 3:301–305

Friedman H (1981) Immunomodulating effects of cimetidine. In: Hersh EM (ed) Augmenting agents in cancer therapy, Raven Press, New York, pp 417–425

Fujita T, Haruyosi A, Naide Y et al. (1988) Antitumour effects of human lymphoblastoid interferon on advanced renal cell carcinoma. J Urol 139:256–258

Garnick MB, Reich SD, Maxwell B et al. (1988) Phase 1/2 study of recombinant interferon gamma in advanced renal cell carcinoma. J Urol 139:251–255

Gaynor ER, Weiss GR, Morgolin KA et al. (1990) Phase 1 study of high dose continuous infusion recombinant interleukin-2 and autologous lymphokine activated killer cells in patients with metastatic or unresectable malignant melanoma and renal cell cancer. J Natl Cancer Inst 82:1397–1402

Geboers AD, deMulder PH, Debruyne FM et al. (1988) Alpha and gamma interferon in the treatment of advanced metastatic renal cell carcinoma. Semin Surg Oncol 4:191–194

Gifford RRM Sr, Hatfield SM, Schmidtke JR (1980) Cimetidine induced augmentation of human lymphocyte blastogenesis by mitogen, bacterial antigen and alloantigen. Transplantation 29:143–148

Glynne-Jones R, Plowman N, Hendry W et al. (1990) Treatment of metastatic renal cell carcinoma with coumarin (1,2-benzopyrene) and cimetidine. Proc Am Soc Clin Oncol 9:139

Grups JW, Frohmuller HG (1989) Cyclic interferon gamma treatment of patients with metastatic renal cell carcinoma. Br J Urol 64:218–220

Herrmann R, Manegold C, Maurer B et al. (1990) Phase 2 trial of coumarin and cimetidine in advanced renal carcinoma. Ann Oncol 1:445–446

Hirsh M, Lipton A, Harvey H et al. (1990) Phase 1 study of interleukin-2 and interferon-alpha 2a as outpatient therapy for patients with advanced malignancy. J Clin Oncol 8:1657–1663

Iigo M, Sakurai M, Tamura T et al. (1988) In vivo antitumour activity of multiple injections of recombinant interleukin-2 alone and in combination with three different types of recombinant interferon on various syngeneic murine tumours. Cancer Res 48:260–264

Isaacs H, Lindemann J (1957) Virus interference 1: the interferon. Proc R Soc Lond [Biol] 147:258

Jones M, Palmer P, Elson P et al. (1992) The clinical effects of interleukin-2 by continuous intravenous infusion for the treatment of renal cancer. Submitted

Kellokumpu-Letinen P, Nordman E (1990) Recombinant interferon-alpha 2a and vinblastine in advanced renal cell cancer: a clinical phase 2 study. J Biol Response Mod 9:439–444

Kempf RA, Grunberg SM, Daniels JR et al. (1986) Recombinant interferon alpha-2 (Intron A) in a phase 2 study of renal cell carcinoma. J Biol Response Mod 5:27–30

Kinney P, Triozzi P, Young D et al. (1990) Phase 2 trial of interferon-beta-serine in metastatic renal cell carcinoma. J Clin Oncol 8:881–885

Kirkwood JM, Harris JE, Vera R et al. (1985) A randomised study of low and high doses of leukocyte alpha interferon in metastatic renal cell carcinoma: the American Cancer Society collaborative trial. Cancer Res 45:863–871

Kish J, Ensley J, Al-Sarraf M et al. (1986) Activity of serine substituted recombinant DNA beta interferon (IFN-beta) in patients with metastatic and recurrent renal cell cancer. Proc Am Assoc Cancer Res 27:184

Koretz MJ, Lawson DH, York RM et al. (1991) Randomised study of interleukin-2 (IL-2) alone verses IL-2 plus lymphokine activated killer cells for treatment of melanoma and renal cell cancer. Arch Surg 126:898–903

Kradin RL, Lazarus DS, Dubinett SM et al. (1989) Tumour infiltrating lymphocytes and interleukin-2 in treatment of advanced cancer. Lancet ii:577–579

Krigel RL, Padavic-Shaller KA, Rudolf AR et al. (1990) Renal cell carcinoma: treatment with recombinant interleukin-2 plus beta-interferon. J Clin Oncol 8:460–467

Krown SE, Einzig Al, Abramson JD et al. (1983) Treatment of advanced renal cell cancer (RCC) with recombinant leukocyte A interferon (rIFN-A). Proc Am Soc Clin Oncol 2:58

Kuebler J, Brown T, Goodman P et al. (1989) Continuous infusion recombinant gamma interferon (Cl gamma IFN) for metastatic renal cell carcinoma (RCC). Proc Am Soc Clin Oncol 8:140

Kumura K, Taguchi T, Urushizaki I et al. (1987) Phase 1 study of recombinant human tumour necrosis factor. Cancer Chemother Pharmacol 20:223–229

Kurzrock R, Gutterman JU, Kantarjian HM et al. (1989) Therapy of chronic myelogenous leukaemia with interferon. Cancer Invest 7:83–91

Kurzrock R, Gutterman JU, Talpaz M (1991) Interferons alpha, beta and gamma: basic principles and preclinical studies. In: DeVita VT, Hellman S, Rosenberg SA (eds) Biologic therapy for cancer. JB Lippincott, Philadelphia, pp 247–274

Kuzmits R, Kokoschka EM, Micksche M et al. (1985) Phase 2 results with recombinant interferons: renal cell carcinoma and malignant melanoma. Oncology 42 (suppl 1):26–30

Lafreniere R, Rosenberg SA (1985) Successful immunotherapy of murine experimental hepatic metastases with lymphokine activated killer cells and recombinant interleukin-2. Cancer Res 45:3735–3741

Lindemann A, Monson JRT, Stahel RA et al. (1990) Low intensity combination treatment with r-interleukin-2 (rh-IL-2) and interferon alpha-2a (rh-IFN-a-2a) in renal cell carcinoma. A multicentre phase 2 trial. Proc Am Soc Clin Oncol 9:150

Linehan WM, Shipley WV, Longo DL (1989) Cancer of the kidney and ureter. In: DeVita VT, Hellman S, Rosenberg SA (eds) Principles and practice of oncology. JB Lippincott, Philadelphia, pp 979–1005

Lotze MT (1991) Interleukin-2: basic principles. In: DeVita VT, Hellman S, Rosenberg SA (eds) Biologic therapy of cancer, JB Lippincott, Philadelphia, pp 123–141

Lotze MT, Grimm EA, Mazumber A et al. (1981) Lysis of fresh and cultured autologous tumour by human lymphocytes cultured in T-cell growth factor. Cancer Res 41:4420–4423

Lotze MT, Matory YL, Ettinghausen SE et al. (1985) In vivo administration of purified human IL-2. Half life, immunologic effects, and expansion of lymphoid cells in vivo with recombinant IL-2. J Immunol 135:2865–2875

Magnusson K, Christophersen IS, Jordel R (1983) Interferon therapy in recurrent renal cell carcinoma. Acta Med Scand 213:221–224

Markowitz A, Talpaz M, Lee K (1989) Phase 1–2 study of recombinant interleukin-2 plus recombinant interferon-alpha 2a in renal cell carcinoma. Proc Am Soc Clin Oncol 8:146

Marshall ME, Mendelsohn L, Butler K et al. (1987) Treatment of metastatic renal cell carcinoma with coumarin (1, 2 benzopyrene) and cimetidine: a pilot study. J Clin Oncol 5:862–866

Marshall ME, Simpson W, Butler K et al. (1989) Treatment of renal cell carcinoma with low dose alpha-interferon. J Biol Response Mod 8:453–461

Marumo K, Murai M, Hayakawa M et al. (1984) Human lymphoblastoid interferon therapy for advanced renal cell carcinoma. Urology 24:567–571

McNichols DW, Seguar JW, deWeerd JH (1981) Renal cell carcinoma: long term survival and late recurrence. J Urol 126:17–23

Montie JE, Bukowski RM, James RE et al. (1982) A critical review of immunotherapy of disseminated renal cell adenocarcinoma. J Surg Oncol 21:5–8

Morales A, Eidinger D (1976) Bacillus Calmette–Guérin in the treatment of adenocarcinoma of the kidney. J Urol 115:377–380

Morant R, Richner J, Evers P et al. (1990) Interleukin-2 (rIL-2) and interferon-alpha combination immunotherapy in patients with metastatic renal carcinoma. Proc Am Soc Clin Oncol 9:141

Morgan DA, Roscetti FW, Gallo RG (1976) Selective in vitro growth of T-lymphocytes from normal bone marrow. Science 193:1007–1008

Mule JJ, Yang JC, Lafreniere R et al. (1987) Identification of cellular mechanisms operational in vivo during the regression of established pulmonary metastases by the systemic administration of high dose recombinant IL-2. J Immunol 139:285–294

Muss HB, Costanzi JJ, Leavitt R et al. (1987) Recombinant alpha interferon in renal cell carcinoma: a randomised trial of two routes of administration. J Clin Oncol 5:286–291

Myers MH, Gloeckler LA (1989) Cancer patient survival rates: SEER program results for 10 years follow-up. CA 39:21–32

Negrier MS, Pourreau CN, Palmer PA et al. (1992) Phase 1 trial of recombinant interleukin-2 followed by recombinant tumour necrosis factor in patients with cancer. J Immunother 11:93–102

Neidhart JA, Murphy SG, Henniek LA et al. (1980) Active specific immunotherapy of stage 4 renal cell carcinoma with aggregated tumour antigen adjuvant. Cancer 46:1128–1134

Neidhart J, Gagen M, Kisner R et al. (1984a) Therapy of renal cell cancer with low (LD), intermediate (ID) and high (HD) dose regimens of human lymphoblastoid interferon (HBLI; Wellferon). Proc Am Soc Clin Oncol 3:60

Neidhart JA, Gagen NM, Young D et al. (1984b) Interferon-alpha therapy of renal cell cancer. Cancer Res 44:4140–4143

Neidhart J, Harris J, Tuttle R (1987) A randomised study of Wellferon (WFN) with or without vinblastine (VBL) in advanced renal cancer. Proc Am Soc Clin Oncol 6:239

Oliver RTD et al. (1989) Unexplained spontaneous regression and alpha-interferon as treatment for metastatic renal carcinoma. J Urol 63:128–131

Osband ME, Shen YJ, Shlesinger M et al. (1981) Successful tumour immunotherapy with cimetidine in mice. Lancet i:636–639

Otto U, Bauer HW, Jager N et al. (1988) Alpha-2 recombinant interferon treatment of metastatic renal cell cancer. Semin Surg Oncol 4:184–191

Palmer P, Vinke J, Philip T et al. (1992) Prognostic factors for survival in patients with advanced renal cell carcinoma treated with recombinant interleukin-2. Ann Oncol 3:174–179

Paolozzi F, Zamkoff K, Doyle M et al. (1989) Phase 1 trial of recombinant interleukin-2 and recombinant beta-interferon in refractory neoplastic diseases. J Biol Response Mod 8:122–139

Papa MZ, Mule JJ, Lafreniere R (1986) The antitumour efficacy of lymphokine activated killer cells and recombinant interleukin-2 in vivo: successful immunotherapy of established pulmonary metastases from weakly and non-immunogenic murine tumour of three distinct histologic types. Cancer Res 46:4973–4978

Patel NP et al. (1978) Renal cell carcinoma: natural history and results of treatment. J Urol 199:722–726

Philip T, Mercatello A, Negrier S et al. (1989) Interleukin-2 with and without LAK cells in metastatic renal cell carcinoma: the Lyon first year experience in 20 patients. Cancer Treat Rev 16 (suppl):91–104

Pichert G, Jost LM, Fierz W et al. (1991) Clinical and immune modulatory effects of alternative weekly interleukin-2 and interferon alpha 2a in patients with advanced renal cell carcinoma and melanoma. Br J Cancer 63:287–292

Porzolt F, Messerer D, Hartman R et al. (1988) Treatment of advanced renal cell cancer with recombinant interferon alpha as a single agent and in combination with medroxyprogesterone acetate. A randomised multicentre trial. J Cancer Res Clin Oncol 114:95–100

Possinger K, Wagner H, Beck R et al. (1988) Renal cell carcinoma. Contr Oncol 30:195–207

Quesada JR, Swanson D, Gutterman JU (1983) Renal cell carcinoma: antitumour effects of leukocyte interferon. Cancer Res 43:940–947

Quesada JR, Reuben J, Mannering JT et al. (1984) Alpha interferon for induction of remission in hairy cell leukaemia. N Engl J Med 310:15–18

Quesada JR, Rios A, Swanson D et al. (1985) Antitumour activity of recombinant derived interferon alpha in metastatic renal cell carcinoma. J Clin Oncol 3:1522–1538

Quesada JR, Talpaz M, Rios A et al. (1986) Clinical toxicity of interferon in cancer patients: a review. J Clin Oncol 4:234–243

Quesada JR, Kurzrock R, Sherwin A et al. (1987) Phase 2 studies of recombinant human interferon gamma in metastatic renal cell carcinoma. J Biol Response Mod 6:20–27

Quesada JR, Evans L, Saks SR et al. (1988) Recombinant interferon alpha and gamma in combination as treatment for metastatic renal cell carcinoma. J Biol Response Mod 7:234–239

Richie JP, Steele GD, Wilson RF et al. (1984) Current treatment of metastatic renal cell carcinoma with xenogenic immune ribonucleic acid. J Urol 131:236–238

Rinehart J, Malspeis L, Young D et al. (1986) Phase 1 trial of interferon-beta-ser in patients with renal cell carcinoma. Cancer Res 46:5364–5367

Rinehart JJ, Young D, Laforge J et al. (1987) Phase 1/2 trial of recombinant gamma-interferon in patients with renal cell carcinoma: immunologic and biologic effects. J Biol Response Mod 6:302–312

Rosenberg SA, Spiess P, Lafreniere R (1986) A new approach to the adoptive immunotherapy of cancer with tumour infiltrating lymphocytes. Science 223:1318–1321

Rosenberg SA, Lotze MT, Muul LM et al. (1987) A progress report on the treatment of 157 patients with advanced cancer using lymphokine activated killer cells and interleukin-2 or high dose interleukin-2 alone. N Engl J Med 316:889–897

Rosenberg SA, Lotze MT, Yang JC et al. (1989) Combination therapy with interleukin-2 and alpha-interferon for the treatment of patients with advanced cancer. J Clin Oncol 7:1863–1874

Rosenstein M, Ettinghausen SE, Rosenberg SA (1986) Extravasation of intravascular fluid mediated by the systemic administration of recombinant interleukin-2. J Immunol 137:1735–1742

Scheithaurer W, Kuerer I, Kutzmits R (1987) Phase 2 trial of recombinant interferon alpha 2a in metastatic renal cell carcinoma. J Biol Regul Homeost Agents 1:81–86

Schnall SF, Davis C, Kirkwood JM et al. (1986) Treatment of metastatic renal cell carcinoma (RCC) with intramuscular (IM) recombinant alpha A (IFN, Hoffman-La Roche). Proc Am Soc Clin Oncol 5:227

Schornagel JH, Verweij J, ten Bokkel Huinink WW et al. (1989) Phase 2 study of recombinant interferon alpha2a with vinblastine in advanced renal cell carcinoma. J Urol 142:253–258

Selby P (1989) The role of alpha interferon in the management of renal cancer. MAC Proceedings 38:1–9

Selby P, Hobbs S, Viner C et al. (1987) Tumour necrosis factor in man: clinical and biological observations. Br J Cancer 56:803–808

Sertoli MR, Brunetti F, Ardizzoni A et al. (1989) Recombinant alpha-2a interferon plus vinblastine in the treatment of metastatic renal cell carcinoma. Am J Clin Oncol 12:43–45

Shearer M, Taylor-Papadimitriou J (1987) Regulation of cell growth by interferon. Cancer Metastasis Rev 6:199–221

Sherman ML, Spriggs DR, Arthur KA et al. (1988) Recombinant tumour necrosis factor administered as a five day continuous infusion in cancer patients. Phase 1 toxicity and effects on lipid metabolism. J Clin Oncol 6:344–350

Siegel JP, Puri RK (1991) Interleukin-2 toxicity. J Clin Oncol 9:694–704

Skillings J, Wierzbicki R, Eisenhauer E et al. (1992) A phase 2 study of recombinant tumour necrosis factor in renal cell carcinoma: a study of the National Cancer Institute of Canada Clinical Trials Group. J Immunother 11:67–70

Smith JW, Urba WJ, Clark JW et al. (1991) Phase 1 evaluation of recombinant tumour necrosis factor given in combination with recombinant interferon-gamma. J Immunother 10:355–362

Spriggs DR (1991) Tumour necrosis factor: basic principles and preclinical studies. In: DeVita VT, Hellman S, Rosenberg SA (eds) Biologic therapy of cancer. JB Lippincott, Philadelphia, pp 354–377

Takaku K, Kumamoto Y, Koisok I et al. (1987) Phase 2 study of recombinant human interferon gamma (S-6810) on renal cell carcinoma. Summary of two collaborative studies. Recombinant Human Interferon Gamma (S-6810) Research Group on Renal Carcinoma. Cancer 60:929–933

Tamura T, Sasaki Y, Shinkai T et al. (1989) Phase 1 study of combination therapy with interleukin-2 and beta-interferon in patients with advanced malignancy. Cancer Res 49:730–735

Thornes RD, Lynch G (1983) Combination of cimetidine with other drugs for treatment of cancer. N Engl J Med 380:591–592

Thornes RD, Edlow DW, Wood S Sr (1968) Inhibition of locomotion of cancer cells by anticoagulant therapy. Effects of sodium warfarin on V2 cancer cells, granulocytes, and macrophages in rabbits. Johns Hopkins Med J 123:305–316

Topelian SL, Rosenberg SA (1991) Adoptive cellular therapy: basic principles. In: DeVita VT, Hellman S, Rosenberg SA (eds) Biologic therapy in cancer. JB Lippincott, Philadelphia, pp 178–196

Topelian SL, Solomon D, Avis FP et al. (1988) Immunotherapy of patients with advanced cancer using tumour infiltrating lymphocytes and recombinant IL-2. J Clin Oncol 6:839–853

Trump DL, Elson PJ, Borden EC et al. (1987) High dose lymphoblastoid interferon in advanced renal cell carcinoma: an Eastern Co-operative Oncology Group study. Cancer Treat Rep 71:165–169

Umeda T, Niijima N (1986) Phase 2 study of alpha interferon on renal cell carcinoma: summary of three collaborative trials. Cancer 58:1231–1235

van de Griend RJ, Ronteltap CPM, Gravekamp C et al. (1986) Interferon-B and recombinant IL-2 can both enhance, but by different pathways, the non-specific cytolytic potential of T3-natural killer cell derived clones rather than that of T3+ clones. J Immunol 136:1700–1707

Vugrin D, Hood L, Taylor W et al. (1985) Phase 2 study of human lymphoblastoid interferon in patients with advanced renal carcinoma. Cancer Treat Rep 68:817–820

Vugrin D, Hood L, Laszlo J (1986) A phase 2 trial of high dose human lymphoblastoid alpha interferon in patients with advanced renal carcinoma. J Biol Response Mod 5:309–314

Waters EW et al. (1979) Aggressive surgical approach to renal cell carcinoma: review of 130 cases. J Urol 122:306–309

West, WH, Tauer KW, Yanneki JR et al. (1987) Constant infusion recombinant interleukin-2 in adoptive immunotherapy of advanced cancer. N Engl J Med 316:398–405

Winkelhake JL, Gauny SS (1990) Human recombinant interleukin-2 as an experimental theraputic. Pharmacol Rev 42:1–10

Yamashita Y et al. (1989) Surgical treatment of renal cell carcinoma associated with pulmonary metastasis. Nippon Gan Chiryo Gakkai Shi 24:759–764 (abstract)

Chapter 15

Conservative Surgery for Renal Cell Carcinoma

A. C. Novick

Introduction

Conservative or nephron-sparing surgery for the treatment of renal tumours dates from the late 1800s. Initial enthusiasm for the procedure abated after significant problems with renal bleeding, urinary fistulae and postoperative mortality were encountered (Novick 1987). Following Robson et al.'s (1969) observations of improved survival after extrafascial nephrectomy, the use of partial nephrectomy in patients with renal cell carcinoma (RCC) fell into disfavour. Recent enthusiasm for conservative surgery has been stimulated by advances in renal imaging, experience with renal vascular surgery for other conditions, improved methods for preventing ischaemic renal damage, the growing incidence of incidentally discovered low stage RCCs (Konnack and Grossman 1985), and good long-term survival reported in patients treated by partial nephrectomy (Topley et al. 1984). Extensive experience has now established that conservative surgery can be performed safely with low morbidity, good preservation of renal function, and long-term cure of RCC in many patients. Although radical nephrectomy remains the procedure of choice for curative treatment of localised RCC, conservative surgery is now indicated when preservation of functioning renal parenchyma is clinically very important.

The role of conservative surgery for RCC is evolving and continued careful evaluation of patient outcome data is needed to defined reasonable limits for this approach. Both the accepted and the controversial aspects of this approach will be reviewed in this chapter.

Current Indications

It is appropriate to consider conservative surgery for the treatment of RCC when preservation of renal function is clinically relevant as in the following situations:

1. Bilateral synchronous renal cell carcinoma
2. Carcinoma in an anatomically or functionally solitary kidney
3. Unilateral carcinoma in patients with a functioning contralateral kidney and any concomitant condition with the potential for adversely affecting future renal function
4. Unilateral carcinoma in patients with a functioning but impaired contralateral kidney

Bilateral synchronous RCC has been a frequent indication for conservative surgery, accounting for 28 of 100 cases in one review (Novick et al. 1989). Our philosophy in these patients has been to attempt to preserve as much functioning renal tissue as possible. This entails performing bilateral partial nephrectomies whenever possible, usually as staged procedures with the less involved side done first. However, when a large tumour on one side precludes partial nephrectomy, a radical nephrectomy is performed on the more involved side with a contralateral partial nephrectomy. In such cases, the partial nephrectomy is performed first as a separate procedure. This sequence obviates the need for temporary dialysis in the immediate postoperative period if acute tubular necrosis (ATN) occurs following partial nephrectomy. This also allows the most flexibility in planning the procedure on the opposite side, and we have occasionally performed a partial rather than a radical nephrectomy on the second side when the initial procedure had resulted in a renal remnant of borderline size to avoid dialysis.

Unilateral RCC in functionally or anatomically solitary kidneys has been a frequent indication for conservative surgery in our experience (Novick et al. 1989). In these cases one does not have the luxury of a functioning contralateral kidney to protect against ischaemic ATN. Therefore, patients must be advised about the potential for temporary or permanent dialysis postoperatively, although this is rarely needed. A renal remnant of at least 20% of one normal kidney is necessary to avoid permanent renal failure.

Unilateral RCC with a functionally impaired contralateral kidney is another indication for conservative surgery. Contralateral functional impairment may be due to renal artery stenosis, hydronephrosis, chronic pyelonephritis, reflux or systemic diseases such as diabetes and nephrosclerosis. The clinical and operative considerations in these patients are similar to those with true solitary kidneys.

Another indication for conservative surgery is represented by patients with unilateral tumours and normally functioning opposite kidneys, but where the opposite kidney is affected by a condition which might threaten its future function such as stones, multiple cysts or renal artery disease. The decision to perform a partial rather than a radical nephrectomy in these patients must be individualised by considering the extent of tumour, the difficulty of partial resection, life expectancy and the ultimate threat to renal function if unilateral total nephrectomy is performed.

Surgical Aspects

A variety of nephron-sparing surgical techniques have been described including enucleation, polar segmental nephrectomy after ligation of the corresponding renal arterial branch, wedge resection, major transerve resection and extra-corporeal partial nephrectomy with autotransplantation. The technical aspects of each of these procedures are described in detail elsewhere (Novick 1987). The basic surgical principles involved in performing partial nephrectomy are:

1. Early vascular control
2. Preservation of function of the operated kidney without ischaemic damage
3. Complete tumour excision with negative surgical margins
4. Watertight closure of the collecting system
5. Careful haemostasis
6. Closure of the renal defect with perirenal fat or haemostatic sponge

The role of ex vivo surgery in the performance of partial nephrectomy for RCC remains controversial. Although there are some large, hypervascular centrally located tumours that can only be excised with an ex vivo approach, such cases are distinctly uncommon. Ex vivo partial nephrectomy with autotransplantation is also associated with a higher incidence of temporary and permanent renal failure which presumably reflects, in part, a more severe ischaemic insult (Novick et al. 1989). Currently, bench surgery is seldom necessary when performing partial nephrectomy for RCC and most cases can be satisfactorily managed in situ.

There is also continuing controversy concerning the value of simple enucleation as a technique for local excision of RCC (Rosenthal et al. 1984; Smith et al. 1984; Marshall et al. 1986). This approach is based on the observation that many RCCs are enveloped by a distinct pseudocapsule of fibrous tissue which would theoretically allow relatively avascular tumour removal with maximal conservation of renal tissue. Some reports have indicated satisfactory short-term clinical results following enucleation with good patient survival and a low rate of local tumour recurrence (Rosenthal et al. 1984). Other studies have suggested an increased risk of leaving residual malignancy in the operated kidney when enucleation is performed (Smith et al. 1984). Careful histopathological studies have demonstrated frequent microscopic tumour penetration of the pseudocapsule which surrounds the neoplasm (Marshall et al. 1986).

Local recurrence of tumour in the operated kidney is a grave complication following partial nephrectomy for RCC and every attempt should be made to prevent this. Since there is currently no method of assuring complete tumour encapsulation prior to surgery, it would seem reasonable to remove a surrounding margin of normal parenchyma with the tumour whenever possible. This provides an added margin of safety against the development of local tumour recurrence and, in most cases, does not appreciably increase the technical difficulty of the operation.

Clinical Results

There have been several reports of excellent long-term cancer-free survival following conservative surgery for localised RCC. The two largest single-centre experiences have been reported from the Cleveland Clinic and the

Mayo Clinic. The Cleveland Clinic series included 100 patients with overall and cancer-specific five-year survival rates of 67% and 84% respectively (Novick et al. 1989). The Mayo Clinic series included 104 patients with overall and cancer-specific five-year survival rates of 80% and 88% respectively (Morgan and Zincke 1990). In the Cleveland Clinic series, survival was significantly greater in patients with stage 1 RCC where the five-year cancer-specific survival rate was 90%. Among patients with stage 1 RCC, the five-year cancer-specific survival rate was greater in unilateral RCC (100%) compared with bilateral synchronous (79%) or bilateral asynchronous (82%) TCC.

The major disadvantage of conservative surgery for RCC is the risk of postoperative local tumour recurrence which has ranged from 6% to 9% (Novick et al. 1989; Morgan and Zincke 1990). Some local recurrences may be a manifestation of undetected multifocal RCC in the renal remnant. The risk of local tumour recurrence after radical nephrectomy has not been determined but is presumably very low.

Renal Cell Carcinoma with Venous Involvement

The role of conservative surgery in patients with localised RCC of higher stage is now well delineated. Selective renal vein venography is a safe technique which can help to identify patients with gross renal vein involvement prior to surgery. This should be obtained in patients with large centrally located tumours or those with a suspicion of a renal vein thrombosis on other imaging studies.

The outcome of this approach has been reviewed in nine patients with RCC in a solitary kidney and intrarenal or main renal venous involvement (Angermeier et al. 1990). Of these nine patients, five were free of disease and had satisfactory renal function after a mean follow-up of 33 months. The remaining four patients died of metastatic RCC including two who had concomitant local recurrences in the renal remnant. Although conservative surgery is technically feasible in this setting, the data suggest an increased incidence of postoperative tumour recurrence. Additional follow-up is needed to better define the potential for extended cancer-free survival in these patients. Therefore, at the present time, conservative surgery should be considered for localised RCC with venous involvement only when radical nephrectomy would render the patient functionally anephric with the requirement for renal replacement therapy.

Renal Cell Carcinoma in Von Hippel–Lindau's Disease

RCC occurs in approximately 45% of patients with von Hippel–Lindau's disease (VHLD). Although it was originally believed to have a less malignant potential than its spontaneous counterpart, RCC in VHLD can metastasise and is a major cause of death in these patients (Horton et al. 1976). Curative treatment for RCC in this setting involves surgical excision with either total or partial nephrectomy.

The rationale for conservative surgery in patients with VHLD is based on their younger age of presentation compared with spontaneous RCC, and the propensity for RCC to be bilateral in this setting (Spencer et al. 1988). However, due to the multicentric nature of RCC in VHLD, these patients are at increased risk for developing local tumour recurrence after conservative surgery (Novick and Streem 1992). Therefore, these patients must be followed-up carefully and advised of the potential need for repeated renal surgery, which may eventually result in total loss of renal function. Previous studies have suggested a 30%–35% risk of tumour progression and death from RCC in VHLD. The risk of progression or death following conservative surgery in these patients is undefined. Consequently, it is not known whether RCC in VHLD is best managed by conservative surgery to preserve function or by immediate bilateral nephrectomy with subsequent renal replacement therapy.

Conservative Surgery with a Normal Contralateral Kidney

The role of conservative surgery in patients with unilateral RCC and a normal contralateral kidney remains controversial. This question is becoming increasingly important with the advent of CT scanning and ultrasound and the growing discovery of unsuspected RCCs. Most of these incidentally discovered tumours are asymptomatic, small, located on the peripheral surface of the kidney and are of low pathological stage (Konnak and Grossman 1985). Surgical excision of such RCCs should be curative in most cases. However, it is not established whether this is best accomplished by partial or total nephrectomy. Several factors argue in favour of radical nephrectomy in this situation.

1. The low risk of contralateral renal loss as defined in long-term follow-up studies of living related donor nephrectomy patients
2. The low risk (1%–2%) of developing metachronous contralateral RCC
3. An approximately 10% local tumour recurrence rate after conservative surgery
4. Occasional cases of unsuspected multifocal RCCs which would not be removed by partial excision

In the case of an incidentally discovered peripheral RCC, conservative surgery can usually be successfully performed with preservation of 85%–90% of renal mass. Ultimately, the correct choice of treatment for small tumours with a normal contralateral kidney will depend on long-term studies which definitively address both the chance of cure after partial nephrectomy and the risk of renal failure after radical nephrectomy. Currently available data suggest that both the risk of local recurrence after partial nephrectomy and the risk of renal failure after radical nephrectomy are small. At the present time, radical nephrectomy should still be considered the accepted treatment for unilateral RCC with a normal contralateral kidney.

Postoperative Follow-up

Patients who undergo conservative surgery for RCC must be followed-up closely in order to detect recurrence of their tumour. Local tumour recurrence is of particular concern and has been reported in 6%–9% of patients (Novick et al. 1989; Morgan and Zincke 1990). CT scanning is presently the most accurate diagnostic method of detecting recurrences, and this should be done at 6-month intervals postoperatively to ensure prompt detection. Patients who develop a local recurrence with no signs of metastasis may be considered for secondary surgical treatment (Novick and Straffon 1987). In some cases, another partial nephrectomy can be done with preservation of renal function. If this is not technically possible, total nephrectomy with initiation of chronic dialysis and subsequent renal allotransplantation is an alternative.

Recent data suggest that patients with less than one kidney are at increased risk for developing proteinuria, glomerular damage and impaired renal function due to glomerular hyperfiltration (Foster et al. 1991; Solomon et al. 1985). We recently evaluated long-term renal function in 14 patients with a solitary kidney who had undergone partial nephrectomy for localised malignancy (Novick et al. 1991). Preoperatively, there was no clinical or histological evidence of primary renal disease. Postoperative renal function remained stable in 12 patients whereas two patients deleloped end-stage renal failure. Nine patients developed proteinuria which was low-grade in four patients (< 750 mg/day) and moderate to severe in five patients (930–6740 mg/day). A statistically significant association was found between increased proteinuria, a lower amount of remaining renal tissue and a longer follow-up interval. A renal biopsy was done in four patients with moderate to severe proteinuria which, in each case, showed focal segmental or global glomerulosclerosis.

These data suggest that patients with $> 50\%$ reduction in overall renal mass are at increased risk of proteinuria, glomerulopathy and progressive renal failure. Structural or functional renal damage in such cases is usually preceded by the appearance of proteinuria. Therefore, the follow-up of patients after partial nephrectomy should include a 24 h urinary protein determination in addition to a serum creatinine level and glomerular filtration rate. Patients who develop proteinuria (> 150 mg/day) may be treated with a low protein diet and a converting enzyme inhibitor agent which, in experimental studies, have prevented glomerulopathy caused by reduced renal mass (Brenner 1983; Meyer et al. 1985).

Conclusions

Conservative surgery provides effective therapy for patients with localised RCC in whom preservation of renal function is a relevant clinical consideration. The technical success rate with this approach is excellent and long-term patient survival free of cancer is comparable with that obtained after radical nephrectomy, particularly for low stage RCC. The major disadvantage of conservative surgery is the risk of postoperative local tumour recurrence which may be reflective of multicentre RCC in some patients. Further long-term outcome data are needed to document the safety and benefits of conservative surgery in patients with unilateral RCC and a normal opposite kidney. The role of conservative surgery in patients with advanced RCC is currently limited but this may change when effective systemic therapy becomes available.

References

Angermeier KW, Novick AC, Streem SB, Montie JE (1990) Nephron-sparing surgery for renal cell carcinoma with venous involvement. J Urol 144:1352–1355

Brenner BM (1983) Hemodynamically mediated glomerular injury and the progressive nature of kidney disease. Kidney Int 23:647–655

Foster MH, Sant GR, Donohoe JF, Harrington JT (1991) Prolonged survival with a remnant kidney. Am J Kidney Dis 17:261–265

Horton WA, Wong V, Eldridge R et al. (1976) von Hippel–Lindau disease: clinical and pathological manifestations in nine families with 50 affected members. Arch Intern Med 136:769–777

Konnack JW, Grossman HB (1985) Renal cell carcinoma as an incidental finding. J Urol 134:1094–1096

Marshall FF, Taxy JB, Fishman EK, Chang R (1986) The feasibility of surgical enucleation for renal cell carcinoma. J Urol 135:231–234

Meyer TW, Anderson S, Rennke HG, Brenner BN (1985) Converting enzyme inhibitor therapy limits progressive glomerular injury in rats with renal insufficiency. Am J Med 79 (Suppl):31–36

Morgan WR, Zincke H (1990) Progression and survival after renal conserving surgery for renal cell carcinoma: experience in 104 patients and extended follow up. J Urol 144:852–858

Novick AC (1987) Partial nephrectomy for renal cell carcinoma. Urol Clin North Am 14:419–433

Novick AC, Straffon RA (1987) Management of locally recurrent renal cell carcinoma after partial nephrectomy. J Urol 138:607–610

Novick AC, Streem SB (1992) Long-term follow up after nephron-sparing surgery for renal cell carcinoma in von Hippel Lindau disease. J Urol 147:1488–1490

Novick AC, Streem SB, Montie JE et al. (1989) conservative surgery in renal cell carcinoma: a single-centre experience with 100 patients. J Urol 141:835–839

Novick AC, Gephardt G, Guz B, Steinmuller D, Tubbs R (1991) Long-term follow up after partial removal of a solitary kidney. N Engl J Med 325:1058–1062

Robson CJ, Churchill BM, Anderson W (1969) The results of radical nephrectomy for renal cancer. J Urol 101:297–301

Rosenthal CL, Kraft R, Zingg EJ (1984) Organ-preserving surgery in renal cell carcinoma: tumour enucleation versus partial kidney resection. Eur Urol 10:222–228

Smith RB, deKernion JB, Ehrlich RM, Skinner DG, Kaufman JJ (1984) Bilateral renal cell carcinoma and renal cell carcinoma in a solitary kidney. J Urol 132:450–454

Solomon LR, Mallick NP, Lawler W (1985) Progressive renal failure in a remnant kidney. Br Med J 291:1610–1611

Spencer WF, Novick AC, Montie JE et al. (1988) Surgical treatment of localised renal cell carcinoma in von Hippel Lindau's disease. J Urol 139:507–509

Topley M, Novick AC, Montie JE et al. (1984) Long-term results following partial nephrectomy for localised renal adenocarcinoma. J Urol 131:1050–1052

Chapter 16

Retroperitoneal Lymphadenectomy in the Management of Testis Cancer

W. F. Hendry

Retroperitoneal lymphadenectomy for early stage testicular cancer is a delightful operation. The surgeon can call upon great anatomical knowledge and display considerable technical expertise, excising apparently normal lymph nodes that just might contain metastatic cancer, whilst carefully preserving the sympathetic nerves that control ejaculation. Morbidity and mortality are low in these fit young men, and most do recover their ejaculation within a year or so. Almost 100% are cured, so where is the problem? Thus runs the logic that continues to condemn so many young men in North America to such major surgery, even after experience at three of the major cancer centres in the world have shown that equally good results can be obtained without this operation, with no interference with ejaculation, by simply following a policy of careful surveillance and only treating relapse when it occurs.

Retroperitoneal lymphadenectomy for postchemotherapy residual masses, on the other hand, can be frightful. The anatomy is often grossly distorted, normal tissues can be inseparably involved, and damage to vital structures may be unavoidable if the mass is to be removed completely. To make matters worse, statistics show that the mass is composed of dead or mature tissue in four out of five cases, in which case the prognosis may not be too bad. The surgeon may wonder whether it is really necessary to pursue the dissection sufficiently far to achieve complete clearance, when the odds are slightly better than those of Russian roulette that leaving a small residuum may not in fact threaten life.

There has always been controversy about the best way to treat lymphatic metastases of testicular tumours, ever since Most (1898) showed that the first nodes to be involved lay far away from the testis, high in the para-aortic region near the renal vessels. Roberts (1902) recognised that "operations for malignant disease should usually include removal of the adjacent lymph nodes" and, after studying Dr Most's work, described an anterior, transperitoneal approach by which the lymph nodes from the renal vessels down to the aortic bifurcation could be removed, and he commented "it is perhaps wise to excise glands on both sides". Unfortunately, his patient developed complications, and a safer but less radical retroperitoneal approach was developed by Bland-Sutton (1909) and Chevassu (1910). This surgical approach was limited to the side of the tumour, and the dissection could not proceed safely above the renal pedicle – recognised by Chevassu as "la zone critique".

The limitations of surgical extirpation of these lymph nodes was pointed out by Jamieson and Dobson (1910), who commented: "it cannot be allowed that either operation . . . warrants the use of the term radical". They showed that the only effective method would be to strip the aorta, vena cava, common iliac vessels, the upper part of the spermatic vessels on both sides and the trunk of the inferior mesenteric artery of all cellulo-fatty tissue on, around and between them from the level of the renal vessels downwards. However, anaesthetic and other limitations imposed on surgery ensured that the unilateral retroperitoneal approach continued to be used in the first half of this century (Hinman 1919; Hinman et al. 1923; Lewis 1948).

Careful pathological studies confirmed that lymph node metastases did not remain ipsilateral, but crossed over to the other side in up to one-third of cases and sometimes extended above the level of the renal vessels (Lowry et al. 1946). With the advent of safe thoracic surgery, a thoracoabdominal approach was described by Cooper et al. (1950) and in four cases greatly improved access to nodes lying above the renal pedicle was obtained, although bilateral node clearance was still difficult. In 1958, Mallis and Patton described in detail an anterior transperitoneal technique, remarkably similar in principle to that originally suggested by Roberts (1902), which did allow direct access to all the nodes below the renal vessels and hence enabled the surgeon to attempt to clear the nodes on both sides from this level downwards. Tavel et al. (1963) used this approach to perform bilateral lymphadenectomy in cadavers, but found that even under these ideal circumstances about one-third of the nodes were still present on subsequent pathological examination, being situated mostly behind the aorta and vena cava. Kaswick et al. (1976) have shown that complete node clearance could be achieved in 11 of 12 cadavers, provided that all the lumbar vessels distal to the renal pedicles were ligated and divided to provided access to the posterior nodes. It was stated that concern over possible devascularisation of the spinal cord was not warranted; provided no lumbar vessels above the renal pedicle were ligated.

Radical retroperitoneal lymphadenectomy has evolved slowly, and with present techniques a reasonably thorough clearance of the nodes can be achieved, bilaterally up to the renal vessels, and this can be extended to the diaphragm on one side by use of a thoracoabdominal approach. The operation is not free from risk, however, and it produces significant morbidity. It is therefore reasonable to examine alternative methods of treatment with care, in order to define with some precision those cases which can be treated effectively by other means and distinguish them from those who might benefit from this operation.

It is now accepted universally that seminomas are so radiosensitive that they can nearly always be cured by radiotherapy. The problem lies with the early stage teratomas, and it is here that the great divergence of opinion has occurred, between those who recommend surveillance and primary chemotherapy for relapse, and others who practise routine retroperitoneal lymphadenectomy. For advanced disease, all are now agreed that chemotherapy should precede surgical excision of residual masses. This chapter will consider in detail the pathological distribution of lymphatic spread and the surgical techniques which have evolved to remove it. The results will be considered in terms of complications and survival rate and compared – as far as possible – with those achieved by surveillance. Finally, there will be an examination of the hypothesis that this operation may be needed only in a highly selected and well-defined subgroup of teratoma patients.

The Pathology and Radiology of Lymphatic Spread

The most detailed information on the frequency and sites of metastases has been provided by Ray et al. (1974), who described their findings in 283 radical lymphadenectomy specimens. The pattern of spread showed distinct differences depending on the side of the primary tumour. Right-sided tumours spread to the paracaval, precaval, interaortocaval, preaortic, right common iliac and proximal external iliac nodes in that order. Ipsilateral nodes were only involved in 85% of cases, ipsilateral and contralateral in 13% and contralateral only in 1.6%. On the left side, para-aortic, preaortic, left common iliac and left external iliac nodes were involved in that order, with subsequent extension to interaortocaval, precaval and paracaval nodes. The spread was ipsilateral in 80% and bilateral in 20%. In no case was spread confined to the contralateral nodes.

As a result of these stuides, Ray et al. (1974) recommended areas for lymphadenectomy as follows. For right-sided tumours, the aorta and vena cava should be cleared below the renal vessels (the upper 2–3 cm only below the renal vessels to the left of the aorta), preserving the inferior mesenteric artery, down to the aortic bifurcation distally, and including the right common iliac and proximal 2 cm of the right external iliac artery. On the left side, the dissection should include the anterior and left side of the cava, both sides of the aorta usually with the inferior mesenteric artery, and extending to the left common iliac and proximal 2 cm of the left external iliac artery.

Surgical/pathological correlation on node histology in this study was 91% if the nodes were positive, and 92% if negative. Clinically detectable metastases above the renal vessels were usually non-resectable, but in the 43 patients in whom thoracoabdominal dissection was done no metastases were found above the renal vessels.

Donohue et al. (1982) carried out extended bilateral retroperitoneal lymph node dissection in 104 consecutive patients with stage II non-seminomatous germ cell tumours following orchidectomy and defined the distribution of nodal metastases. With right-sided tumours, 93% had extended to the interaortocaval nodes, and with left-sided tumours, 88% extended to preaortic and left para-aortic nodes. Suprahilar nodes were involved with 13%–33% of right-sided and 16%–42% of left-sided tumours. It was concluded that contralateral nodes were likely to be negative in low stage, but were commonly positive in high stage disease.

It may be concluded that, if radical lymphadenectomy is done, it should be bilateral up to the level of the renal vessels in all cases. Extension of the dissection above the renal vessels up to the diaphragm may be required, but ideally this should be recognised before operation so that a thoracoabdominal incision may be used.

The Surgical Approach for Radical Lymphadenectomy

There are several possible routes to the retroperitoneal lymph nodes, and each approach has advantages and limitations.

Retroperitoneal

This operation was used originally as an extension of the orchidectomy, to permit the testicle, the cord, the testicular vessels and the lymph nodes to be removed as a monobloc dissection. The incision varied slightly (Hinman 1919; Hinman et al. 1923), but usually extended from the tenth or twelfth rib, obliquely downwards to the internal inguinal ring. After dividing the muscles of the abdominal wall, the peritoneum was reflected forwards to allow the dissection to be carried up to the renal pedicle. This was a very safe operation and Lewis reported no mortality in 169 cases in 1948, at a time when eight patients in his series of 250 cases died of complications of radiotherapy. The node dissection was limited to the side of the tumour, and it was difficult to extend the exposure if the nodes appeared to be extensively involved. Of the 169 cases described by Lewis 10% were found to be inoperable.

Thoracoabdominal

This was developed from the retroperitoneal approach, by extending the incision through the bed of the tenth rib as far back as the posterior axillary line (Cooper et al. 1950), in order to obtain clearance of ipsilateral nodes above the renal vessels. Skinner and Leadbetter (1971) have shown that a bilateral para-aortic node dissection could also be completed up to the renal vessels with extension up to the diaphragm on the side of the incision, and they described 58 cases without operative mortality.

Anterior Transperitoneal

Once the abdomen has been opened by a long midline incision extending from xiphisternum to pubis, access to the para-aortic nodes is obtained by one of two methods. The first method was described by Mallis and Patton (1958). The transverse colon is placed on the chest between moist packs and the small bowel is packed away on the right side. The posterior peritoneum is then incised between the aorta and the vena cava, and the incision is extended down to the bifurcation of the ipsilateral iliac artery and up to the level of the renal vessels. In an alternate approach, described by Staubitz et al. (1969), the ascending colon and duodenum are mobilised and reflected to the left until both renal pedicles are exposed superiorly. The entire small bowel, ascending and transverse colon are then exteriorised to allow free access to the great vessels. This gives excellent exposure of the vena cava and right kidney.

The ureters mark the lateral extent of the dissection on each side. The ipsilateral testicular artery and vein are always included in the dissection and traced down as far as the internal ring. The inferior mesenteric artery can be sometimes preserved, but it should be divided if it is surrounded by involved nodes. This improves access to the left side of the aorta. The dissection proceeds up as far as the renal pedicle, and a second thoracoabdominal or thoracic operation may be necessary if there are metastases present above this level.

Complications

The surgical excision of involved lymph nodes adjacent to the great vessels is difficult and dangerous, and significant complications have been reported including death from massive haemorrhage, ischaemic necrosis of the aorta, renal vein thrombosis, nephrectomy, ureteric division or fibrosis requiring lysis, retroperitoneal lymphocyst, chylous ascites, pancreatitis, intestinal ischaemia or obstruction due to adhesions and wound infection, dehiscence or hernia. The overall complication rate in two large series has been reported as 11% (Lindsey and Glenn 1976) and 12% (Staubitz et al. 1974).

Ejaculatory impotence commonly occurs after bilateral lymphadenectomy. Bracken and Johnson (1976) reported a significant decrease in semen volume in 42 of 50 patients, although 7 of 12 patients who wanted to were able to produce pregnancies. Six of 44 patients reported diminished sex performance and nine had decreased sex drive. In contrast, 29 patients irradiated for seminoma all reported little or no change in performance or drive and two-thirds of those who wanted to were able to produce pregnancies.

Leiter and Brendler (1967) considered that loss of ejaculation was due to interruption of lumbar sympathetic outflow, which passes via the presacral plexus to provide motor innervation to the vasa and vesicles. Damage usually occurs either at the level of the lumbar sympathetic ganglia or at the presacral (hypogastric) plexus. Although many patients report improvement with the passage of time, sometimes the disability may be permanent (Nijman et al. 1987). Jewett et al. (1988) identified and preserved the retroperitoneal sympathetic nerves while performing lymphadenectomy, and showed that a nerve-sparing procedure was possible in 20 of 30 consecutive patients. Of these 20 patients, 18 (90%) ejaculated normally, including eight who had bulky metastases. However, the meticulous dissection of these nerve roots added approximately 1 h to the operative time. A nerve-sparing technique has now been widely adopted by those surgeons who prefer this approach to surveillance for stage I disease (Richie 1990; Jewett 1990).

Results in Early Stage Disease

The cure rate is the same for stage I disease, whether para-aortic lymphadenectomy is done or not. The advocates of the operation point out that it prevents relapse in the retroperitoneum, but this does not free the patient from the need for careful follow-up, or from the possibility that chemotherapy may be required. The latest results from the MRC study of surveillance in clinical stage I teratoma indicate that 75% of patients require no further treatment. Of those that do relapse, 60% do so in the retroperitoneum. The 4-year survival rate including mortality from all causes was 98% (Mead et al. 1992).

Comparison with results obtained by para-aortic lymphadenectomy is difficult, since "surgical" stage A implies that pathological examination of the nodes revealed no metastases. Relapse in the retroperitoneum in such cases is exceptionally uncommon (Bredael et al. 1983). If the lymph nodes are positive (stage B) the likelihood of relapse depends on the number that are involved. Although this is of prognostic significance, equally useful information can be derived from detailed examination of the pathology of the excised testis: vascular or lymphatic invasion, the presence of undifferentiated cells, and the absence of yolk sac elements are predictive of a high risk of relapse when three or four risk factors are present (Mead et al. 1992).

There seems little point in submitting the patient to a 2.5–5 h (median 3.5 h) thoracoabdominal operation (Richie 1990) to obtain this prognostic information, and to spare 10% or so the need for well-tolerated chemotherapy, even though only 10% or so now lose ejaculation with modern nerve-sparing techniques. It remains our belief that with a careful surveillance policy equally good results are obtained, with no interference with ejaculation or fertility. The difficulties of running a successful surveillance policy have been described by Pizzocaro et al. (1987), but this method has been used successfully at two major cancer centres – the Royal Marsden Hospital in London (Hoskin et al. 1986) and the Memorial Sloan-Kettering Cancer Center in New York – and several other hospitals (Sogani 1991).

If there is evidence of localised nodal disease in the retroperitoneum on CT scanning (stage 2A disease) the case for preliminary chemotherapy is overwhelming (Peckham and Hendry 1985; Socinski et al. 1988) since up to 75% of these patients will relapse after surgery alone. Not only will effective chemotherapy eliminate the need for surgery in 73% of those with stage 2A and in 61% with 2B disease (Horwich et al. 1994), the extent of the dissection will be much less in those who are left with a residual mass (see below). Obvious though these conclusions may seem, routine para-aortic lymphadenectomy continues to be recommended as standard initial treatment in early stage disease in the USA (Hesketh and Krane 1990).

Surgery in Late Stage Disease, Postchemotherapy

After completion of chemotherapy, a residual mass is left behind in almost one-quarter of cases (Tait et al. 1984) and CT scanning is more than 95% accurate in defining its site, size and extent (Kennedy et al. 1985). Initially it was hoped that radiotherapy would eliminate any active tumour remaining after chemotherapy. However, comparative studies showed that there was still residual undifferentiated tumour in 20% after planned chemotherapy and radiotherapy, compared to 24% after chemotherapy alone (Hendry et al. 1981). Furthermore, side effects after radiotherapy following chemotherapy were not inconsiderable, and so this treatment modality was abandoned at our centre, although it is still used by others (Read et al. 1986). It became our policy to recommend excision of all substantial residual masses one month or so after completion of chemotherapy. Since the likelihood of residual active tumour was shown to be related to the size of the mass (Hendry et al. 1981), we set a lower limit of 2 cm transverse diameter; only rarely has active tumour been found in nodes smaller than this (Dexeus et al. 1989).

It should be appreciated that the persistence of a mass on CT scanning was never regarded as a failure of chemotherapy. It was always made clear to patients with metastatic disease, before commencing chemotherapy, that surgical excision might be necessary for any potentially malignant tissue that did not disappear. As a result, patients coming to our Joint Testicular Tumour Clinic for assessment for surgery arrive with minds well prepared, with no sense of disappointment or feeling that all has not gone as well as expected. This positive approach makes the surgeon's job much easier than it is with patients referred in from some other units, when an air of despondency surrounds the discussion of the forthcoming operation. It is generally only necessary to explain to our patients that the lump has to be removed (a) to get rid of it, and (b) to make sure that the chemotherapy has completely eliminated the cancer. Most testicular tumour patients are young and adapt well psychologically to their disease, provided it is explained adequately (Cassileth and Steinfeld 1987), although inevitably a few have long-term psychosocial problems if treatment results in alteration in sexual function (Tamburini et al. 1989).

Preparation for excision of residual masses therefore commences at presentation, and by the time chemotherapy is completed it is fairly clear which patients are likely to require surgery. An appointment is made at this time for joint consultation with surgeon and oncologist. All relevant recent X-rays and scans are made available, up-to-date marker results are obtained, and the patient is told the purpose of the meeting. Close relatives are welcome to attend.

Planning and Preparation

The surgeon needs to know exactly where the masses are, and their size. Adjacent structures may be at risk of damage, or may have to be removed along with the mass, and this can only be assessed by careful reference to the scans. Not only is this essential for the surgeon to plan the operative approach, but the patient and his relatives must be advised of the likely extent of the surgery, and warned of any likely effect on other organs. In particular, failure to warn the patient of potential loss of a major organ such as a kidney, or interference with ejaculation, could be interpreted as negligence. Nonetheless, a positive matter-of-fact approach should be taken, and although potential risks should not be ignored or glossed over, they need not be dwelt upon. The patient should be advised to stop smoking.

In 70% of cases, the residual masses are in the para-aortic lymph nodes in the retroperitoneum, in 18% they are in the chest, and in 12% they are above and below the diaphragm (Tait et al. 1984). In the latter group the thoracic surgeon and the urologist should meet to discuss whether it is possible to remove all the tumours at once, through a thoracoabdominal incision, or whether a staged approach is preferable. In general, we have found that it is better not to be overambitious, hoping to remove everything in one operation, since access and hence safety may be compromised. Our approach is that masses above the diaphragm are always best dealt with by a thoracic surgeon, whereas those in the neck may require a separate operation by a third surgical specialist.

In planning the surgical approach to retroperitoneal or other abdominal masses, it is very helpful indeed to have a "scanogram" – this is a freehand drawing of the tumour showing its relation to the great vessels, and in particular to the renal vessels and kidneys (Fig. 16.1). The first decision that must be made is whether an anterior, long midline incision will provide adequate access. Analysis of 231 para-aortic lymphadenectomies at the Royal Marsden Hospital over a 10-year period indicated that this incision was used in 85% of cases (Hendry et al. 1993). It has the great advantage that it provides excellent direct access to the great vessels, with equally good exposure on either side: as a result even very large masses can be completely excised, provided they are below the renal vessels. Occasionally the vena cava itself may be involved (Ahlering and Skinner 1989; Jacqmin et al. 1989); this should be recognised in advance so that adequate arrangements can be made for blood transfusion, and a vascular surgeon may be invited to the operation. Similarly, if a liver metastasis is present it may be sensible to involve a surgeon who is experienced at hepatic resection. Particular attention must be paid to the kidneys: the metastatic tumour commonly causes ureteric obstruction, and although some renal function may return after chemotherapy there may be significant postobstructive atrophy of one or even both kidneys. The residual mass may be inseparably stuck onto the kidney, its vessels or the ureter, and in our experience nephrectomy had to be done in 11% of cases; it is therefore essential in all cases to make sure that the contralateral kidney function is adequate.

A thoracoabdominal approach is essential if simultaneous excision of supradiaphragmatic masses is to be carried out. Excellent access is provided to retrocrural nodes, and this incision may be chosen for massive tumours which are predominantly on one side.

Decision on optimum approach, possible involvement of adjacent organs, the need for additional surgical expertise, transfusion requirements and any postchemotherapy lung function defects that might lead to anaesthetic or postoperative difficulties should all be addressed at the planning visit in outpatients, in a calm considered atmosphere and not left to the last moment

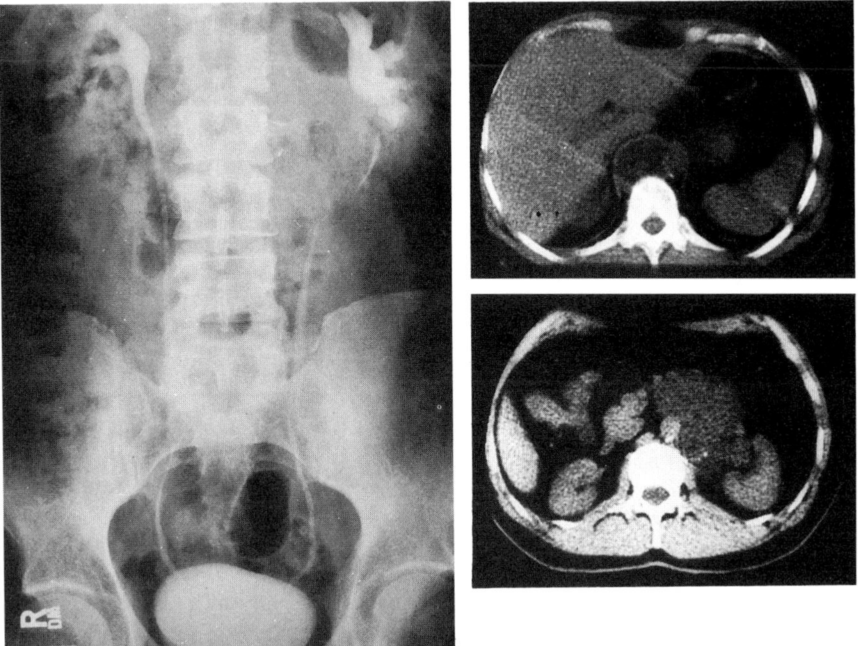

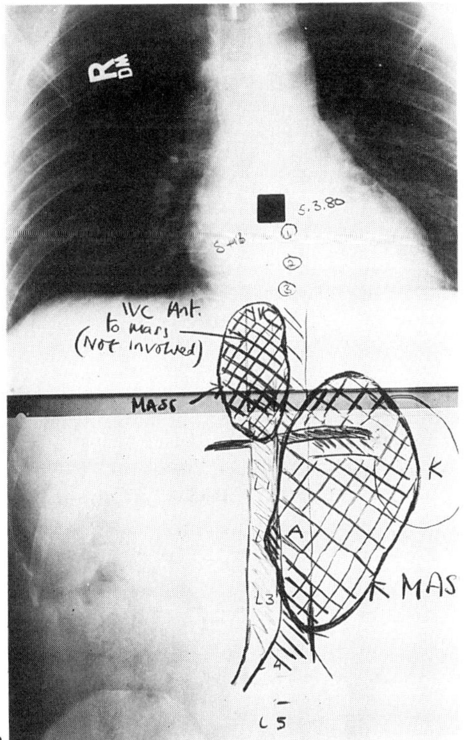

Fig. 16.1. a Intravenous urogram showing displacement of left kidney and upper left ureter. b CT scan showing mass in the hilum of left kidney with additional mass high in the retrocrural region. c Scanogram making the situation clear that there are two separate masses requiring excision. A left thoracoabdominal approach provided good access.

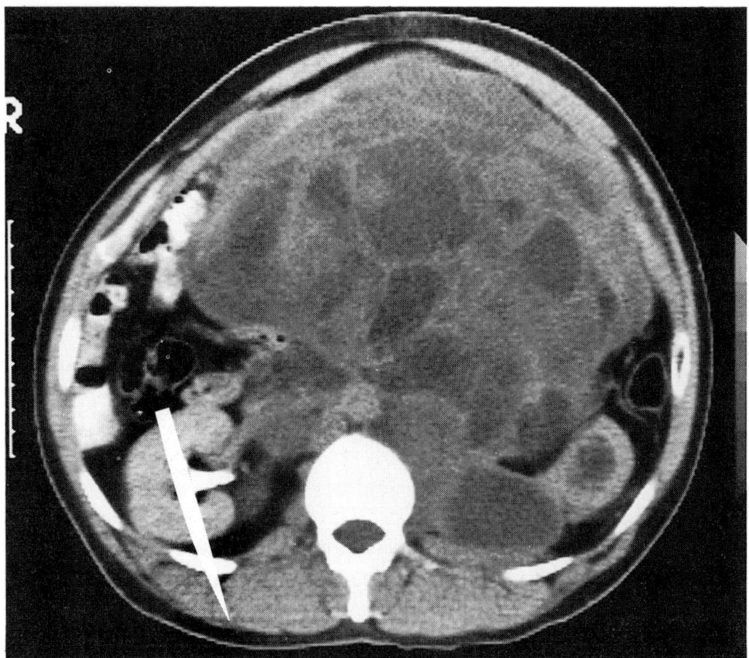

Fig. 16.2. CT scan showing massive teratoma which was completely removed through an anterior approach.

before surgery. Many of these masses are large – 25% being over 10 cm diameter in our experience (Hendry et al. 1993) – and they may present a formidable appearance. Perhaps the most difficult decision is to know when the case is inoperable. Massive tumours below the renal vessels can be excised (Fig. 16.2), and most nodal deposits above this level, but occasionally a case is encountered in which tumour encases the coeliac axis and superior mesenteric vessels, extending into the small bowel mesentery. Surgery has little to offer such cases, and these patients should not be subjected to the additional suffering associated with unnecessary laparotomy.

The Operation

The operation is usually scheduled to take place 4–6 weeks after completion of chemotherapy. The patient is admitted 48 h prior to operation, to allow preoperative blood tests, chest X-ray, cross-matching, bowel preparation and physiotherapy to be arranged. Prophylactic broad-spectrum antibiotics are started preoperatively.

The classical technique of para-aortic lymphadenectomy was well described by Mallis and Patton (1958), and the basic principles remain the same in excision of residual masses in this region. Once the boundaries of the residual mass have been defined and freed from surrounding normal tissues, work can commence on patiently and delicately dissecting the mass from the great vessels. It is generally best to free it from the vena cava first, and then the aorta. If the vena cava is damaged it can be repaired by oversewing, or even ligated above and below the site of injury with no ill effect. Extensive injury to the aorta is more serious and may require grafting. Some tumours seem to induce softening of the aortic wall, perhaps by myxoid degeneration, and the surgeon should be prepared to control the aorta above the renal vessels while inserting an aortic graft. The renal vessels may be surrounded by tumour, and great care must be exercised in approaching the origin of the renal arteries. The left kidney is not uncommonly inseparable from the tumour mass, and provided contralateral renal function is adequate, it should be removed with the mass rather than risk leaving tumour behind in the renal hilum (Fig. 16.3).

A thoracoabdominal approach is used if the mass extends above the renal vessels, or if it is massive and predominantly unilateral (Skinner 1977). The incision is made along the most prominent rib over the middle of the lymph node mass (usually the 8th, 9th or 10th) and extends from the midaxillary line to the midline, and then down the midline as far as necessary. The chest may be entered above the rib, or after excising it, and the abdomen opened widely in the same line; the diaphragm is incised as necessary. The colon is mobilised, with or without the spleen on the left, or the duodenum on the right, and the lateral and upper margins of the tumour mass are defined. The colon is allowed to fall back into place while the great vessels are exposed and dissected out as described above. It is essential that the tumour mass is freed from the great vessels, including dissection and division of the lumbar

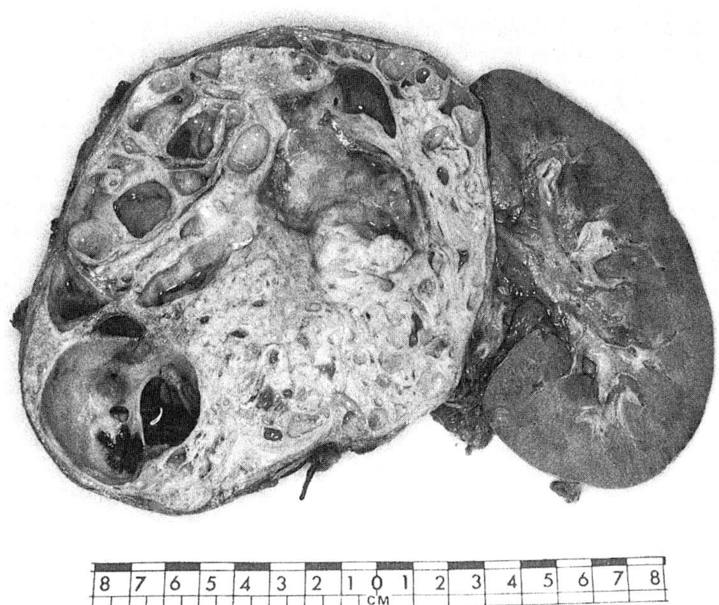

Fig. 16.3. A large deposit of differentiated teratoma involving the left renal hilum. This was removed together with the kidney in order to obtain complete clearance.

vessels if necessary, before mobilisation of the main tumour mass is attempted. Ipsilateral nephrectomy may be required, and involvement of the vena cava may occasionally be encountered.

Postoperative Care

The patient is nursed in an intensive care or high dependency unit for the first 48 h. Blood replacement and fluid losses are monitored by arterial and central venous monitoring. Urine output is carefully recorded. Early active physiotherapy encourages chest expansion and limb movement. Paralytic ileus is common, and intravenous fluids and nasogastric suction are required for a few days. Antibiotics are discontinued as soon as the patient is mobile and arterial and venous lines, and urinary catheter are removed. Most patients go home 10–14 days after operation, and are advised to limit their physical activity for a month.

If para-aortic lymphadenectomy is combined with thoracic surgery, such as removal of lung metastasis, the patient should be kept in intensive care for a few days postoperatively. The combination of preoperative bleomycin therapy, perhaps with smoking, and a long thoracoabdominal operation can predispose to adult respiratory distress syndrome, which may carry a high mortality and may require active therapy.

Results in Late Stage Disease After Chemotherapy

Among 231 para-aortic lymphadenectomies operated on by the author at the Royal Marsden Hospital between 1976 and 1990, there was residual undifferentiated teratoma (MTU) in 48 (21%), differentiated teratoma (TD) in 131 (57%), and only fibrosis/necrosis in 52 (22%) (Hendry et al. 1993). Residual MTU was found in 13% of 54 masses 3 cm or less in diameter, 25% of 118 measuring 4–8 cm in diameter and 20% of 59 large masses 9 cm or greater in diameter (not significant). There was residual MTU in 24% of the 17 who had received radiotherapy in the preceding 3 months, compared to 21% of the 214 who had not (not significant). There was residual MTU in 14% of the 152 men with normal serum markers within one month of surgery, compared to 58% of 36 with raised markers ($\chi^2 = 29.3$; $P<0.001$). There was residual MTU in 16% of 182 who had complete excision, 30% of 36 who had a difficult and possibly incomplete excision, and 55% of 11 who had incomplete excision ($\chi^2 = 9.76$; $P = 0.002$). Residual MTU was found in 12% of 182 patients undergoing "elective" excision, compared to 53% of the 49 who had "salvage" surgery ($\chi^2 = 37$; $P<0.001$).

A total of 47 patients relapsed 1–136 (median 8.2) months after surgery: 16 relapsed in sites outside the abdomen, 12 in the abdomen only, six in the abdomen and elsewhere, and 13 with elevation of markers only. Of these 25 (53%) ultimately died, despite treatment with further chemotherapy.

Overall, 80% of patients were alive 5 years after surgery (95% confidence limits 73%–85%). Five-year survival rates (with 95% confidence limits) by stage at presentation were as follows: stage I 94% (65–99); stage II 84%

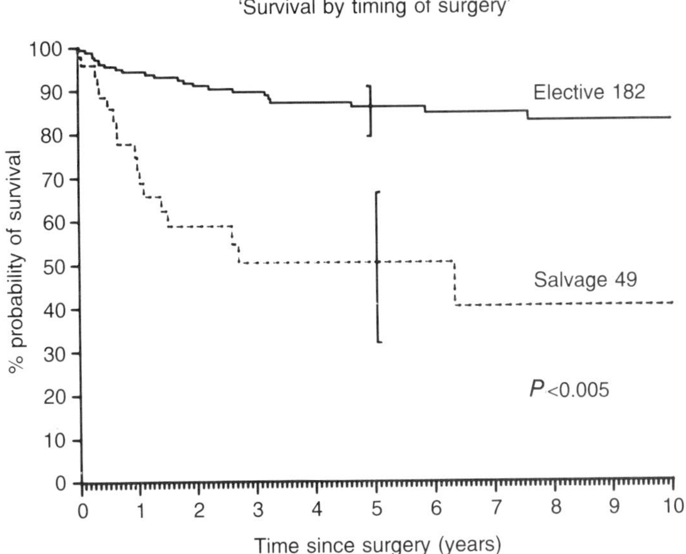

Fig. 16.4. Survival after elective postchemotherapy para-aortic lymphadenectomy compared to survival after salvage lymphadenectomy following second-line chemotherapy. (From Hendry et al. (1993), with permission.)

(74–92); stage III 69% (43–85); and stage IV 76% (64–85). These differences are not statistically significant. Survival was significantly better among those who had "elective" as compared to "salvage" surgery (Fig. 16.4), and in those who had normal serum markers at the time of surgery compared to those whose markers were elevated (Fig. 16.5). Survival was significantly worse in those who had residual MTU in the excised specimen compared to the rest (Fig. 16.6).

Survival was significantly better in those whose masses were excised completely compared to those whose excision was difficult and possibly incomplete, and those whose excision was incomplete, all of whom died (Fig. 16.7). This trend was confirmed in those with residual MTU in the excised specimen. There was no significant correlation between survival and the size of the mass.

Multivariate analysis was performed looking at completeness of excision, pathology of excised mass, elective versus salvage surgery, whether or not serum markers were elevated at surgery, size of mass and year of presentation (before or after 1984). The following were found to be independent prognostic variables: completeness of excision ($P<0.001$), pathology (MTU versus the rest) ($P<0.001$), elective versus salvage surgery ($P<0.01$) and year of treatment ($P = 0.03$). Serum markers at the time of surgery and size were not found to be of any additional prognostic value once pathology and completeness of excision were taken into account.

Most patients tolerated the surgery well, even though the mass was very large in some cases. However, two patients died within one month of surgery (operative mortality 0.9%), one from respiratory failure and one

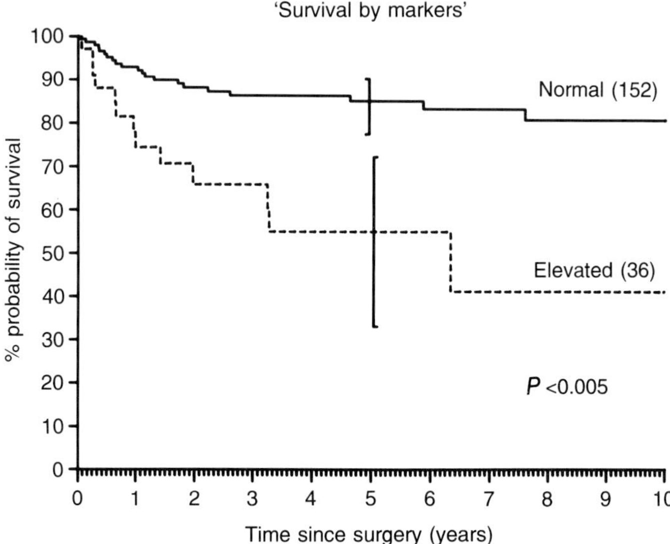

Fig. 16.5. A comparison of survival after para-aortic lymphadenectomy following chemotherapy comparing those with normal markers with those with elevated markers at the time of surgery. (From Hendry et al. (1993), with permission.)

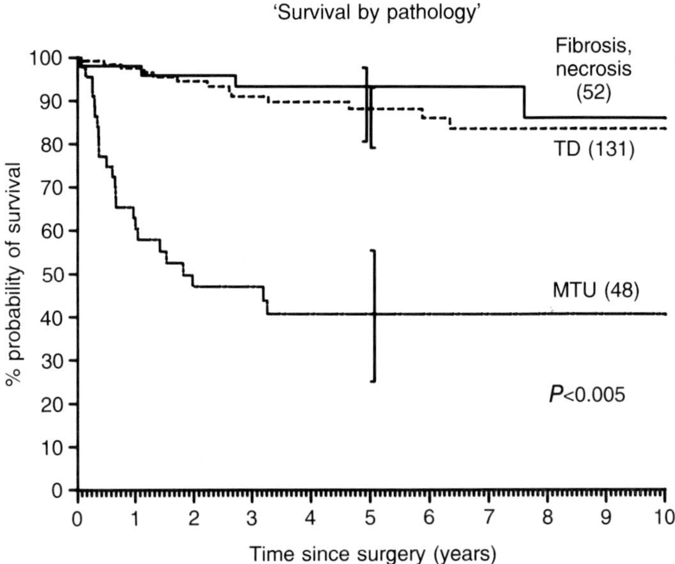

Fig. 16.6. Survival after para-aortic lymphadenectomy following chemotherapy for metastatic teratoma by pathology of excised mass. Survival was significantly worse when there was undifferentiated teratoma in the excised specimen. (From Hendry et al. (1993), with permission.)

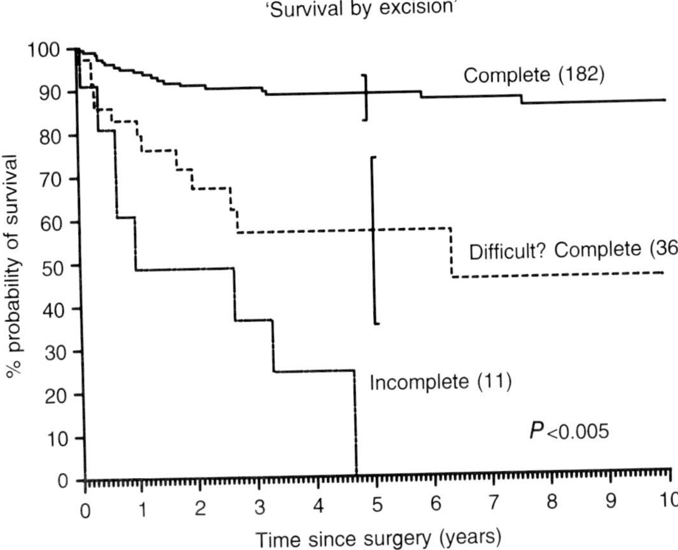

Fig. 16.7. Survival after para-aortic lymphadenectomy following chemotherapy for metastatic testicular teratoma related to completeness of surgical excision. (From Hendry et al. (1993), with permission.)

from secondary haemorrhage. Two patients died subsequently of causes possibly related to the surgery – one of pulmonary embolism at 12 weeks after further chemotherapy, and one of renal failure 14 months after injury to a renal artery. One other patient became hypertensive after damage to a renal artery.

In 29 (12.5%) patients the ipsilateral kidney was removed with the lymph node mass. The aorta or iliac artery was resected and grafted in 10 (4%), and the vena cava was resected and tied off without ill effect in seven (3%). A ureter was involved in three, bowel in nine and liver in four patients. Ejaculation was noted to be absent postoperatively in 42 (24%) of 175 patients in whom accurate information was available. Loss of ejaculation occurred significantly more often after bilateral (46%) compared to unilateral (14%) lymphadenectomy, and was also related to increasing size of the excised mass (<4 cm 4%; 4–8 cm 19%; >8 cm 60%). Adoption of a nerve-sparing operative technique led to a significant reduction in postoperative ejaculatory dysfunction (pre-1984, 37%; post-1984, 19%). Once lost, few patients regained ejaculation and we have had little success with adrenergic drug therapy, although others have reported restoration of ejaculation with ephedrine 25–75 mg (Lynch and Maxted 1983), imipramine 25–50 mg (Nijman et al. 1982), electroejaculation (Bennett et al. 1987; Ohl et al. 1991; Denil et al. 1992). It is therefore important to recognise patients at high risk of loss of ejaculation early in the course of their treatment so that seminal analysis and cryopreservation of semen in suitable cases can be arranged (Hendry et al. 1983).

The incidence of residual MTU in this series is similar to that reported from other centres (Table 16.1). Since it is impossible to distinguish radiologically those with MTU from the rest, we recommend excision of all substantial residual masses one month or so after completion of chemotherapy. What size is substantial? We have excised all masses greater than 2 cm diameter, and although MTU was found in only 13% of masses less than 3 cm diameter in our series, it has been recorded in a mass only 1.7 cm diameter (Dexeus et al. 1989). We therefore examine carefully all masses 1–2 cm diameter and select those for surgery that do not continue to shrink with time. Herr et al. (1991) recommended exploration of all cases with an initial mass greater than 3 cm diameter irrespective of the postchemotherapy X-ray findings.

Heading the list of factors associated with poor prognosis are incomplete excision of the residual mass, and presence of undifferentiated tumour. These two factors are related, since tissue with persistent active malignancy is undoubtedly more difficult to remove; however, complete clearance of residual masses which do turn out to contain active disease is clearly of therapeutic benefit, as shown by the results of the multivariate analysis which indicated that these two factors were independently significant.

There was residual MTU in 14% of those with normal serum markers, after chemotherapy, and so neither this finding, nor the mere size of the mass, should lull the oncologist into believing that surgery is unnecessary. On the other hand, raised serum markers at the time of surgery was highly predictive of the presence of undifferentiated tumour in the residual mass, and of subsequent relapse and death. Nevertheless, it can be seen that 50% of such patients were long-term survivors after excision of their residual masses with follow-on chemotherapy, when otherwise their prognosis would have been poor. Benefit from surgical excision was also observed prior to the advent of effective chemotherapy in 1976 (Hendry et al. 1980).

Donohue (1988) also found that survival was significantly worse after salvage, as compared to elective surgery after primary chemotherapy, probably reflecting the lower complete remission rate after salvage chemotherapy (Loehrer et al. 1988). The presence of sarcoma in the excised tissue was recognised as a particularly bad sign (Ahlgren et al. 1984; Ulbright et al.

Table 16.1. Comparison of histological findings in excised residual masses following chemotherapy at Royal Marsden Hospital (RMH) 1976–1990 (Hendry et al. 1992) with those reported from elsewhere

Author and year	Number	Histology of residual mass (%)		
		Fibrosis/ necrosis	TD	MTU
Bracken et al. (1983)	60	25(42)	14(23)	17(28)
Staehler et al. (1989)	65	23(35)	25(39)	17(26)
Harding et al. (1989)	42	15(36)	14(33)	9(21)
Williams et al. (1989)	25	13(52)	9(36)	3(12)
Herr et al. (1991)	122	57(47)	48(39)	17(14)
Kulkarni et al. (1991)	67	18(27)	29(43)	20(30)
Donohue et al. (1991)	529	143(27)	246(47)	140(26)
RMH 1976–1990	231	52(22)	131(57)	48(21)

1984) and this coincides with our experience (four of seven patients died). Donohue (1988) also observed that those who had greater than 90% reduction of measured tumour volume in metastases from MTU all had necrosis/fibrosis in their resected specimens; however, it remains to be seen whether this will become established as such a good prognostic feature that surgical excision can be omitted (Herr et al. 1991).

The number of reports of late relapse in the retroperitoneum is growing steadily (Carr et al. 1981; Geier et al. 1983; Maatman et al. 1984; Chan et al. 1985; Kuzmits and Ludwig 1986; Gelderman et al. 1989). The unstable nature of teratomatous metastases, even those composed of differentiated tissue (TD), was recognised by Logothetis et al. (1982) and termed the "growing teratoma syndrome", a term also used by Jeffery et al. (1991). The difficulties inherent in treating patients once relapse has occurred makes prevention a preferable alternative. Excision of residual masses allows early recognition of adverse prognostic features, and elimination of unstable or frankly malignant tissue. We are not alone (Staehler et al. 1989; Herr et al. 1991; Donohue, 1989) in believing that this policy is preferable to the "wait-and-see" approach recommended by others (Levitt et al. 1985; Read et al. 1986).

References

Ahlering TE, Skinner DG (1989) Vena caval resection in bulky metastatic germ cell tumours. J Urol 142:1497–1499

Ahlgren AD, Simrell CR, Tricke TJ, Ozols R, Barsky SH (1984) Sarcoma arising in a residual testicular teratoma after cytoreductive chemotherapy. Cancer 54:2015–2018

Bennett CJ, Seager SWJ, McGuire EJ (1987) Electroejaculation for recovery of semen after retroperitoneal lymph node dissection: case report. J Urol 137:513–515

Bland-Sutton J (1909) An improved method of removing the testicle and spermatic cord in malignant disease. Lancet 109:1406–1409

Bracken RB, Johnson DE (1976) Sexual function and fecundity after treatment for testicular tumours. Urology 7:35–38

Bracken BR, Johnson DE, Frazier OH, Logothetis CJ, Trindade A, Samuels ML (1983) The role of surgery following chemotherapy in Stage III neoplasms. J Urol 129:39–43

Bredael JJ, Vugrin D, Whitmore WF (1983) Recurrences in surgical stage I nonseminomatous germ cell tumours of the testis. J Urol 130:476–478

Carr BI, Gilchrist KW, Carbone PP (1981) The variable transformation in metastasis from testicular germ cell tumours: the need for selective biopsy. J Urol 126:52–54

Cassileth BR, Steinfeld AD (1987) Psychological preparation of the patient and family. Cancer 60:547–552

Chan SYT, Ford G, Sikora K (1985) Late relapse in testicular teratoma after chemotherapy. Lancet ii:773–774

Chevassu M (1910) Le traitement chirurgical des cancers du testicule. Rev Chir 41:628–666

Cooper JF, Leadbetter WF, Chute R (1950) The thoracoabdominal approach for retroperitoneal gland dissection: its application to testis tumours. Surg Gynecol Obstet 90:486–496

Denil J, Ohl DA, Menge AD, Keller LM, McCabe M (1992) Functional characteristics of sperm obtained by electroejaculation. J Urol 147:69–72

Dexeus FH, Shirkhoda A, Logothetis DJ et al. (1989) Clinical and radiological correlation of retroperitoneal metastases from nonseminomatous testicular cancer treated with chemotherapy. Eur J Cancer Clin Oncol 25:35–43

Donohue JP (1988) Indications and results of surgery after chemotherapy of testicular tumours (NSGC-T and seminoma). Prog Clin Biol Res 269:451–459

Donohue JP (1989) The case for retroperitoneal lymphadenectomy after chemotherapy for selected patients with nonseminomatous tumours of the testis. In: Carlton CE (ed) Controversies in urology. Yearbook Publishers, Chicago, pp 225–229

Donohue JP, Zachary JM, Maynard BR (1982) Distribution of nodal metastases in nonseminomatous testis cancer. J Urol 128:315–320

Donohue JP, Foster RS, Rowland RG, Bihrie R, Einhorn L (1991) Post chemotherapy surgery for advanced testis cancer. Abstract: 22nd Congress, Societe Internationale d'Urologie, Seville, Spain, p 131

Geier LJ, Volk SA, Weldon D, Redmond J (1983) Late relapse in testicular cancer after chemotherapy. Lancet i:1049

Gelderman WA, Oosterhuis JW, Koops HS, Oldhoff J, Sleijfer DT (1989) Late recurrence of mature teratoma in nonseminomatous testicular tumours after PVB chemotherapy and surgery. Urology 33:10–14

Harding MJ, Brown IL, Macpherson SG, Turner MA, Kaye SB (1989) Excision of residual masses after platinum based chemotherapy for non seminomatous germ cell tumours. Eur J Cancer Clin Oncol 25:1689–1694

Hendry WF, Barrett A, McElwain TJ, Wallace DM, Peckham MJ (1980) The role of surgery in the combined management of metastases from malignant teratomas of testis. Br J Urol 53:38–44

Hendry WF, Goldstraw P, Husband JE, Barrett A, McElwain TJ, Peckham MJ (1981) Elective delayed excision of bulky para-aortic lymph node metastases in advanced nonseminoma germ cell tumours of testis. Br J Urol 53:648–653

Hendry WF, Stedronska J, Jones CR, Blackmore CA, Barrett A, Peckham MJ (1983) Semen analysis in testicular cancer and Hodgkin's disease: pre and post-treatment findings and implications for cryopreservation. Br J Urol 55:769–773

Hendry WF, A'Hern RP, Hetherington JW, Peckham MJ, Dearnaley DP, Horwich A (1993) Para-aortic lymphadenectomy after chemotherapy for metastatic non-seminomatous germ cell tumours: prognostic value and therapeutic benefit. Br J Urol 71:208–213

Herr HW, Toner GC, Geller NL, Bosl GJ (1991) Patient selection for retroperitoneal lymph node dissection after chemotherapy for nonseminomatous germ cell tumours. Eur Urol 19:1–5

Hesketh PJ, Krane RJ (1990) Prognostic assessment in nonseminomatous testicular cancer: implications for therapy. J Urol 144:1–9

Hinman F (1919) Radical operation for teratoma testis, with report of 5 cases. Surg Gynecol Obstet 28:495–508

Hinman F, Gibson TE, Kutzman AA (1923) The radical operation for teratoma testis. An analysis of 79 cases, 10 of which are personal. Surg Gynecol Obstet 37:429–451

Horwich A, Norman A, Fisher C, Hendry W F, Nicholls J, Dearnaley D P (1994) Primary chemotherapy for stage II nonseminomatous germ cell tumours of the testis. J Urol 151:72–78

Hoskin P, Dilly S, Easton D, Horwich A, Hendry W, Peckham MJ (1986) Prognostic factors in stage I nonseminomatous germ cell testicular tumours managed by orchidectomy and surveillance: implications for adjuvant chemotherapy. J Clin Oncol 14:1031–1036

Jacqmin D, Bertrand P, Anssieau JP, Dufour P, Bollack C (1989) Involvement of the caval vein lumen by a metastasis of a nonseminanomatous testicular tumour. Eur Urol 16:233–234

Jamiesen JK, Dobson JF (1910) The lymphatics of the testicle. Lancet i:493–495

Jeffery GM, Theaker J, Lee AHS, Blaquiere RM, Smart CJ, Mead GM (1991) The growing teratoma syndrome. Br J Urol 67:195–202

Jewett MAS (1990) Nerve sparing technique for retroperitoneal lymphadenectomy in testis cancer. Urol Clin North Am 17:449–456

Jewett MAS, Kong Y-SP, Goldberg SD et al. (1988) Retroperitoneal lymphadenectomy for testis tumour with nerve sparing for ejaculation. J Urol 139:1220–1224

Kaswick JA, Bloomberg SD, Skinner DG (1976) Radical retroperitoneal lymph node dissection: how effective is removal of all retroperitoneal nodes. J Urol 115:70–72

Kennedy CL, Husband JE, Bellamy EA, Peckham MJ, Hendry WF (1985) The accuracy of CT scanning prior to para-aortic lymphadenectomy in patients with bulky metastases from testicular teratoma. Br J Urol 57:755–758

Kulkarni RP, Reynolds KW, Newlands ES et al. (1991) Cytoreductive surgery in disseminated non seminomatous germ cell tumours of testis. Br J Surg 78:226–229

Kuzmits R, Ludwig H (1986) Late relapse in testicular cancer from a residual tumour. Lancet i:1207–1208

Leiter E, Brendler H (1967) Loss of ejaculation following bilateral retroperitoneal lymphadenectomy. J Urol 98:375–378

Levitt MD, Reynolds PM, Sheiner JH, Byrne MJ (1985) Nonseminomatous germ cell testicular tumours – masses after chemotherapy. Br J Surg 72:19–21

Lewis LG (1948) Testis tumours: report on 250 cases. J Urol 59:763–772

Lindsey CM, Glenn JF (1976) Germinal malignancies of the testis: experience, management and prognosis. J Urol 116:59–62

Loehrer PJ, Laver R, Roth BJ, Williams SD, Kalasinski LA, Einhorn LH (1988) Salvage therapy on recurrent germ cell cancer: ifosfamide and cisplatin plus either vinblastine or etoposide. Ann Intern Med 109:540–546

Logothetis CJ, Samuels ML, Trindale A, Johnson DE (1982) The growing teratoma syndrome. Cancer 50:1229–1236

Lowry EC, Beard DE, Hewitt LW, Barner JL (1946) Tumour of the testicle: analysis of one hundred cases, a preliminary report. J Urol 55:373–384

Lynch JH, Maxted WC (1983) Use of ephedrine in post-lymphadenectomy ejaculatory failure: a case report. J Urol 129:379

Maatman T, Bukowski RM, Montie JE (1984) Retroperitoneal malignancies several years after initial treatment of germ cell cancer of the testis. Cancer 54:1962–1965

Mallis N, Patton JF (1958) Transperitoneal bilateral lymphadenectomy in testis tumour. J Urol 80:501–503

Mead GM, Stenning SP, Parkinson MC et al. (1992) The second Medical Research Council study of prognostic factors in nonseminomatous germ cell tumours. J Clin Oncol 10:85–94

Most (1898) Ueber maligue Hodengeschwulste und ihre Metastasen. Arch Pathol Anat 154:138–177

Nijman JM, Jager S, Boer PW, Kremer J, Oldhoff J, Koops HS (1982) The treatment of ejaculation disorders after retroperitoneal lymph node dissection. Cancer 50:2967–2971

Nijman JM, Koops HS, Oldhoff J, Kremer J, Jager S (1987) Sexual function after bilateral retroperitoneal lymph node dissection for nonseminomatous testicular cancer. Arch Androl 18:225–267

Ohl DA, Denis J, Bennett CJ, Randolph JF, Menge AC, McCabe M (1991) Electroejaculation following retroperitoneal lymphadenectomy. J Urol 145:980

Peckham MJ, Hendry WF (1985) Clinical stage II nonseminomatous germ cell testicular tumours. Results of management by primary chemotherapy. Br J Urol 57:763–768

Pizzocaro G, Zanoni F, Salvioni R, Milani A, Piva L, Pilotti S (1987) Difficulties of a surveillance study omitting retroperitoneal lymphadenectomy in clinical stage I nonseminomatous germ cell tumours of the testis. J Urol 128:1393–1396

Ray B, Hajdu SI, Whitmore WF (1974) Distribution of retroperitoneal lymph node metastases in testicular germinal tumours. Cancer 33:340–348

Read G Johnson RJ, Wilkinson PM (1986) The role of radiotherapy after chemotherapy in the management of persistent paraaortic nodal disease in nonseminomatous germ cell tumours. Br J Cancer 53:623–628

Richie, JP (1990) Clinical stage I testicular cancer; the role of modified retroperitoneal lymphadenectomy. J Urol 144:1160–1163

Roberts JB (1902) Excision of the lumbar lymphatic nodes and spermatic vein in malignant disease of the testicle. Ann Surg 36:539–549

Skinner DG (1977) Advances in the management of nonseminomatous germinal tumours of the testis. Br J Urol 49:553–560

Skinner DG, Leadbetter WF (1971) The surgical management of testis tumours. J Urol 106:84–93

Socinski MA, Garnick MB, Stomper PC, Fung CY, Richie JP (1988) Stage II nonseminomatous germ cell tumours of the testes: an analysis of treatment options in patients with low volume retroperitoneal disease. J Urol 140:1437–1441

Sogani PC (1991) Evolution of the management of stage I nonseminomatous germ-cell tumours of the testis. Urol Clin North Am 18:561–573

Staehler G, Wiesel M, Clemm C, Gokel JM, Marchner M (1989) Significance of salvage lymphadenectomy in the therapeutic concept of advanced nonseminomoatous germ cell tumours. Urol Int 44:84–86

Staubitz WJ, Magoss IV, Grace JT, Schenk WG (1969) Surgical management of testis tumours. J Urol 101:350–355

Staubitz WJ, Early KS, Magoss IV, Murphy GP (1974) Surgical management of testis tumour. J Urol 11:205–209

Tait D, Peckham MJ, Hendry WF, Goldstraw P (1984) Post chemotherapy surgery in advanced nonseminomatous germ cell testicular tumours: the significance of histology with particular reference to differentiated (mature) teratoma. Br J Cancer 50:601–609
Tamburini M, Filiberti A, Barbieri A et al. (1989) Psychological aspects of testicular cancer therapy: a prospective study. J Urol 142:1487–1490
Tavel FR, Osius TG, Parker JW et al. (1963) Retroperitoneal node dissection. J Urol 89:241–245
Ulbright TM, Loehrer PJ, Roth LM, Einhorn LH, Williams SD, Clark SA (1984) The development of non-germ cell malignancies within germ cell tumours. A clinico-pathological study of 11 cases. Cancer 54:1824–1833
Williams SN, Jenkins BJ, Baithun WI, Oliver RTD, Blandy JP (1989) Radical retroperitoneal node dissection after chemotherapy for testicular tumours. Br J Urol 63:641–643

Index